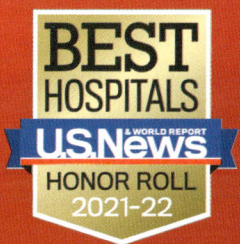

#1 IN NEW YORK

THE BEST HOSPITAL IN NEW YORK FOR OVER 20 YEARS

Here's to our doctors, nurses, staff and patients.
Because of you, we are one of the nation's best hospitals.

NewYork-Presbyterian

NewYork-Presbyterian Hospital as ranked by U.S. News & World Report 2021–22

Weill Cornell Medicine | **NewYork-Presbyterian** | **COLUMBIA**

CONTENTS

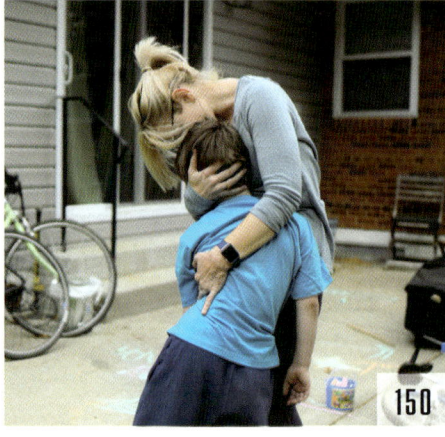

103 Eating the Mediterranean Way
One expert's view of the pleasures of following the 2021 top diet overall.

CHAPTER FOUR

Children's Health

150 A Focus on Mental Health
Children's hospitals step up to improve access to care.

158 Why Your Child's Weight Really Matters
An expert from Cleveland Clinic Children's explains how addressing excess weight gain early can prevent serious conditions in adulthood. Plus: How to pack a healthy lunch.

162 The Health Effects of So Much Screen Time
Migraines, eye strain and sleep issues are a few of the possible costs doctors are seeing.

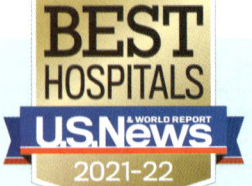

The U.S. News Rankings

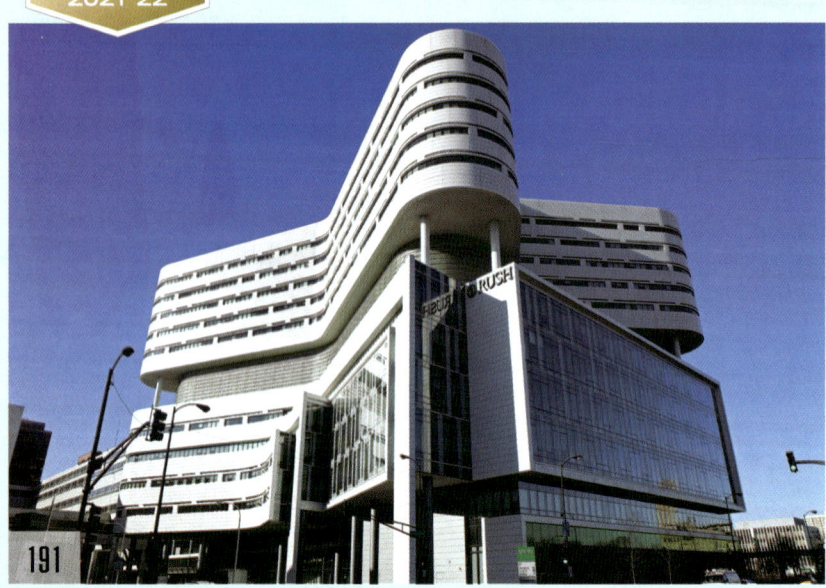

CHAPTER THREE

Best Hospitals

108 The Honor Roll
Twenty elite medical centers get a special nod.

110 A Guide to the Rankings
How U.S. News identified standouts in 15 specialties

114 Cancer

118 Cardiology & Heart Surgery

124 Diabetes & Endocrinology

126 Ear, Nose & Throat

130 Gastroenterology & GI Surgery

131 Geriatrics

132 Gynecology

134 Neurology & Neurosurgery

136 Orthopedics

140 Pulmonology & Lung Surgery

142 Rehabilitation

144 Urology

146 Ophthalmology, Psychiatry, Rheumatology

CHAPTER FIVE

Best Children's Hospitals

168 The Honor Roll
These children's hospitals got the highest marks.

173 A Key to the Rankings
How we identified 89 outstanding children's hospitals

178 Cancer

180 Cardiology & Heart Surgery

182 Diabetes & Endocrinology

184 Gastroenterology & GI Surgery

186 Neonatology

188 Nephrology

190 Neurology & Neurosurgery

191 Orthopedics

192 Pulmonology & Lung Surgery

194 Urology

CHAPTER SIX

Best Regional Hospitals

198 Getting Great Care Near Home
Read about how U.S. News identified and ranked top hospitals in each state.

200 The Rankings:
See how nearby hospitals performed in areas of specialty care and in common procedures and conditions.

218 Best Regional Children's Hospitals:
A region-by-region ranking based on performance in 10 specialties

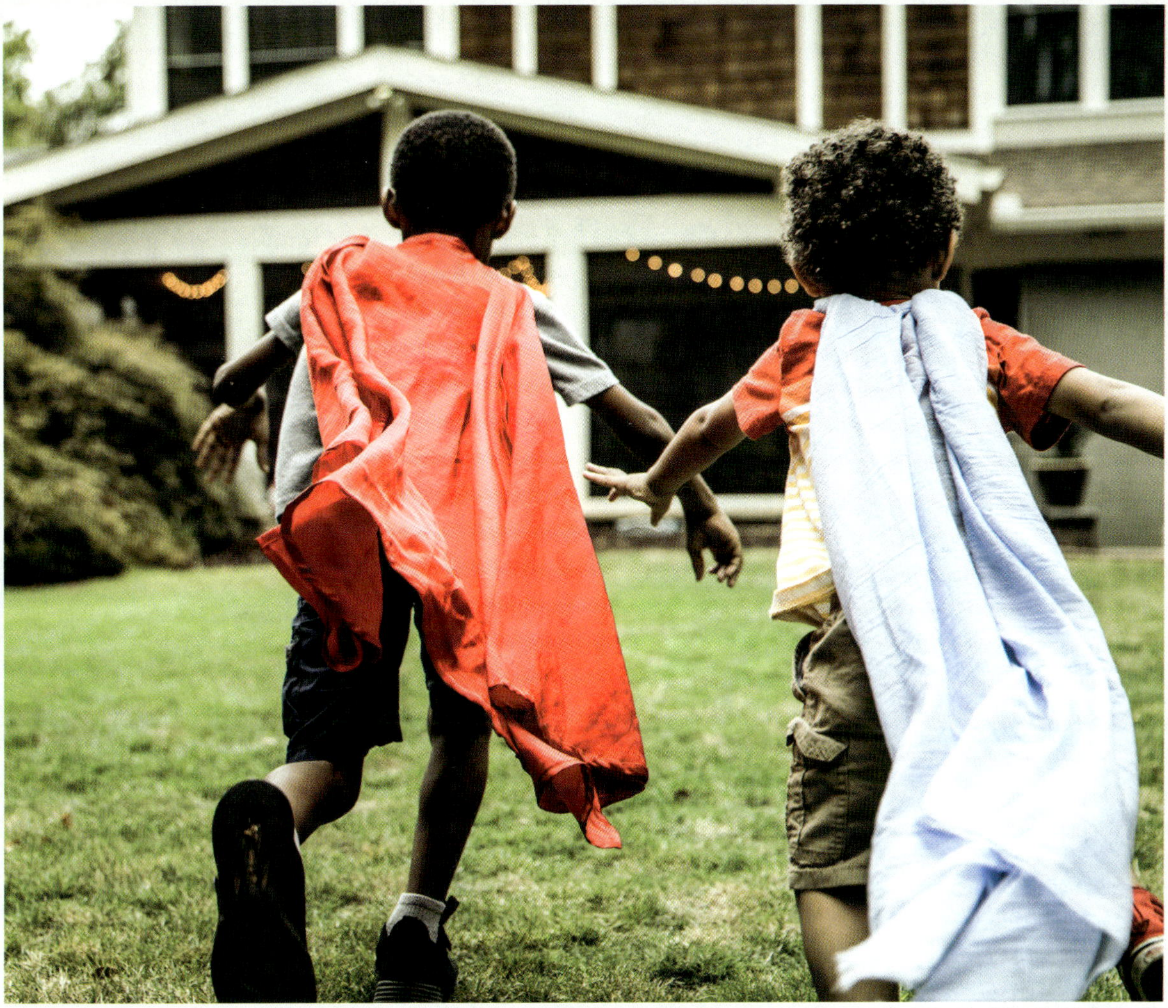

The #1 children's hospital in Texas.

For 13 years in a row, U.S. News & World Report has recognized us as one of the best children's hospitals in the Nation and #1 in Texas. Our best is something we strive for each day, caring for our patients—not looking back at what we accomplished but towards what we can do tomorrow.

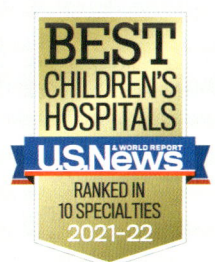

Where *Tomorrow* gets better.

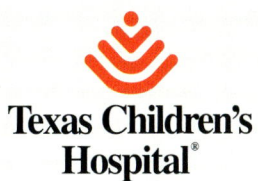

See why we're #1 at **TexasChildrens.org/best** or schedule an appointment at 832-824-4800

© 2021 Texas Children's Hospital. All rights reserved.

ON THE WEB

Here's What's @usnews.com
You'll find a wealth of advice on staying well and finding care

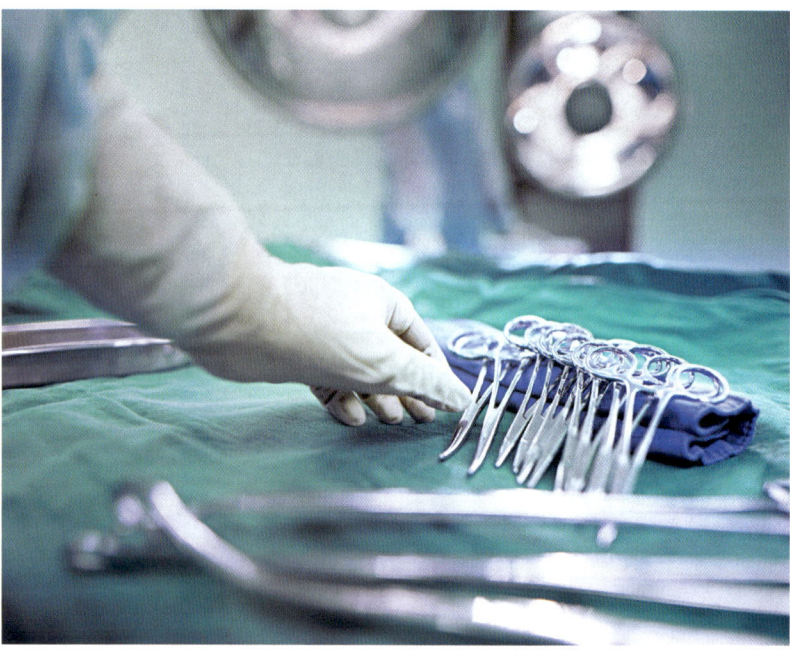

NUTRITION & LIFESTYLE

Best Diets
A look at some of the most popular and most researched diets, with reviews by a panel of health experts. Discover the top diets for weight loss, diabetes management and heart health, as well as the best plant-based and commercial diets.
usnews.com/bestdiets

Eat + Run
Doing what it takes to stay in shape can be tough to manage. We regularly serve up expert advice to support you.
usnews.com/eat-run

INSURANCE

Best Medicare Advantage Plans
State-by-state ratings of insurers offering Medicare Advantage and Medicare Part D plans, plus tips on choosing one of these plans vs. original Medicare.
usnews.com/medicare

PANDEMIC EXPERIENCES

Hospital Heroes
A series spotlighting the extraordinary efforts that have been mounted by health professionals in the trenches fighting the historic coronavirus pandemic
usnews.com/hospital-heroes

BEST HOSPITALS HONOR ROLL

A Visual Tour of the Top 20
See the best of the Best Hospitals – 20 medical centers that lead the pack in a host of specialties, procedures and conditions, excelling in both breadth and depth of care.
usnews.com/hospitalphototour

BEST HOSPITALS

In Specialties, Procedures & Conditions
We've evaluated more than 4,500 hospitals on up to 17 common procedures and conditions, including hip replacement, knee replacement, heart bypass surgery, colon cancer surgery, diabetes and stroke, as well as 15 medical specialties from cancer care to orthopedics to cardiology and heart surgery.
usnews.com/best-hospitals

SENIOR CARE

Best Nursing Homes
We've analyzed government data and published ratings of more than 15,000 facilities nationwide.
usnews.com/nursinghomes

PHARMACIST PICKS

Top Recommended Health Products
Which over-the-counter products do pharmacists prefer? Check out Top Recommended Health Products to make your next trip to the drugstore easier.
usnews.com/tophealthproducts

PHYSICIAN SEARCH TOOL

Doctor Finder
A searchable directory of more than 900,000 doctors. Patients can find and research doctors who have the training, certification, practical experience and hospital affiliation they want – and can see ratings based on other patients' experience. With free registration, physicians can update the profile patients see.
usnews.com/doctors

I've got cancer

but I also have researchers who will stop at nothing until there's a cure.

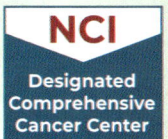 The National Cancer Institute recognizes only the nation's most elite cancer centers as Comprehensive Cancer Centers for their groundbreaking research, innovative clinical trials, scientific leadership, resources, and impact on their community. Rutgers Cancer Institute of New Jersey in partnership with RWJBarnabas Health is New Jersey's only NCI-designated Comprehensive Cancer Center. But with 12 locations across the state, NCI-designated cancer care is never far from home. Visit rwjbh.org/beatcancer or call 844-CANCERNJ.

RUTGERS
Cancer Institute of New Jersey
RUTGERS HEALTH

RWJBarnabas HEALTH

Let's beat cancer together.

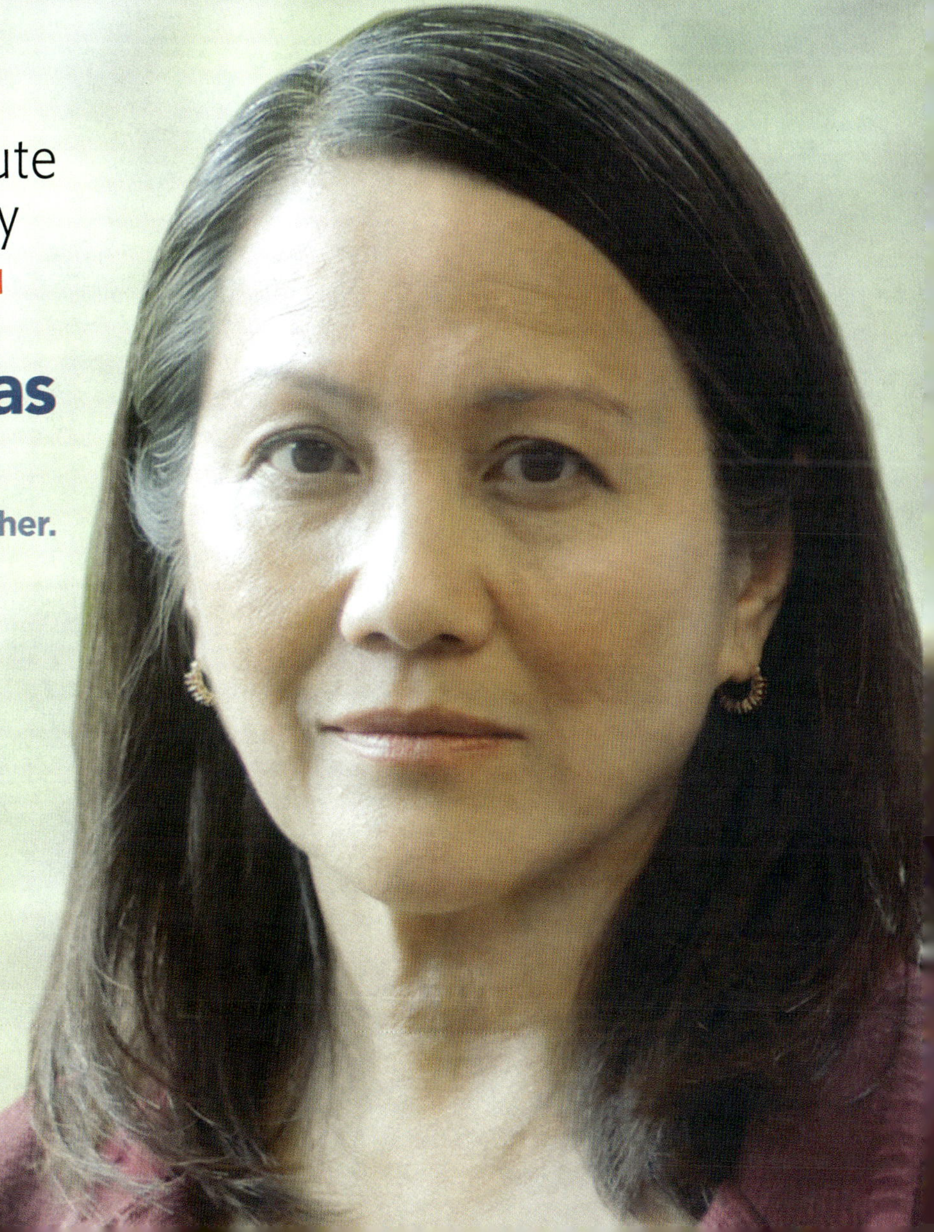

Top 10 in the Nation

UCSF MEDICAL CENTER IS RANKED IN 14 SPECIALTIES

CANCER | CARDIOLOGY & HEART SURGERY | DIABETES & ENDOCRINOLOGY
EAR, NOSE & THROAT | GASTROENTEROLOGY & GI SURGERY | GERIATRICS
GYNECOLOGY | NEUROLOGY & NEUROSURGERY | OPHTHALMOLOGY | ORTHOPEDICS
PSYCHIATRY | PULMONOLOGY | RHEUMATOLOGY | UROLOGY

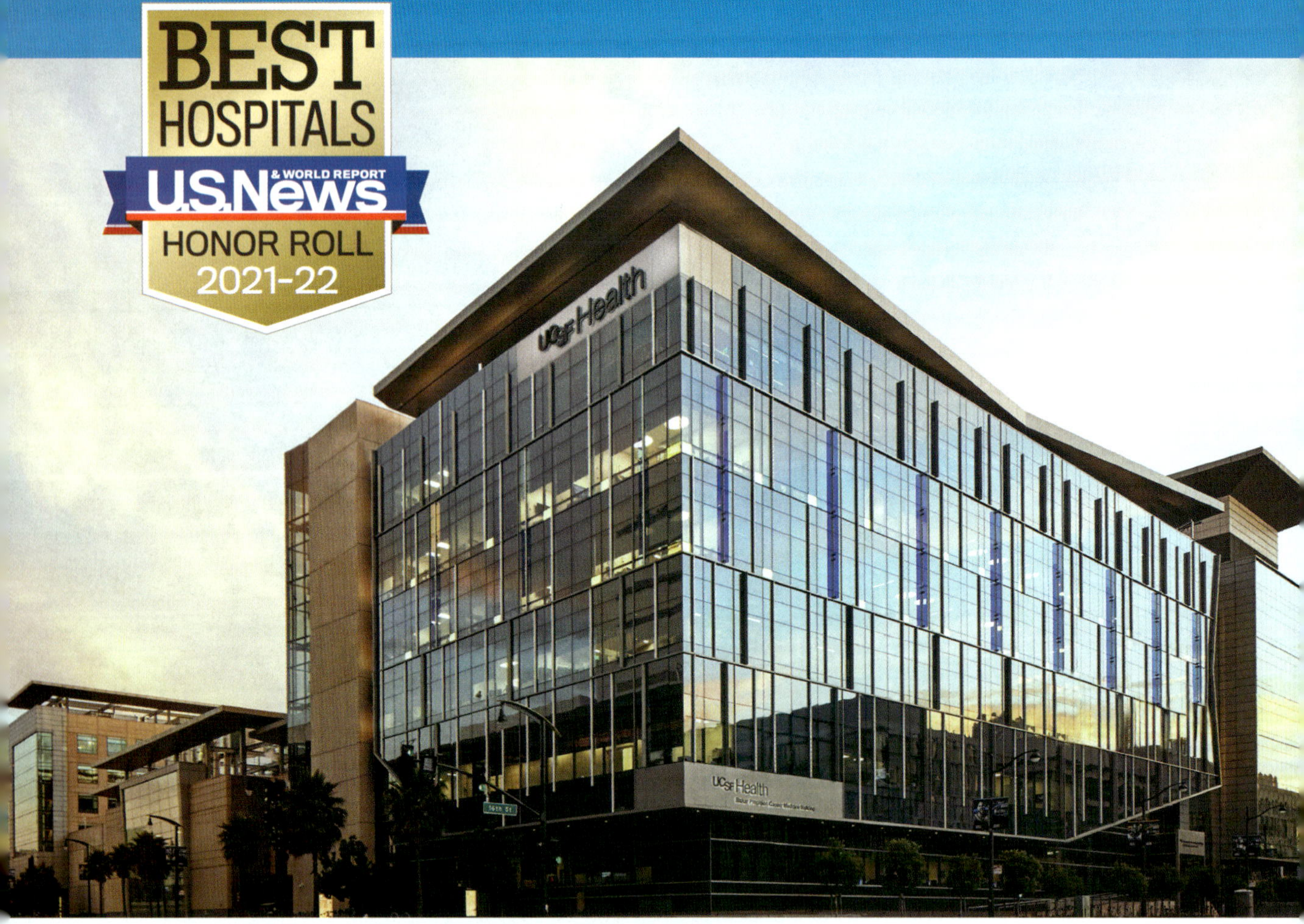

BEST HOSPITALS — U.S. News & World Report — HONOR ROLL 2021-22

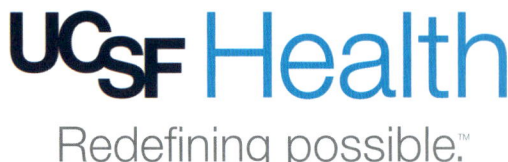

Redefining possible.™

CHAPTER 1

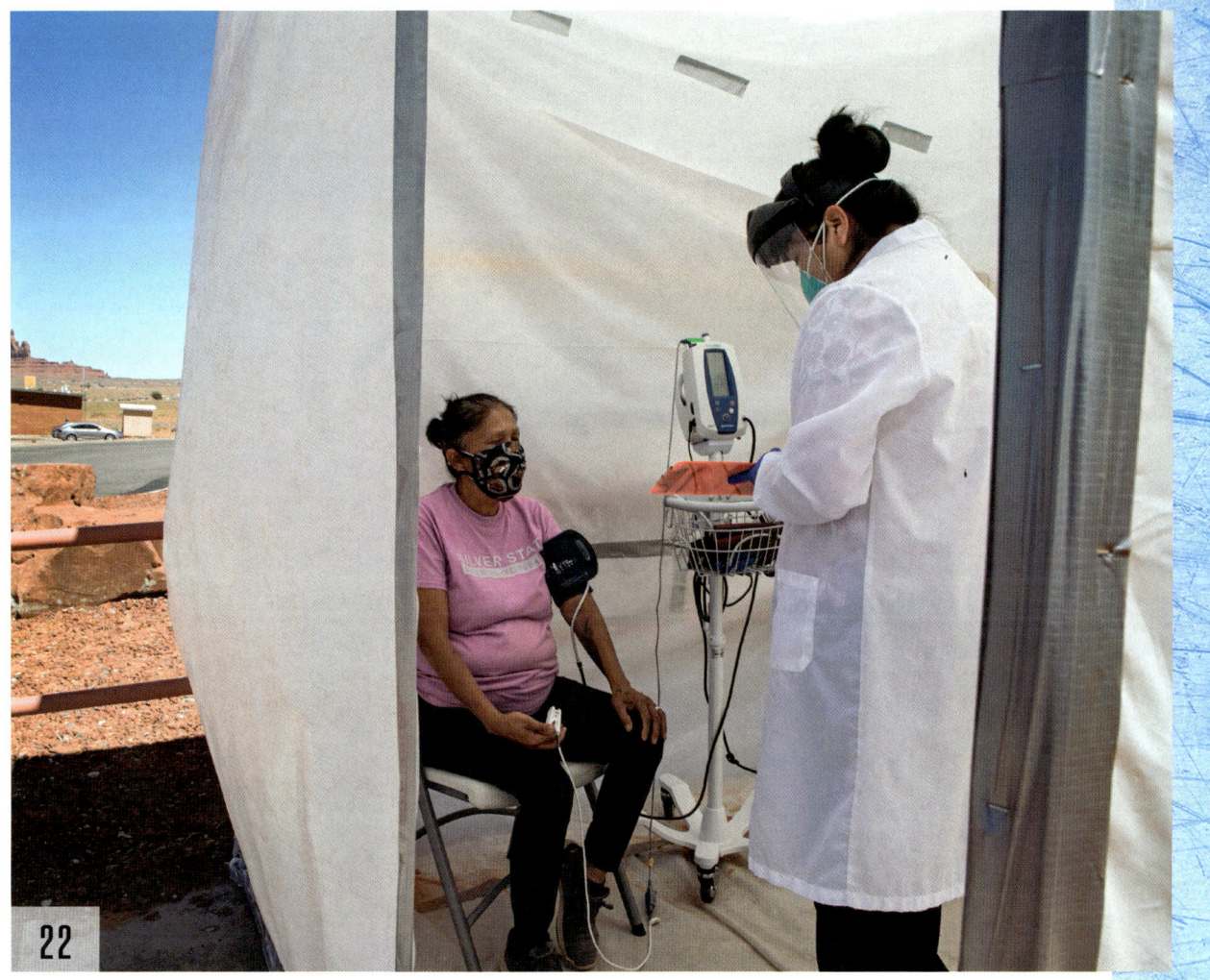

On Medicine's Front Lines

Coping with COVID's Aftermath **12**

Photo Essay: A Look Back **22**

Virtual Care's Post-pandemic Role **30**

An Urgent Mission: Closing Health Gaps **52**

A Roundtable on Cancer Advances **58**

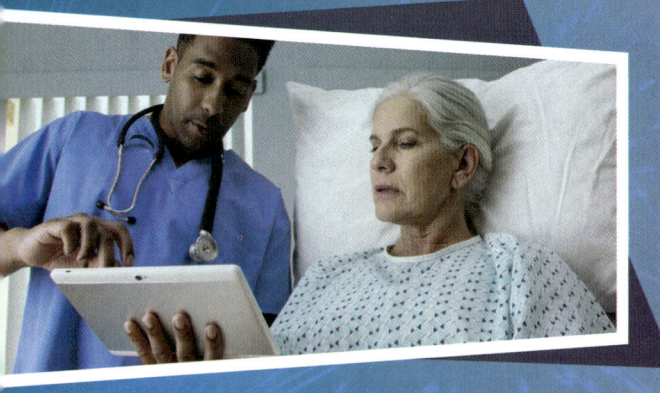
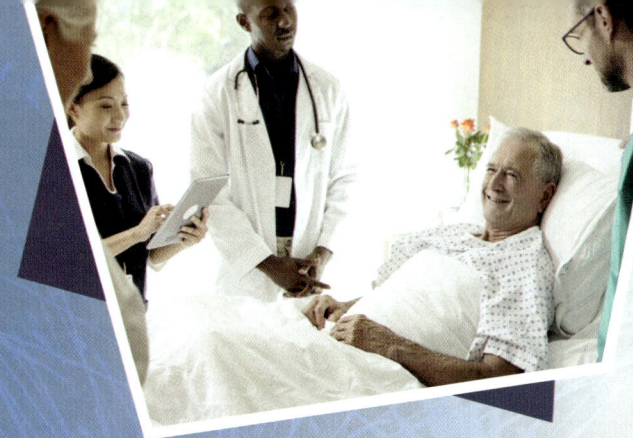

Celebrating Great Achievements

The American College of Cardiology (ACC) applauds those hospitals and health care facilities that have achieved a HeartCARE Center designation and the work of the HeartCARE Center champions who provide leadership in earning this great distinction.

Each of the institutions demonstrates a commitment to world-class cardiovascular care through community engagement coupled with quality improvement in care delivery and implementation of disease and procedure-specific accreditation programs. Additionally, the constant support of many qualified and dedicated physicians and cardiovascular care team members, including credentialed Fellows and Associates of the ACC, is essential to each hospital and facility's ongoing HeartCARE Center achievement.

We recognize their collaborative efforts, purposeful focus, and passion for excellence in working to deliver exceptional care and optimal outcomes for cardiovascular patients.

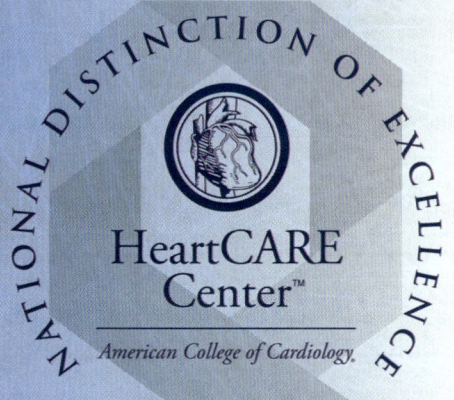

Please visit *cvquality.acc.org/hcc* to learn how hospitals can achieve ACC's HeartCare Center recognition.

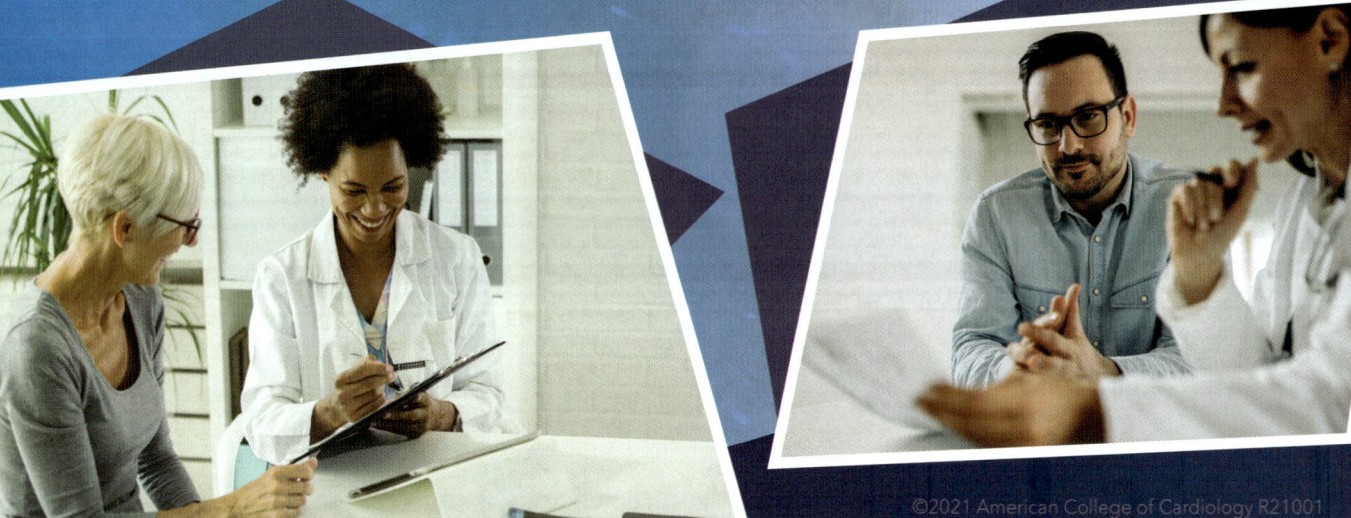

©2021 American College of Cardiology R21001

NORTHEAST

Christiana Care Health System
Wilmington, DE
Jennifer Oldham, MSN, RN, AACC
Neil Wimmer, MD, FACC

Lahey Hospital and Medical Center
Burlington, MA
Shauna Holden*, NP-C
Frederic Resnic, MD, FACC

Lawrence General Hospital
Lawrence, MA
Kathy Caredeo, RN, AACC
Sunit Mukherjee, MD, FACC

JFK Medical Center
Edison, NJ
Charyl Asuncion, AGPCNP-BC, MSN, AACC
Saleem Husain, MD, FACC

St. Elizabeth Medical Center
Utica, NY
Wendy Cooley, BSN, RN-BC, AACC
Michael Kelberman, MD, FACC

Conemaugh Memorial Medical Center
Johnstown, PA
Shannah D Boyer, CCRN, RN, AACC
Cyril Nathaniel, MD, FACC

Einstein Medical Center
Philadelphia, PA
Yolanda Nixon Huertas, ACNP-BC, CRNP, MSN, AACC
Sumeet Mainigi, MD, FACC

Regional Hospital of Scranton
Scranton, PA
Debra Jadick, NP, AACC
Srihar Sampath-Kumar, MD, FACC

Chester County Hospital
West Chester, PA
Ralph G Smith, IV, RN, AACC
Timothy Boyek, MD, FACC

SOUTH

AdventHealth Ocala
Ocala, FL
Lynn Smith, RN, AACC
Robert Feldman, MD, FACC

AdventHealth Tampa Pepin Heart Institute
Tampa, FL
Esther Fernandez, ARNP, AACC
Charles Lambert, MD, PhD, MBA, FACC

Baptist Health Lexington
Lexington, KY
Megan Switzer, NP, AACC
Azhar Aslam, MBBS, FACC

Baptist Health Paducah
Paducah, KY
Blair Brockman, NP, AACC
Michael Faulkner, MD, FACC

Our Lady of the Lake Regional Medical Center
Baton Rouge, LA
Dawn Denicola, FNP-C, AACC
Bryan Hathorn, MD, FACC

CHRISTUS St. Patrick Hospital
Lake Charles, LA
Anna Landry, NP, AACC
Michael Turner, MD, FACC

Norton Audubon
Louisville, KY
Melissa Wright, APRN, AACC
Ibrahim Fahsah, MD, FACC

Frye Regional Medical Center
Hickory, NC
Seth A Call, PA-C, AACC
Vincent Patrone, MD, FACC

CarolinaEast Medical Center
New Bern, NC
Laura Peters, BS RT, AACC
Alex Kirby, MD, FACC

Hillcrest Hospital South
Tulsa, OK
Michelle Bierig, RCS, RDCS, AACC
Edward Martin, MD, FACC

Spartanburg Regional Healthcare System
Spartanburg, SC
Jennifer Smith, MSN, RN, AACC
Nalin Srivastava, MD, FACC

Lexington Medical Center
West Columbia, SC
Dawn Crumpton, RN-BSN, AACC
Robert Malanuk, MD, FACC

The Hospitals of Providence Sierra Campus
El Paso, TX
Laura Wilson, AGACNP-BC, AACC
Edward Assi, DO, FACC

Baylor St. Luke's Medical Center
Houston, TX
Lisa Wall, AGPCNP-BC, NP-C, AACC
Emerson Perin, MD, FACC

CHI St. Luke's Health
Lufkin, TX
Jamie Huckabee, FNP-C, AACC
Neil Wimmer, MD, FACC

Woodland Heights Medical Center,
Lufkin, TX
Richard Fennell, BSN, CCRN, AACC
Vivek Mangla, MD, FACC

Methodist Texsan Hospital
San Antonio, TX
Michael Hendricks, MBA, RN, AACC
Obinna Isiguzo, MBBS, FACC

CHRISTUS Mother Frances Hospital, Tyler, TX
Jamie Moore, RN, AACC
Oscar Paniagua, MD, FACC

Mon Health Medical Center
Morgantown, WV
Denise Palmer, RN, AACC
Bradford Warden, MD, FACC

Camden-Clark Medical Center
Parkersburg, WV
Peggy Sisson, CCRN, AACC
David Gnegy, MD, FACC

MIDWEST

Indiana University Health Methodist Hospital
Indianapolis, IN
Andrea Price, CPHQ, RCIS, AACC
Richard Kovacs, MD, MACC

Lutheran Hospital of Indiana
Fort Wayne, IN
Amanda Lutter, AGPCNP-BC, AACC
Vijay Chilakamarri, MD, FACC

Bryan Medical Center
Lincoln, NE
Sarah Schroeder, NP, AACC
John Steuter, MD, FACC

WEST

Adventist Health and Rideout Hospital
Marysville, CA
Eric Cooper, BSN, MPA, NE-BC, RN-BC, AACC
Rajinder Singh, MBBS, FACC

Medical Center of Aurora
Aurora, CO
Linda Pilon, CCRN, MSN, NE-BC, AACC
Charlie Fuenzalida MD, FACC

UCH-Memorial Hospital
Colorado Springs, CO
Dawn Lovejoy, RN, AACC
Mark Boulware, MD, FACC

Rose Medical Center
Denver, CO
Lauren Meehan, MSN, AACC
Michael Wahl, MD, FACC

Saint Mary's Regional Medical Center,
Reno, NV
Rachael Coe, RN-BC, AACC
Devang Desai, MBBS, FACC

* AACC application in process

To find a hospital or facility that participates in ACC's quality improvement efforts or to find the right hospital to meet your needs, please visit
www.cardiosmart.org/find-your-heart-a-home.

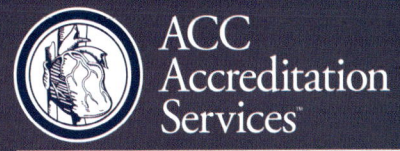

ON MEDICINE'S FRONT LINES

Weighing a Heavy Toll

The hit to the nation's health goes far beyond the effects of the virus itself

by **Arlene Weintraub**

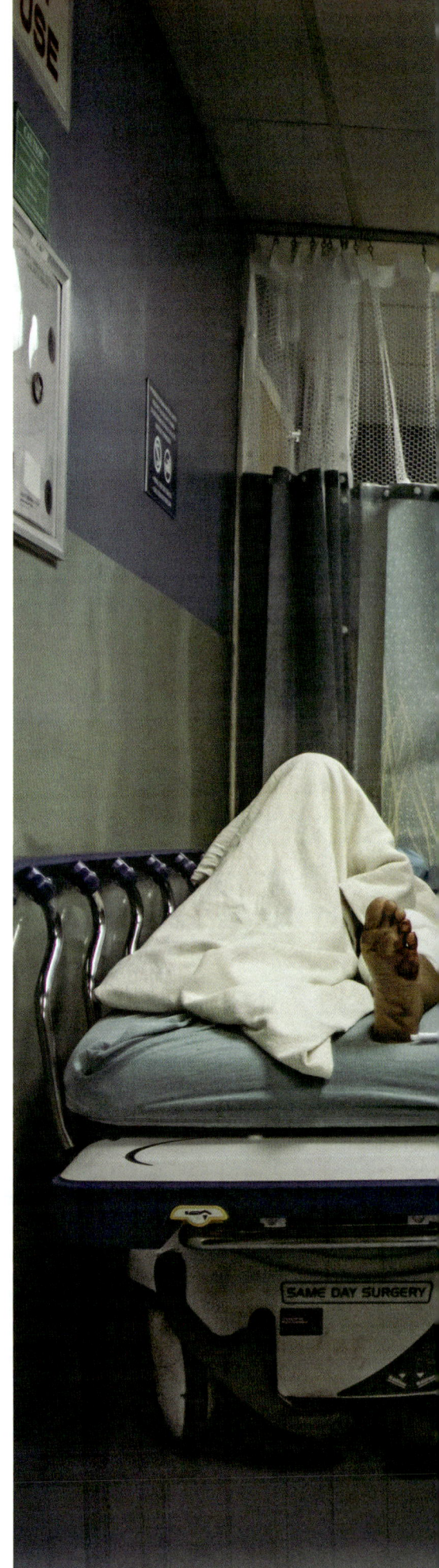

A PATIENT WAITS FOR A ROOM AT PROVIDENCE CEDARS-SINAI TARZANA IN CALIFORNIA LAST JANUARY.

AS SCHOOL CLOSINGS brought on by the COVID-19 pandemic stretched into the fall of 2020, Tucson Medical Center Chief Executive Officer Judy Rich faced a staffing problem. The hospital was overrun with COVID patients, yet many members of the medical staff – nurses especially – could not work extra shifts to help handle the influx.

"I heard from our nurses that they couldn't pick up extra time because they were so overwhelmed helping their children with school," says Rich, a registered nurse who has worked in hospital administration for more than 30 years. Discovering that local school districts had no plans to reopen for in-person learning, Rich turned to Higher Ground, a Tucson organization that provides after-school programs such as tutoring. Higher Ground set up a space inside the hospital where staffers' children, from kindergarten through fifth grade, could gather for "school" and play, logging into their remote learning programs and having meals and recess together.

"I could leave her there and know she would be okay, even if I had to extend my hours," says Grace Dellomes-Botor, a nurse and manager of patient care services in the cardiac unit who was "floated" to help care for COVID patients when cardiac care was put on hold. That meant coping

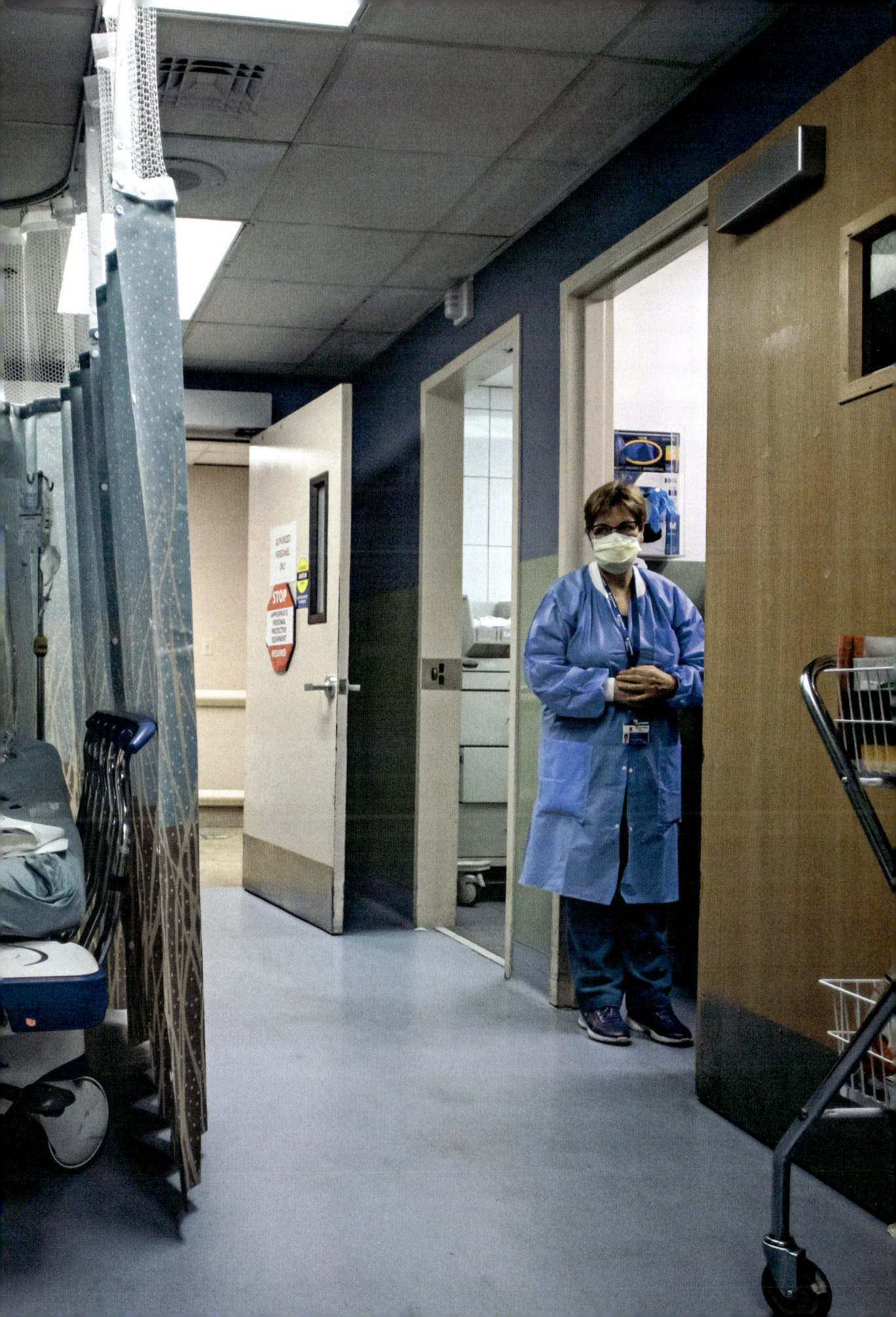

ON MEDICINE'S FRONT LINES

not only with often-critical people but also with uncertainty about when she might need care for her 6-year-old daughter. The Higher Ground staff "helped her with her homework, they had activities. She had social interaction that she was missing at home." TMC's program was so popular – more than 50 children enrolled – that the hospital offered a day camp version over the summer.

The on-site school helped alleviate an urgent concern Tucson Medical Center, like most hospitals, has dealt with as a result of COVID: worsening staff burnout. "We have struggled with the issue of burnout forever, but nothing has been close to what we've been through with COVID," Rich says. "The constant requests to work more shifts, more hours, longer hours – it was just beyond all of our capabilities."

An epidemic of exhaustion and mental health woes among health workers is one example of the heavy toll the pandemic has taken on the nation's health care system and on Americans' health as a whole. As the virus swept the country and all but COVID-related care came to a screeching halt, hospitals experienced large – and in some cases crippling – financial shortfalls. And beyond the severe effects of the coronavirus itself, which largely explain a dramatic 1.5-year drop in life expectancy in the U.S. population between 2019 and 2020, the crisis created yawning gaps in care needed by people with cancer

A Rethinking of Hospital Design

HEN JASON Schroer, director of health at HKS, an international architecture firm based in Dallas, saw hospitals being deluged with COVID-19 patients, he empowered his teams across the globe to provide pro bono design services to help hospitals manage the flood. That work ran the gamut from putting up temporary walls to creating triage centers to converting convention centers into field hospitals. "This is a pivotal moment that will impact how hospitals will be designed going forward," Schroer says.

Because it's financially prohibitive to build new hospitals to accommodate the next pandemic, which might not occur for decades, the ability to convert existing spaces quickly is the focus today for architects, engineers and designers. Orlando Regional Medical Center in Florida had a head start, having been influenced by the 2014-2016 U.S. Ebola outbreak to open a new area of the emergency department, designed by HKS, in 2015. Flexible pods that normally are used for patients with less severe conditions and injuries can, at the flip of a switch, be converted to negative airflow rooms where the air pressure is lower than the air pressure outside the room. When doors are opened, contaminated air doesn't flow out. Instead, fresh filtered air flows in, and exhaust systems remove contaminated air, filtering it before it's pumped outside. The 12 negative pressure airflow rooms can easily be converted to 25 single rooms with separate entrances. During the current first true test, the negative airflow rooms have made staff feel safer while treating patients, says Patrick Cassell, director of emergency services.

Surge ready. As has been seen, even corridors, lobbies and conference rooms may be needed for patient care in a pandemic, Schroer notes. "That means we should think about placing infrastructure such as oxygen and medical gases, pipes and wiring in alternative spaces that can be hidden from view, but easily accessible behind wall panels," he says. Being "surge ready" means having water, electric, and medical hookups available to convert even parking lots and adjacent structures into field hospitals, says Bill Scrantom, the Americas health care leader at Arup, a global engineering and consulting firm.

Anterooms between hallways and patient rooms, where caregivers can wash their hands, sterilize equipment and put on and remove protective gear, create greater separation between clean and contaminated air. But because costs typically prevent all rooms from being "designed to the highest contagion standard," Schroer says, health systems need to strike a balance between rooms designed to be convertible for treating pandemic patients and rooms dedicated to normal operations.

Providing adequate room airflow and proper disinfection of surfaces is key to preventing the spread of infection. Scrantom points out that direct ultraviolet light will kill germs on surfaces, but can be used only when rooms are empty because it can cause skin burns and eye injuries. Antimicrobial surfaces like copper and silver provide limited defense against viruses like COVID-19, so regular disinfecting regimes are crucial.

Proper airflow. Air filtration systems continually clean the air, while ventilation systems bring in fresh air. Air should be constantly circulating in order to dilute concentrations of pathogens, and although plastic barriers can help protect people from direct sneezes and coughs, they can also obstruct good airflow. Placing infectious patients in closed2 rooms under negative pressure isn't absolutely required for COVID-19, but could be vital for the next novel coronavirus.

"Establishing one-way circulation for infectious patients from building entry to patient room is also important," Scrantom says. "This keeps uninfected individuals out of harm's way

and heart disease and other serious conditions, resulting in delayed diagnoses and treatments that could have life-altering consequences for years to come.

Caught short. The underresourcing of the system and lack of preparedness that quickly became apparent as the virus spread have been big contributing factors. The U.S. has just 19 hospitals per million people, placing it low on the list of wealthy countries in terms of hospital density, and has fewer physicians per 1,000 people than comparable countries, according to the Peterson-Kaiser Family Foundation Health System Tracker. One survey of 53 hospitals undertaken before the pandemic by researchers at the University of Pittsburgh found near universal concern about lack of pandemic preparedness.

The good news is that hospitals have learned valuable lessons from the experience, experts say, and have implemented changes during the pandemic that should improve health care delivery. "What we've been through is the largest public health crisis in the last century," says Richard Pollack, president and chief executive officer of the American Hospital Association. "What we learned is that we have a health infrastructure that has been underresourced and needs a lot of rebuilding. Hospitals have stepped in to fill the gap."

Many health systems, already concerned about burnout before COVID, have ramped up efforts to support their

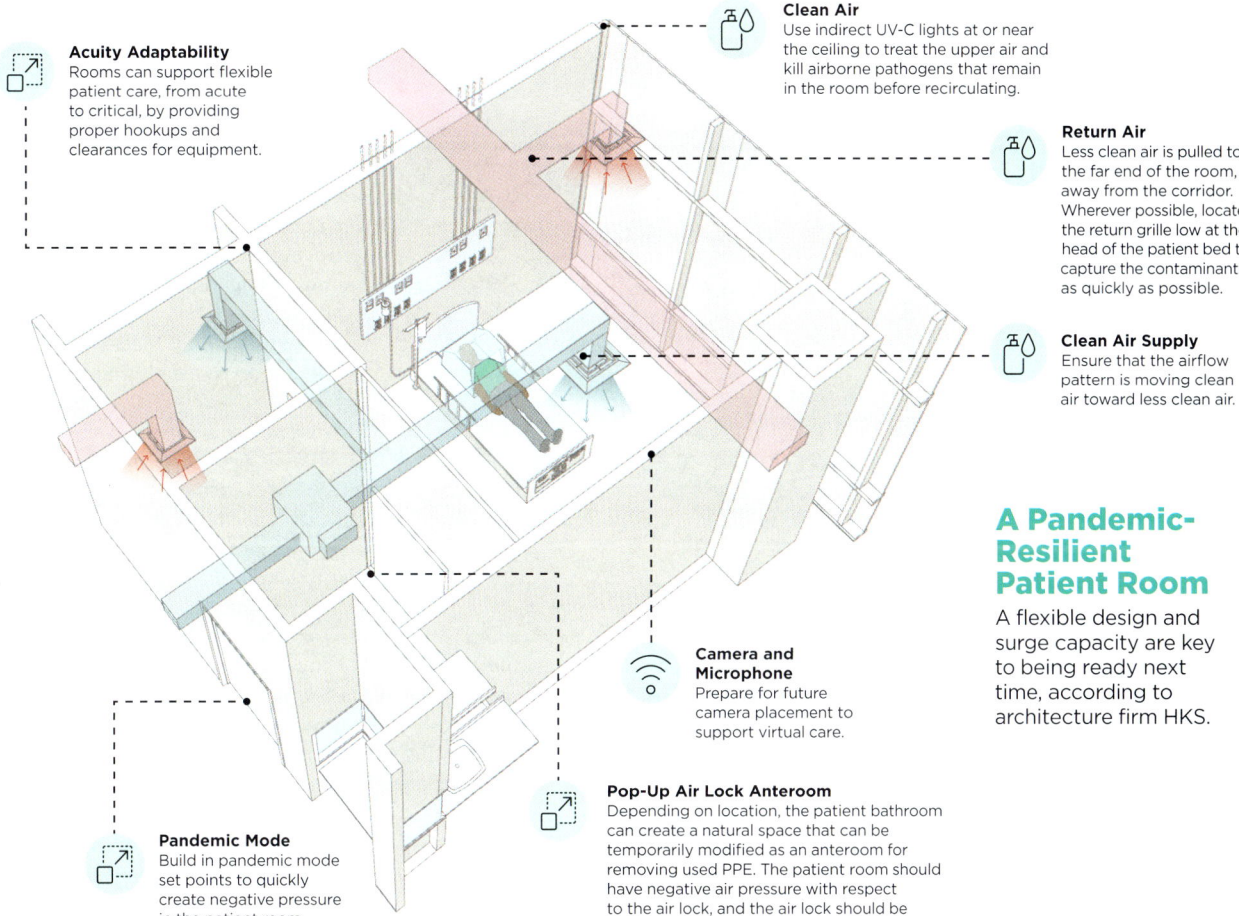

A Pandemic-Resilient Patient Room

A flexible design and surge capacity are key to being ready next time, according to architecture firm HKS.

and keeps the containment pathway well understood for cleaning."

Since physical interaction between patients and hospital staff should be limited to avoid infection spread, patient rooms and nurse stations will be designed with virtual care technology, experts say. Caregivers will be able to closely monitor and communicate with patients without always having to enter the room. Scrantom says hospitals will also be equipped to monitor less ill patients in their homes.

Finally, much attention is being paid to finding ways for health care workers to relax and relieve stress. Schroer says offering access to rooms with windows that overlook gardens is a good start. "Ideally, we'd like to see designated spaces to recharge" that allow staffers to turn down sound or lighting and have privacy for reflection. "It's important," he says, that "we focus on healing the healers." –*Barbara Sadick*

ON MEDICINE'S FRONT LINES

staffs, driven by a flood of reports of mental health problems among health care workers during the crisis. A poll published last October by the American College of Emergency Physicians and Morning Consult found that 72% of emergency physicians were suffering from increased burnout since the start of the pandemic (although almost half felt uncomfortable seeking any mental health care). Researchers at the Icahn School of Medicine at Mount Sinai in New York found that 39% of more than 3,300 staff members were suffering from COVID-related depression, anxiety or post-traumatic stress disorder.

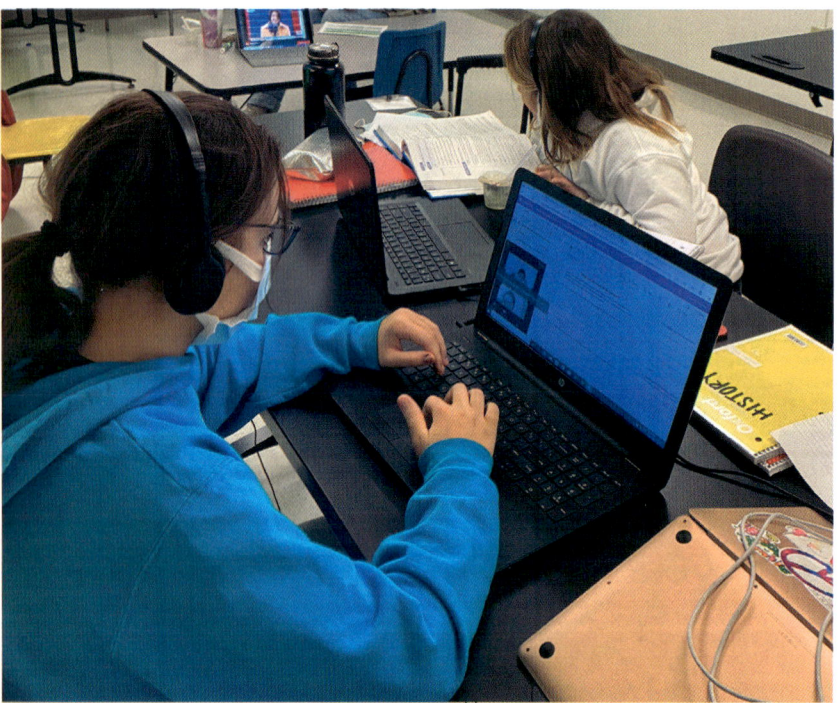

CHILDREN IN THE HIGHER GROUND PROGRAM AT TUCSON MEDICAL CENTER ENGAGE IN REMOTE STUDY.

In response, just months into the pandemic, Mount Sinai launched the Center for Stress, Resilience, and Personal Growth, a retreat in the hospital where staffers can get help dealing with their mental and emotional strain. The center offers resilience workshops, one-on-one counseling and referral to additional mental-health services if needed.

"We've had over 800 visits to the CSRPG and only a 1 percent no-show rate, so people are very engaged," says Dr. Deborah Marin, the center's director. And after the pandemic? "We plan to continue offering these services, and we have support from the highest levels of this institution," she says. "It's about enhancing the well-being of our health system."

Benson Kahiu, a clinical nurse manager on the neuroscience medical-surgical unit, took a five-week resilience workshop after suffering months of insomnia and stress brought on by 10- to 12-hour days and frequent weekends spent managing his unit. "I learned that instead of jumping out of bed in the morning, I should take a couple of deep breaths and plan my day ahead," Kahiu says. "We talked about listening to the birds as we walked to work, focusing on the little things." Incorporating such meditation techniques into his daily routine lowered his stress levels and helped him cope, he says.

Mount Sinai's study on COVID-19 stress found that workers who reported receiving a high level of support from hospital leadership faced the lowest risk of depression, anxiety or PTSD. That's no surprise, says Dr. Lotte Dyrbye, a professor of medicine and medical education at the Mayo Clinic who studies physician well-being. "To really tackle burnout, you need commitment from the top leadership at the organization and leaders at all levels," Dyrbye says.

At Mayo, that means constantly monitoring staff for signs of burnout and implementing improvements in processes that are designed to take some of the burden off physicians and nurses. Examples include rebalancing workloads, promoting better teamwork and improving electronic health records.

Broad health hit. Meanwhile, as providers postponed routine screenings and elective surgeries, the overall physical and emotional health of the population as a whole has also suffered. This phenomenon has highlighted the need – and spurred efforts – to find innovative ways to prevent disruptions in the future.

Take cancer patients. Two-thirds of radiation oncologists surveyed in February said cancer patients were showing up for treatment with more advanced-stage disease than was typically seen, and 73% of physicians reported a drop-off in routine screenings, according to the American Society for Radiation Oncology. "People didn't get their mammograms, colonoscopies, skin screenings, and that's probably going to be an issue for the next decade," says the society's board chair Dr. Thomas Eichler, a radiation oncologist at Sarah Cannon Cancer Institute in Richmond, Virginia. In fact, National Cancer Institute director Dr. Ned Sharpless projected that there would be 10,000 excess deaths just from breast and colorectal cancer over the next 10 years because of missed screenings.

Eichler expects that one result will be an acceleration of a trend that had already been taking off in rural communities: mobile cancer screening. Stony Brook University Cancer Center in New York, for example, sends a van throughout Long Island offering mammography to all women age 40 and older, no prescription needed.

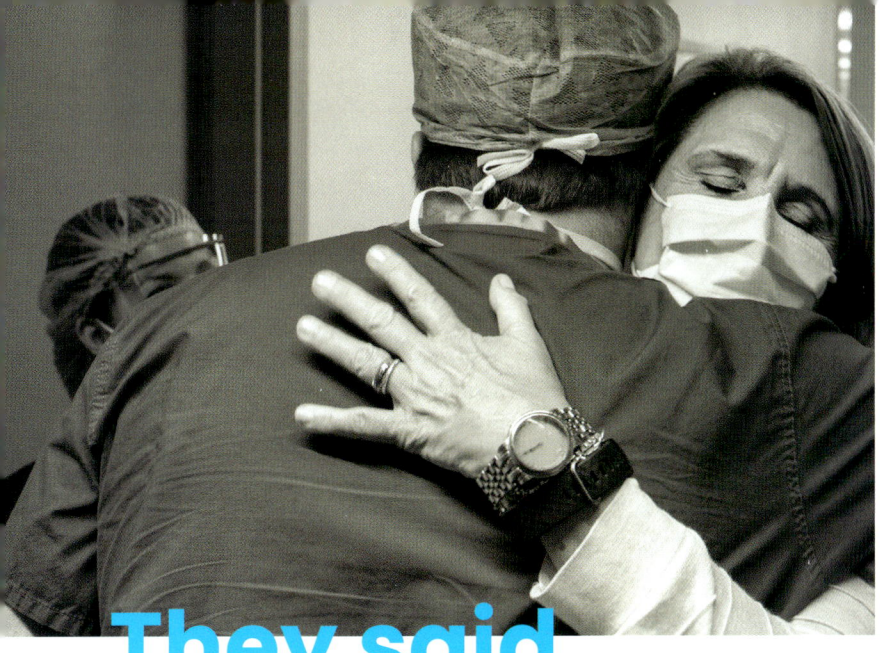

They said it couldn't be done. We didn't listen.

We've done hard things before, we do them all the time.

For most cancer patients, the usual options are surgery, chemotherapy, or radiation. So we're working on ways to get the immune system to deploy billions of cancer-killing cells and help more patients survive.

When some people experienced mysterious COVID symptoms and had nowhere to go, our team created the first Center for Post-COVID Care.

It wasn't that long ago we had to open up your whole chest for heart surgery. Now we're pioneering a bypass that goes through a few tiny incisions. With this surgery, we can get you back on your feet in weeks instead of months.

So if anyone ever tells you there's no other way—don't listen.

| WE FIND A WAY

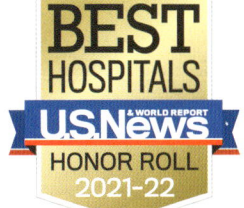

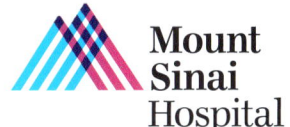

ON MEDICINE'S FRONT LINES

"If the patient isn't going to go to the hospital, then the hospital needs to go to the patient," Eichler says.

Interrupted heart care. People with heart disease also lost access to diagnostic procedures. A survey of 909 inpatient and outpatient centers published in January found that the volume of procedures such as echocardiograms and stress tests fell 64% between March 2019 and April 2020. There was a subsequent increase in deaths from cardiovascular disease, particularly in minority communities. A study published in May by researchers at Beth Israel Deaconess Medical Center in Boston found a 19% relative increase in heart disease deaths among Black, Asian and Hispanic people between 2019 and 2020, compared with a 2% increase among white people.

"There was a proportion of the population that didn't get the diagnostic tests they needed and therefore didn't get appropriate interventions," says Dr. Rishi Wadhera, a cardiologist at Beth Israel Deaconess and an assistant professor of medicine at Harvard Medical School. He hopes that in the future, public health initiatives will encourage people with heart disease to continue to seek out care, conveying the message "that hospitals are safe places to receive care, even in a pandemic." And the messaging needs to reach vulnerable populations, he says.

As for mental health issues brought on by the pan-

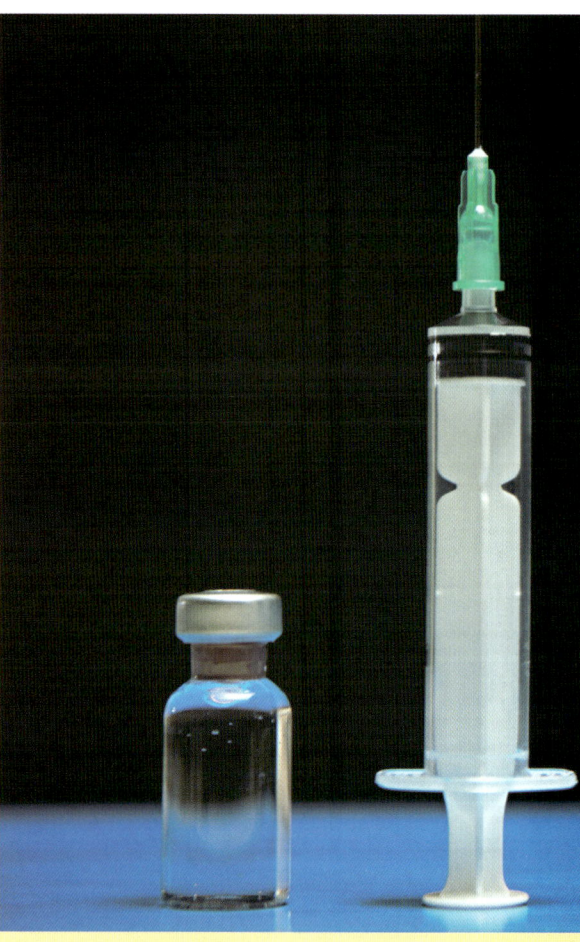

The Future of mRNA Vaccines

IN DECEMBER 2020, scientists in South Africa sequenced the genome of a variant of SARS-CoV-2 that was causing an aggressive new strain of COVID-19 to start spreading around the world. Just two months later, vaccine maker Moderna said it was ready to test two booster shots to its original COVID vaccine – both designed to tackle the new variant.

The new mRNA technology behind the Moderna and Pfizer-BioNTech COVID-19 vaccines is being hailed as a gamechanger in the future battle against infectious diseases, and even against some cancers. That's largely because of how quickly mRNA vaccines can be developed in response to new invaders – and then tweaked if those invaders mutate to try to escape an immune attack. "There are hundreds and hundreds of diseases for which mRNA could be useful," says Dr. Drew Weissman, a professor of medicine at the University of Pennsylvania whose lab has developed several mRNA vaccines that are on the verge of human testing.

Next up: the flu. Making an mRNA vaccine entails taking a piece of a virus's DNA strand – in the case of COVID, it's the part that makes the spike protein that gives the virus that studded appearance – and using it to teach the immune system to recognize and eliminate the virus. The vaccine causes cells to make the target protein, prompting the immune system to eliminate the virus anytime it appears in the body.

One target for which the technology is considered especially promising: influenza. Manufacturing the seasonal flu vaccine currently is a laborious six-month-or-longer process that involves growing what are predicted to be the dominant virus strains in eggs, harvesting and inactivating them, and then making vaccine doses at huge scale. If an unexpected strain pops up, the vaccine can't be changed on a dime to cover it. An mRNA vaccine that teaches the body to

demic, the Kaiser Family Foundation found that 4 in 10 adults reported symptoms of anxiety or depression, as compared to 1 in 10 in 2019. That correlated with a 12% increase in substance abuse, a 36% increase in sleep disorders and other problems. The Centers for Disease Control and Prevention found a 31% rise in emergency-room visits by 12- to 17-year olds suffering from mental health issues between April and October 2020. And some people who lost loved ones to the virus could be suffering from "prolonged grief disorder," a recently recognized condition in which intense, disabling grief makes it difficult for those who are mourning to adjust to the permanence of the loss, says Dr. Naomi Simon, a psychiatry professor at NYU Grossman School of Medicine and director of the Anxiety, Stress and Prolonged Grief Program at NYU Langone. "When you consider the nature of the death, and the bereaved not getting a chance to say goodbye or come together with family or friends, there's a risk that many people will have stress-related psychological issues over time," Simon says.

A promising effect of all the disruption, and good news for patients with chronic illnesses physical and mental, is that health systems across the country have embraced telehealth (story, Page 30). In the privately

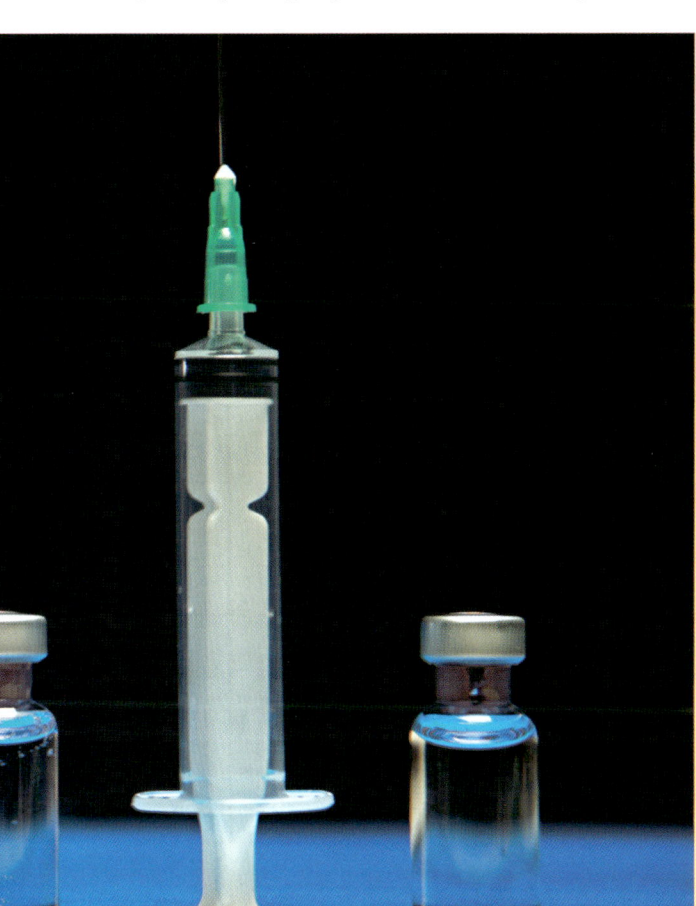

recognize hemagglutinin A or B, the proteins on the surface of flu viruses, could be developed much faster and adjusted quickly, Weissman says.

In January, Moderna said it was developing three mRNA vaccines covering four seasonal flu viruses, and the company has recently begun human testing.

Weissman and a range of companies, including mRNA vaccine developer CureVac, are using the technology to try to develop a universal flu vaccine – a single shot that could cover most strains of the influenza A virus that emerge over time. Rather than target the "head" of the hemagglutinin protein, which tends to mutate every year, the vaccine would be designed to elicit an immune response to the less changeable "stem" or "stalk" region, explains Weissman.

Other targets. Moderna and BioNTech are also working on mRNA vaccines to prevent HIV, a virus that mutates quickly. The idea is to use the technology to elicit broadly neutralizing antibodies, immune proteins that target the virus and keep it at bay even as it changes, says Dr. Rajesh Gandhi, an infectious diseases physician at Massachusetts General Hospital and co-director of the Harvard Center for AIDS Research.

And mRNA technologies could be applied to develop vaccines against other viruses that can hide out in the body for years, often producing no symptoms but raising the risk of other diseases. Epstein-Barr virus, or EBV, has been linked to an increased risk of multiple sclerosis and some cancers, for example. In February 2020, just before the pandemic diverted the biopharma industry's attention, Moderna announced it was starting clinical trials of an mRNA vaccine to prevent EBV.

"There is increasing evidence that infectious agents may be a trigger for some of the major diseases of mankind," says Dr. Anthony Komaroff, a professor of medicine at Harvard Medical School. "A vaccine given early in life could have an enormous protective effect."

Other diseases for which mRNA vaccines are now in development include Zika, yellow fever and tuberculosis. Therapeutic mRNA vaccines designed to stimulate an immune response to cancer are also being explored in melanoma, prostate cancer, lung cancer and many other tumor types. Says Ghandi: "We're on the threshold of a new revolution in vaccinology." –*Arlene Weintraub*

ON MEDICINE'S FRONT LINES

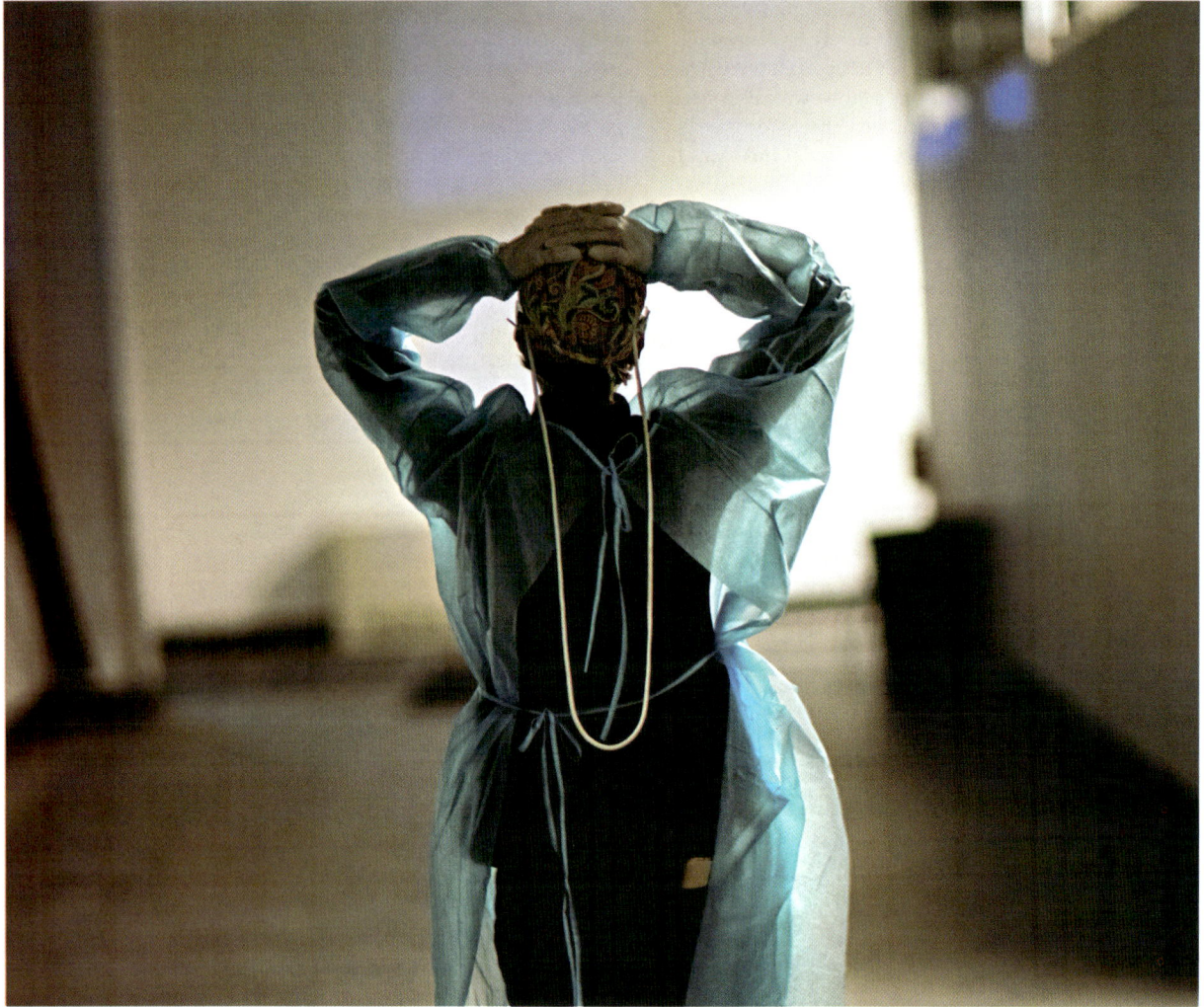

NIGHT SHIFT IN A CRANSTON, RHODE ISLAND FIELD HOSPITAL LAST FEBRUARY, WITH MANY BEDS AT LAST EMPTY.

insured working-age population, remote visits accounted for nearly 24% of health care interactions during the early part of the pandemic, up from less than 1% in 2019, according to a study by researchers at the Johns Hopkins Bloomberg School of Public Health published in March.

Telehealth is here to stay, predicts Cynthia Cox, vice president at Kaiser Family Foundation and director of the Peterson-Kaiser Health System Tracker. "It has a lot of potential to solve a lot of problems in the health care system, from access to cost. Now we just need to learn how to work with it and use it to its best potential."

Financial stresses. Hospitals are undertaking these efforts under extreme financial pressure, however. The AHA estimates that hospitals lost more than $323 billion in 2020, as they were forced to end nonessential care. Half of hospitals could be operating with negative margins by the end of 2021, far more than before the pandemic, according to research firm Kaufman Hall.

Clearly, resources will need to be found as the country undertakes the massive challenge of making sure the health system is ready for the next – inevitable – emergency, from designing more resilient hospitals (box, Page 14) to rapidly developing drugs and vaccines (box, Page 18). The AHA has been pushing the federal government to chip in on hospital infrastructure expansion efforts, with some success. The American Jobs Plan, introduced in March, allocates $18 billion in government funding for modernizing veteran's hospitals. The bill proposes another $50 billion in infrastructure investments, including improvements to community hospitals and other health facilities.

"The four 'S's' of disaster preparedness – staff, stuff, space and systems – all came to light during the pandemic, from issues related to personal protective equipment to hospitals needing to use tents to the absolute lack of staffing," says Dr. David Wallace, professor of critical care medicine at the University of Pittsburgh School of Medicine. "But most hospitals learned. And they're now thinking about the next one." ●

Calm Down.*

***Bad advice for a heart attack — and mental health**

Mental health issues are as real as any heart attack. And just like heart attacks, mental health issues can become even more difficult to manage if not treated early. As one of the nation's top mental health providers, our renowned clinicians offer unparalled care to support you and your family through any challenge – at any stage in life. With more than 160 programs to fit your needs, Sheppard Pratt is here to help.

Take the first step at sheppardpratt.org/treatit.

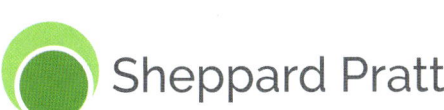

Hospitals | Communities | Schools | Residential | Telehealth

ON MEDICINE'S FRONT LINES

Looking Back

Photo Editing by **Lydia Chebbine**

THE STRESSES that have so challenged the nation's hospitals these past 18 months have uncovered some serious shortcomings in the system, to be sure. But they also have revealed health care providers' enormous dedication, compassion and resilience. The following pages revisit a few moments, from around the country, of these difficult times.

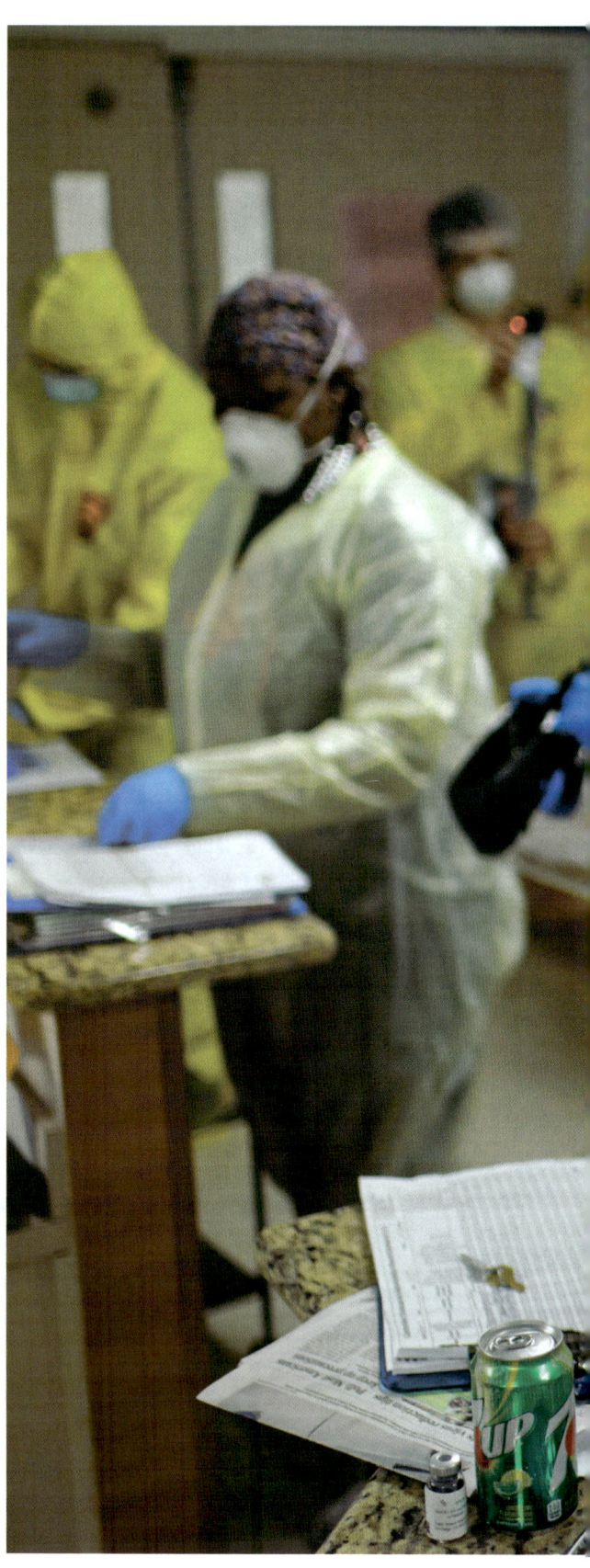

HOUSTON – JULY 2, 2020 | **AS CASES EXPLODED IN TEXAS, A STAFFER AT UNITED MEMORIAL MEDICAL CENTER RECEIVED A SHOULDER RUB FROM A COLLEAGUE BEFORE HEADING INTO THE COVID-19 UNIT.**
MARK FELIX – AFP VIA GETTY IMAGES

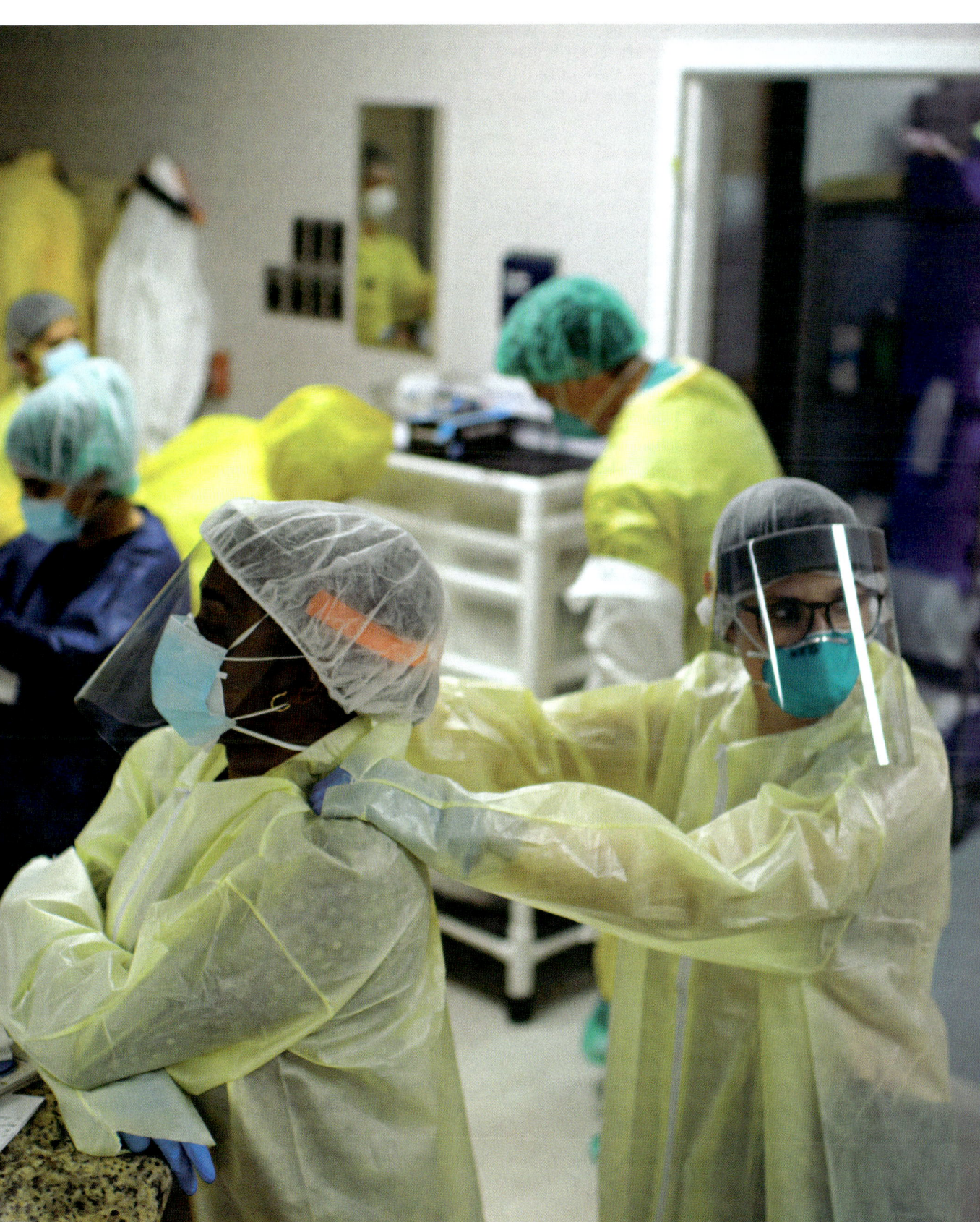

ON MEDICINE'S FRONT LINES

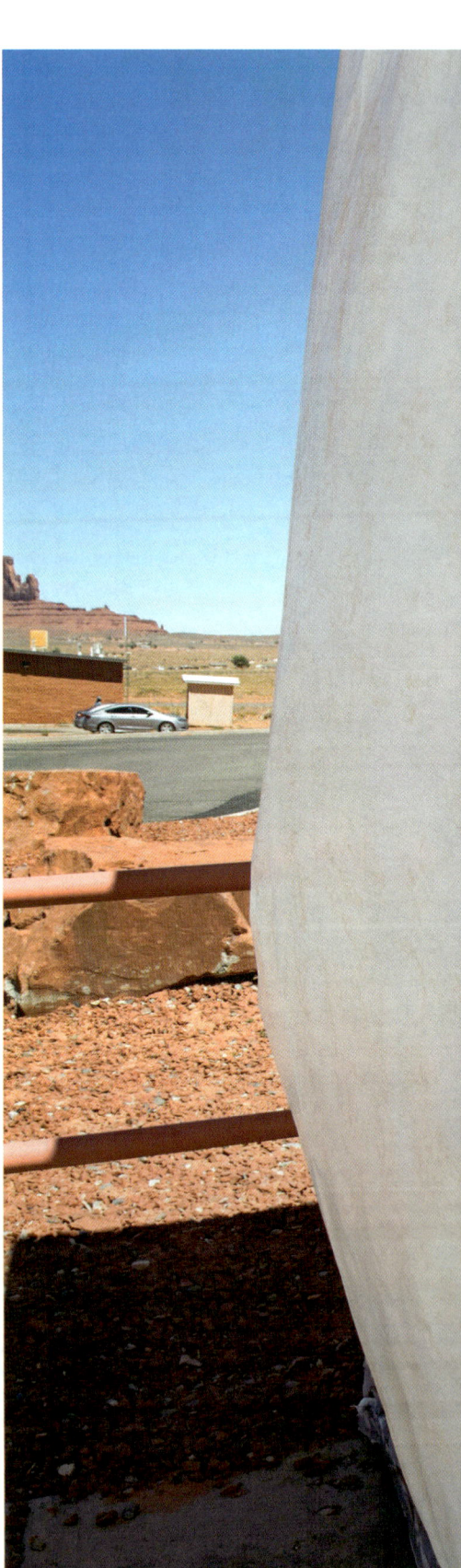

MONUMENT VALLEY, ARIZ. – MAY 21, 2020 | **A NURSE AT A COVID-19 TESTING CENTER IN THE HARD-HIT NAVAJO NATION CHECKED THE VITALS OF A WOMAN COMPLAINING OF VIRUS SYMPTOMS.**
MARK RALSTON – AFP VIA GETTY IMAGES

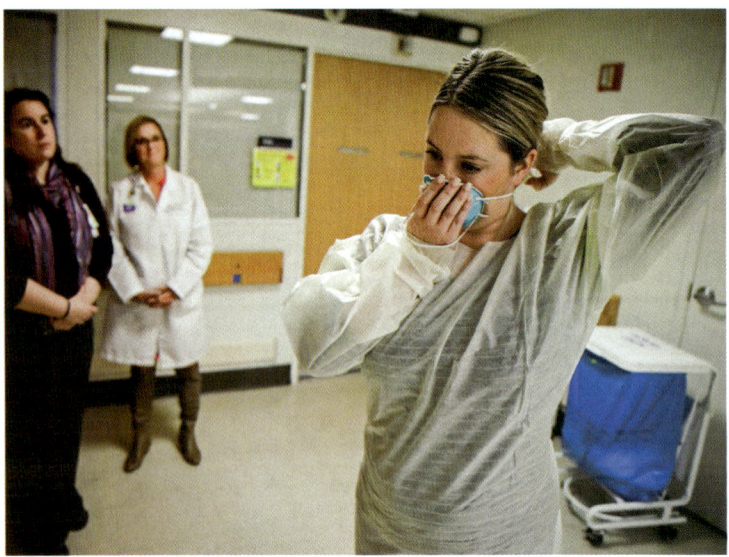

BOSTON - FEBRUARY 27, 2020 | **EARLY IN THE PANDEMIC, AS BOSTON PREPARED FOR WIDESPREAD INFECTION, STAFFERS AT MASSACHUSETTS GENERAL HOSPITAL WATCHED A DEMONSTRATION OF HOW TO WEAR PROTECTIVE GEAR.**
ERIN CLARK – THE BOSTON GLOBE VIA GETTY IMAGES

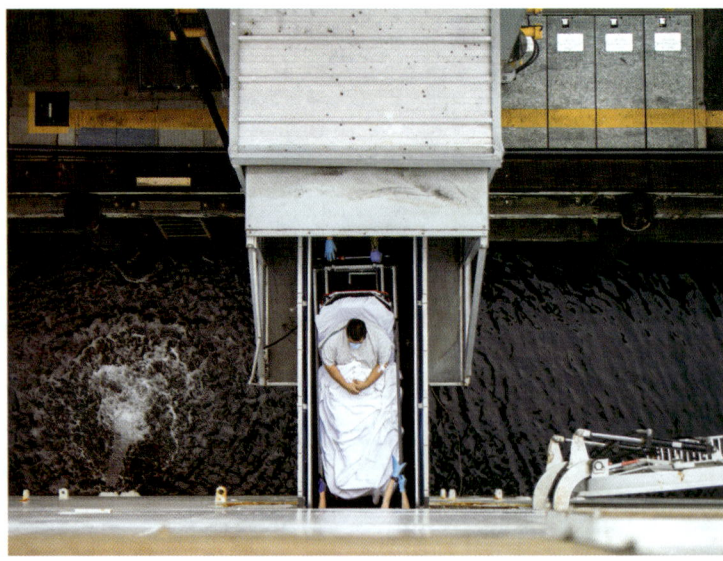

LOS ANGELES – APRIL 6, 2020 | **SAILORS BROUGHT A PATIENT ABOARD THE HOSPITAL SHIP USNS MERCY, WHICH WAS DEPLOYED TO SUPPORT LOCAL HOSPITALS BY TAKING CARE OF NON-COVID PATIENTS AND FREEING UP BEDS.**
RYAN BREEDEN – U.S. NAVY VIA GETTY IMAGES

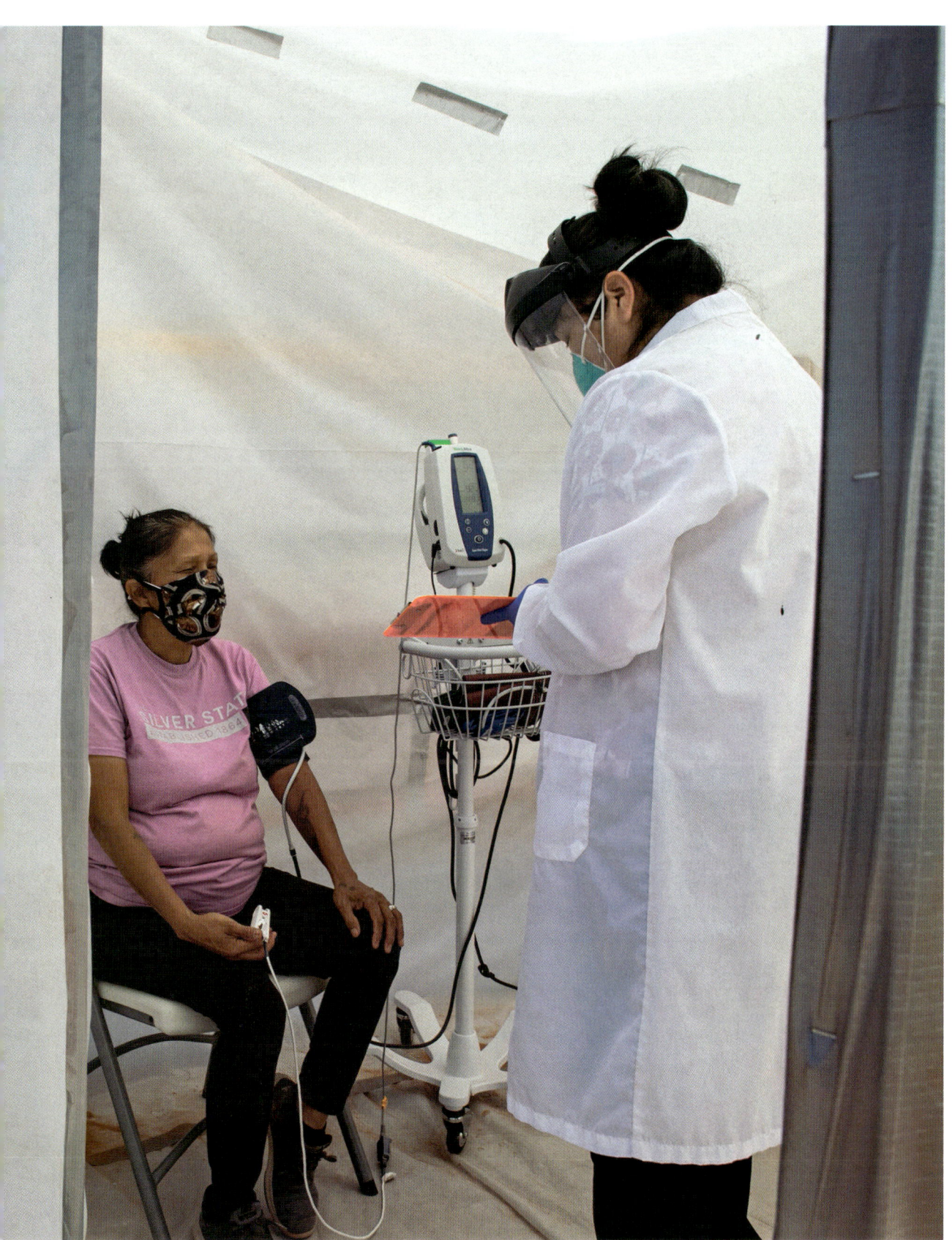

ON MEDICINE'S FRONT LINES

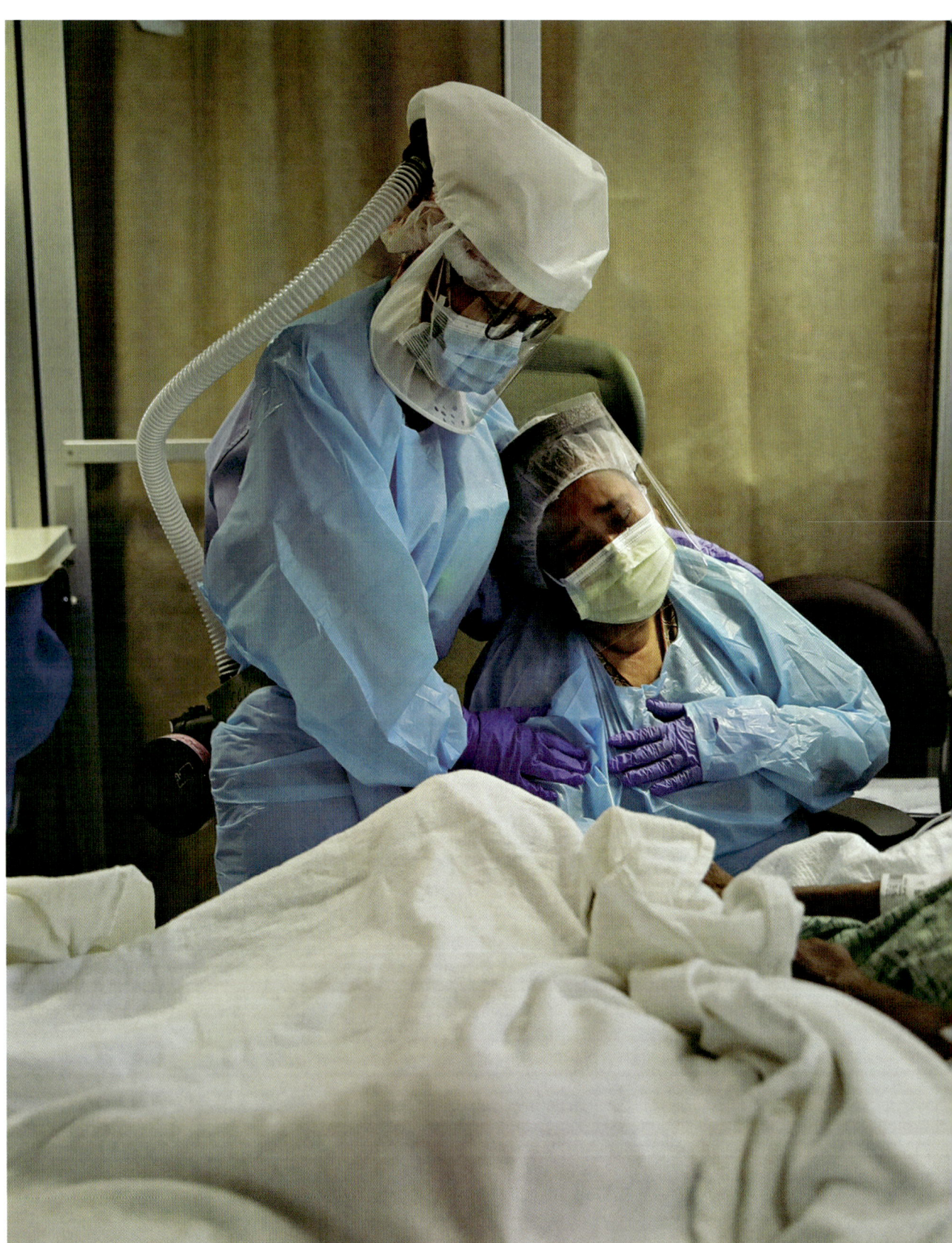

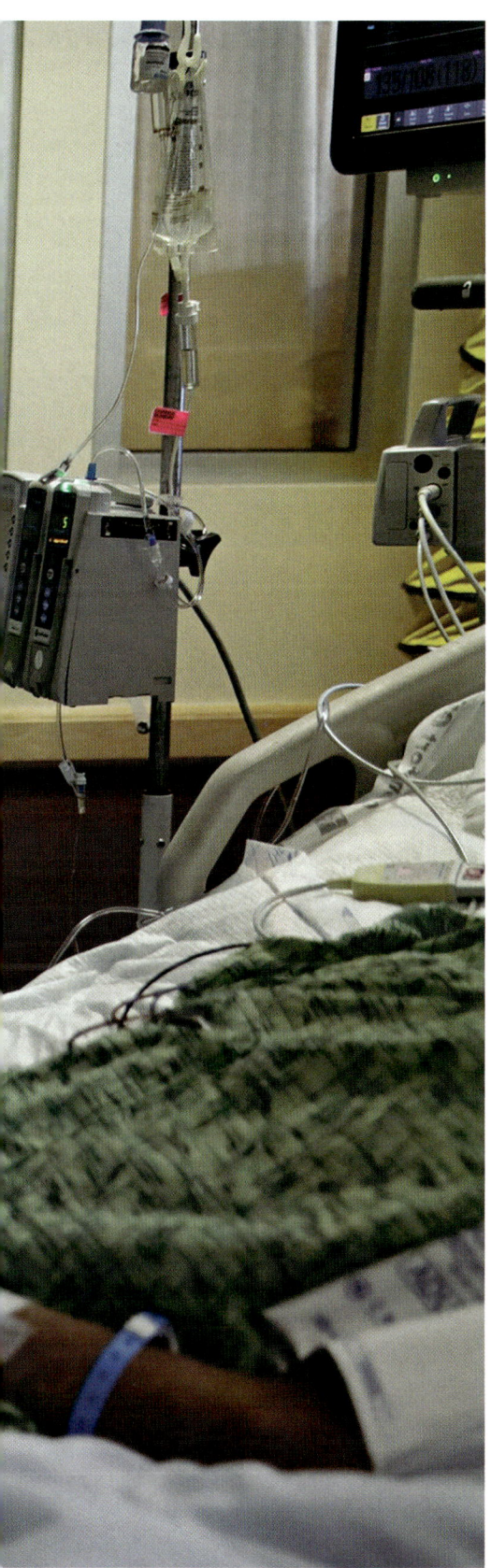

FULLERTON, CALIF. – JULY 31, 2020 | **ST. JUDE MEDICAL CENTER NURSE MICHELE YOUNKIN COMFORTED ROMELIA NAVARRO AT THE BEDSIDE OF HER DYING HUSBAND, ANTONIO NAVARRO.**
JAE C. HONG – AP

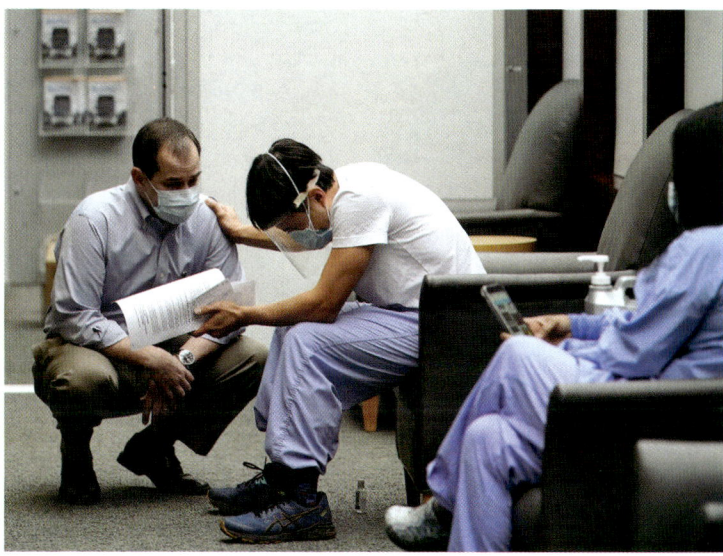

SEATTLE – DECEMBER 15, 2020 | **DR. THUAN ONG (CENTER), WHOSE TEAM AT UW MEDICINE WAS THE FIRST TO TREAT COVID PATIENTS AT LONG-TERM CARE FACILITIES IN THE AREA, SPOKE OF THEM, REMEMBERING PARTICULARLY THOSE WHO HAD DIED, WITH CHIEF MEDICAL OFFICER DR. TIM DELLIT.**
ELAINE THOMPSON – AP

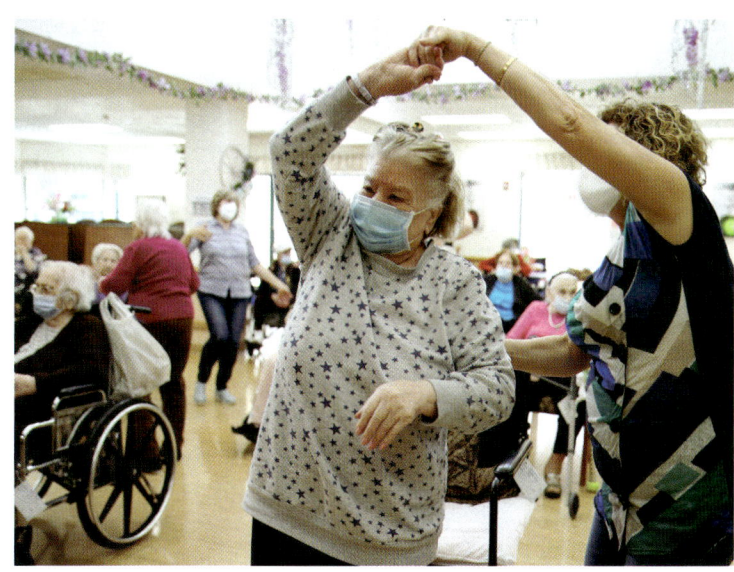

LOS ANGELES – APRIL 1, 2021 | **VACCINATED RESIDENTS OF THE ARARAT NURSING FACILITY CELEBRATED AT AN EASTER CONCERT AS RESTRICTIONS EASED.**
MARIO TAMA – GETTY IMAGES

ON MEDICINE'S FRONT LINES

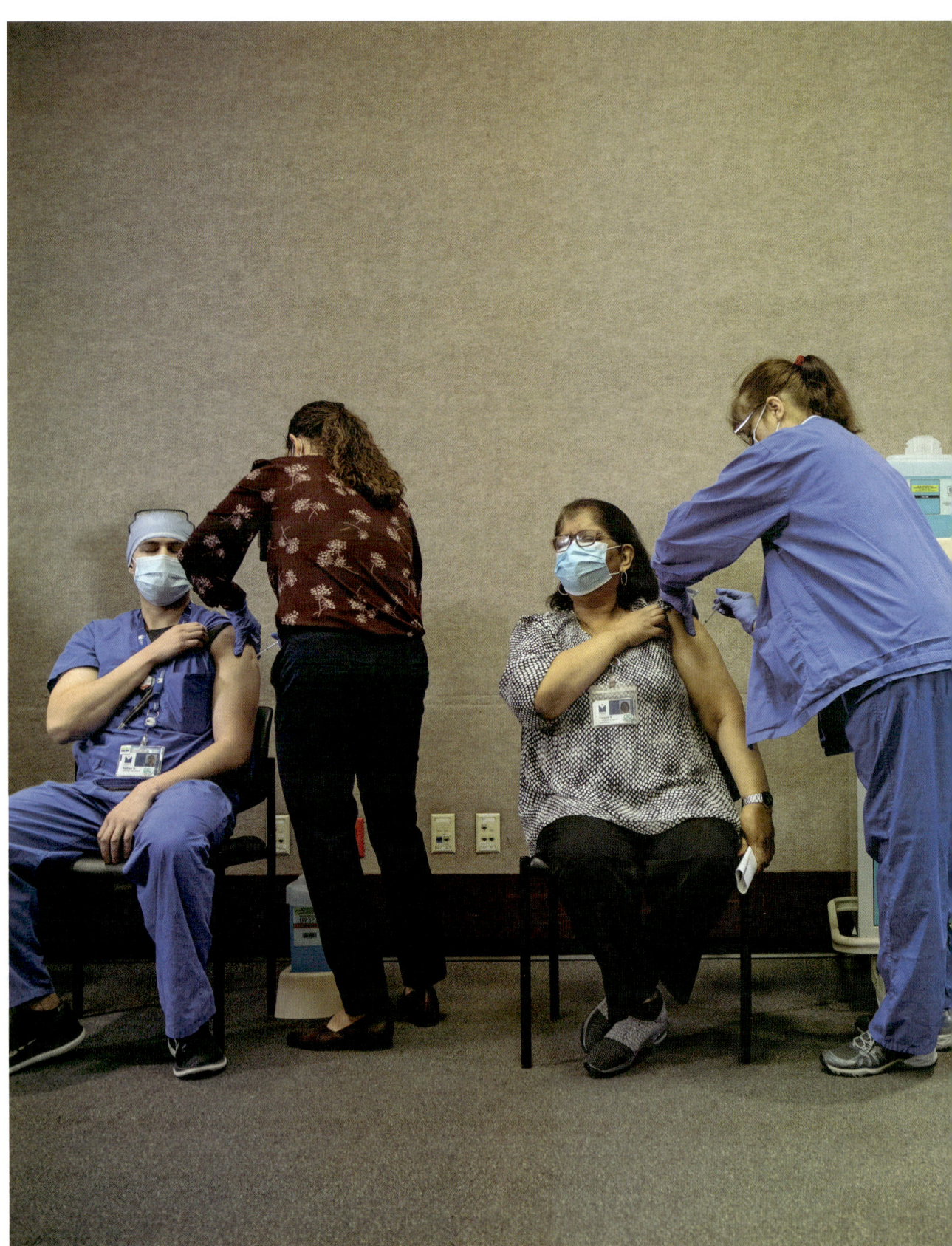

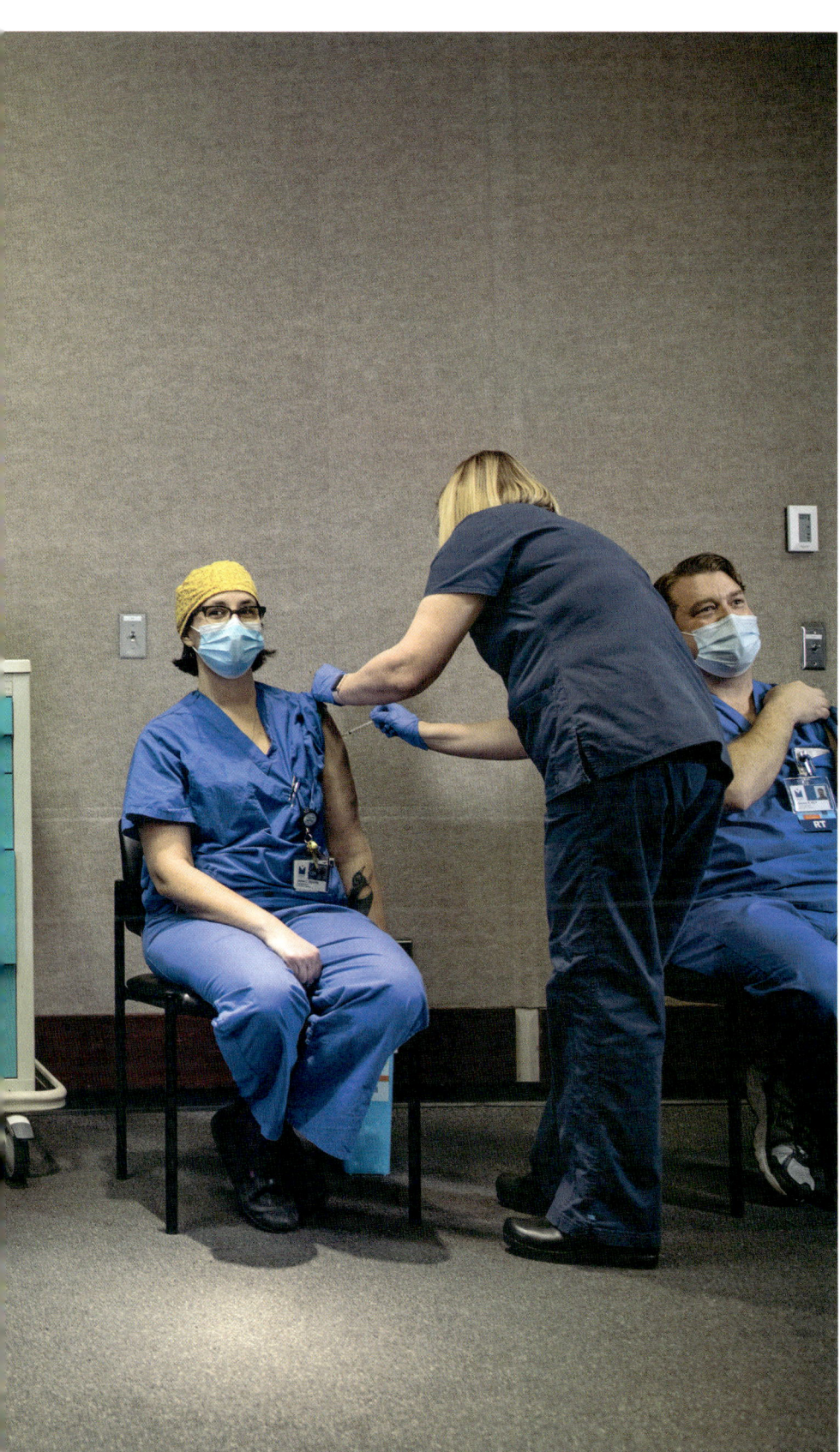

PORTLAND, ORE. – DECEMBER 16, 2020 | **ON THE FIRST DAY OF VACCINATIONS IN OREGON, HEALTH CARE WORKERS AT LEGACY EMANUEL MEDICAL CENTER LINED UP TO RECEIVE A DOSE OF THE PFIZER-BIONTECH VACCINE.**
PAULA BRONSTEIN – GETTY IMAGES

ON MEDICINE'S FRONT LINES

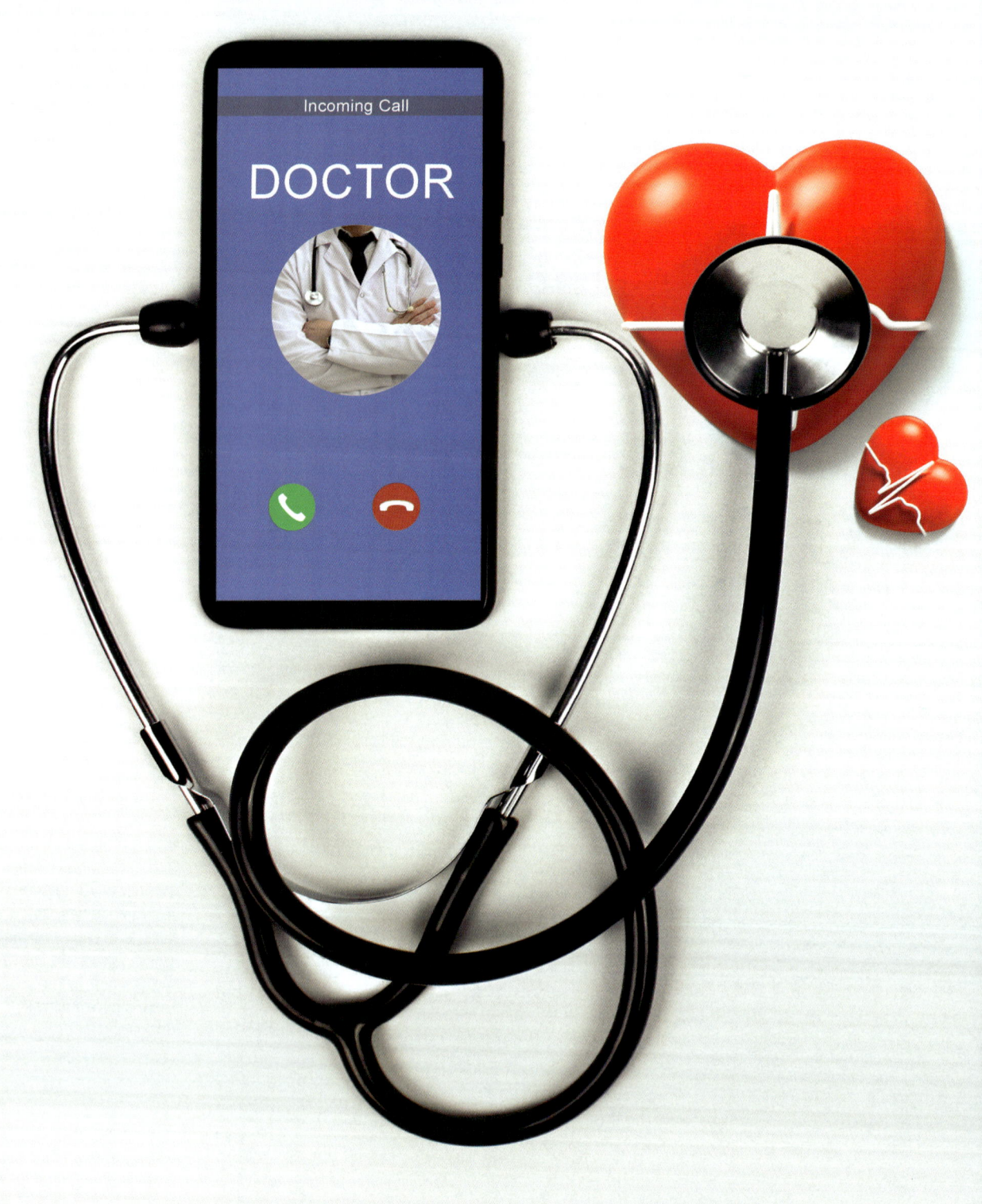

The Post-Pandemic Role of Virtual Care

After 2020's rapid shift to telemedicine, experts think as much as half of care could be delivered remotely

by **Margaret Loftus**

AMY SHIDELER had barely put down roots in Northeast Ohio last fall when she tested positive for COVID-19. Aside from a friend who lived 30 miles away, her support system had yet to be built, and her parents, in Indiana, were recovering from the virus themselves. Beset by fatigue and fever, she worried about being alone, especially since she had a history of asthma. "It was a very isolating feeling."

But a new home monitoring program at Cleveland Clinic, where Shideler is employed as a social worker manager, made her feel less alone. Each day, she used the MyChart app on her smartphone to log her symptoms, temperature and oxygen level, which were then assessed by care coordinators at the clinic. Within 10 minutes of reporting shortness of breath one morning, she was called by a nurse and connected to a physician, who immediately prescribed a new inhaler. In all, the medical center's virtual team evaluated her three times for symptoms that might otherwise have sent her to the emergency room. "I felt very cared for," she says. "It was comforting to know I was going to get what I needed right where I was."

AT CLEVELAND CLINIC, VIRTUAL VISITS SKYROCKETED FROM ABOUT 37,000 IN 2019 TO 1.2 MILLION LAST YEAR.

Caring for patients where they are has long been the promise of telemedicine, but it took unexpected and explosive demand last year to make the promise real. Cleveland Clinic, whose telehealth work pre-pandemic amounted to second opinion and urgent care video calls, went from some 37,000 virtual visits in 2019 to 1.2 million in 2020. Virtual care company Teladoc Health facilitated 10.6 million visits last year, a 156 percent increase over 2019.

As normalcy returns, what should patients expect of virtual care in the future? Demand has leveled off, but experts predict that telemedicine – from doctor and psychotherapist visits to remote monitoring of chronic conditions – has established its place as a key mode of care delivery. "Now that people have been exposed to it, it's going to be a part of everything that we do," says Dr. Steven Shook, a neurologist and lead for virtual health at Cleveland Clinic. Consulting firm McKinsey estimated last year that up to $250 billion of the U.S. health care industry has the potential to become virtual, up from a pre-COVID revenue of $3 billion annually; providers estimate that as much as 50 percent of care could be delivered remotely.

The extent to which the industry grows depends largely on whether or not Congress makes

ON MEDICINE'S FRONT LINES

permanent changes to rules that allowed for the expansion of telehealth services, such as more favorable reimbursement rates and allowing remote care without geographic restrictions. At press time, sustaining expanded telehealth services had wide bipartisan support, but it's the eventual fine print – for example, the rates at which various telehealth services are reimbursed compared to those in clinical settings – that will shape the future.

Home as clinic. To that end, a group of providers that includes Intermountain Healthcare, Ascension, and Amazon Care recently formed a coalition – called Moving Health Home – to advocate for policy changes to designate the home as a site of clinical care. Members argue that advances in medical record-sharing, remote monitoring technologies and digital therapeutics have made it possible to deliver even acute care in the home in many cases. Salt Lake City-based Intermountain, for example, treats patients at home with everything from heart failure to some types of cancer with a combination of technology and visits from an interdisciplinary caregiving team.

Consumers, for the most part, like the idea. McKinsey found that 76 percent of consumers are now interested in using virtual care, compared to 11 percent prior to COVID.

'I don't think we can go back to where we were.'

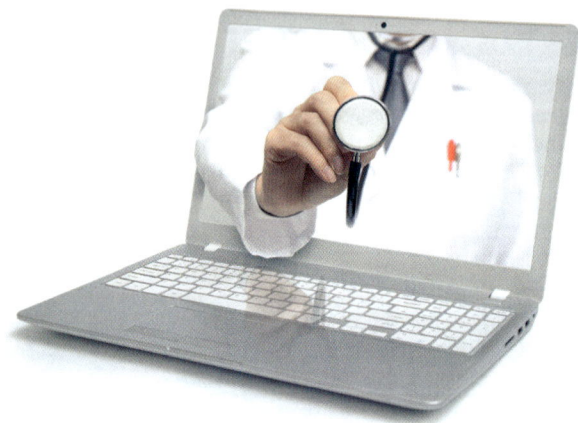

To be sure, any visits that require hands-on evaluation, such as orthopedics, are limited in their telehealth potential. On the other end of the spectrum, the possibilities for behavioral health are wide open: Mental health visits through Teladoc Health grew more than 500 percent in 2020 alone.

Another promising area: chronic diseases such as diabetes, which drive 80 percent of the health care costs in the U.S. Before COVID, Dr. Rachel Caskey, an internal medicine and pediatrics physician at UI Health in Chicago, only very rarely used telehealth. Today, she manages many of her patients with chronic conditions remotely by, for example, having those with diabetes rely on a glucometer to keep track of their blood sugar and people with hypertension use a blood pressure cuff to take their own measurements. "Coming into a clinic every three months can be onerous, so a quick 20-minute call is no problem," she says. "I'm finding at least every other visit can be replaced." Likewise, at the Medical University of South Carolina, diabetes patients are monitored through cellular-connected glucometers, which beam data via a secure cloud to a team of nurses who can adjust insulin.

The coronavirus itself became a case study for remote monitoring. In one study, UI Health partnered with the digital health care company physIQ to send COVID patients home fitted with a biosensor patch to collect data on heart and respiratory rates and arrhythmias, as well as movement. The sensor, which is connected to an Android device – essentially a burner phone – sends the data to a team of nurses who check in with patients once a day. The goal is to mine the collective data for markers that precede a decline of a patient's condition. "This kind of technology can and should be given to patients with lots of other chronic conditions," says Dr. David Chestek, one of the investigators and interim chief medical information officer at UI Health.

Predictive value. Indeed, a study last year by physIQ and four VA hospitals found that such analytics accurately predicted hospitalization for heart failure patients. And because these patients often have other health issues, it also predicted adverse events such as pneumonia and renal failure.

For all its technological promise, telemedicine has the potential to foster a more patient-centered health care system, proponents argue. Consider that much of routine care has been delivered in 15-minute increments once a year, says Dr. James McElligott, the medical director for the Center of Telehealth at MUSC. "It's all about one point in time, but that's not how health and wellness work." McElligott thinks telehealth will provide the opportunity to check in more often with patients where they live, with more of a focus on their functioning and wellness. "A big page has turned," he says. "I don't think we can go back to where we were." ●

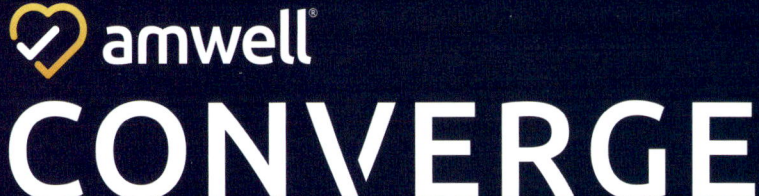

amwell CONVERGE

Further Advancing Digital Connectivity with Next Generation Telehealth Platform

Virtual care in a single meeting place.

 Simplicity   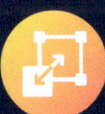 Extensibility

 Reliability    Integration

 Efficiency   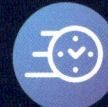 Support

Visit **www.amwell.com** to learn more.

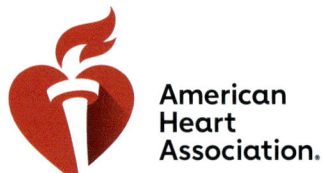

BRANDFUSE

Be Confident in Consistent Care

Here's how to find heart and stroke care measured by the American Heart Association near you.

Access to high-quality care is something that everyone should have, especially in today's times. Each year, the American Heart Association recognizes hospitals across the country that demonstrate commitment to following up-to-date, research-based guidelines for the treatment of heart disease and stroke.

These hospitals have maintained unrelenting standards in the midst of adversity to ensure all patients have access to the best practices and lifesaving care. Read more about the recognition categories from the American Heart Association and find a participating hospital near you.

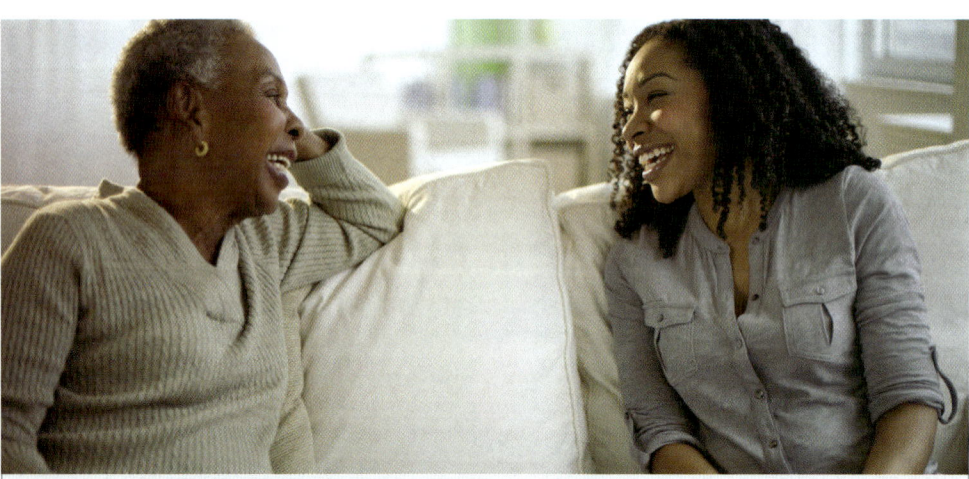

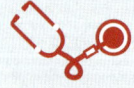 Heart disease and stroke are the No. 1 and No. 5 causes of death in the United States, respectively.

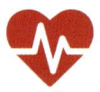 Every 40 seconds, someone in America has a stroke or heart attack.

 American Heart Association gives hospitals up-to-date treatment guidelines with its Get With The Guidelines program.

 More than 2,500 hospitals participate in AHA's GWTG initiative, a 20-plus year effort to bring research-based care to heart and stroke patients.

ADOBE STOCK

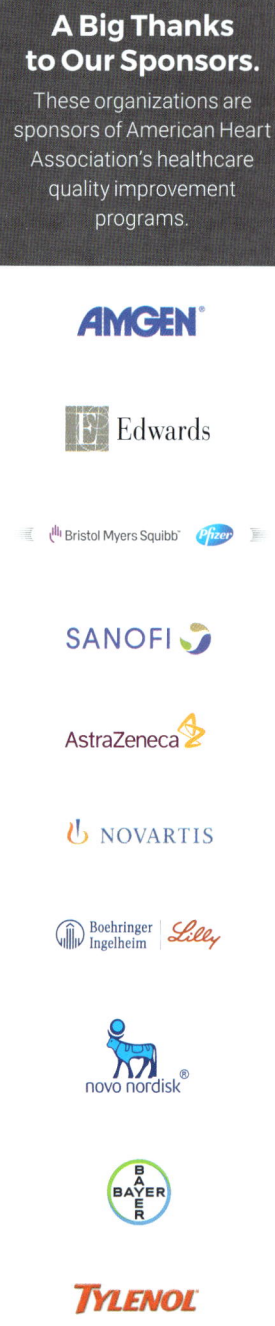

A Big Thanks to Our Sponsors. These organizations are sponsors of American Heart Association's healthcare quality improvement programs.

This content is produced by or on behalf of our sponsor; it is not written by and does not necessarily reflect the view of U.S. News & World Report editorial staff. Learn more at mediakit.usnews.com.

SPONSORED CONTENT

Key to the Awards

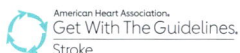 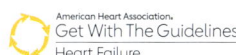 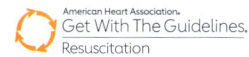 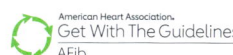 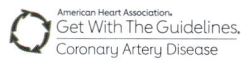

Gold Plus Achievement
These hospitals are recognized for two or more consecutive calendar years of 85% or higher adherence on all achievement measures applicable and 75% or higher adherence with additional select quality measures in heart failure, and/or stroke.

Silver Plus Achievement
These hospitals are recognized for one calendar year of 85% or higher adherence on all achievement measures applicable and 75% or higher adherence with additional select quality measures in heart failure, and/or stroke.

Gold Achievement
These hospitals are recognized for two or more consecutive calendar years of 85% or higher adherence on all achievement measures applicable to each program.

Silver Achievement
These hospitals are recognized for one calendar year of 85% or higher adherence on all achievement measures applicable to each program.

*These hospitals received Get With The Guidelines-Resuscitation awards from the American Heart Association for two or more patient populations.

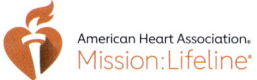 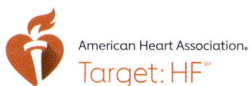 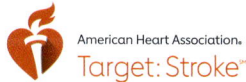

STEMI: Gold Plus Receiving and Silver Plus Receiving
These hospitals are recognized, in addition to their baseline gold or silver award, for 50% or higher adherence to First Door-to-Device time of 120 minutes or less for transferred STEMI patients.

STEMI: Gold Receiving or Silver Receiving
These hospitals are recognized, in addition to their baseline gold/silver award, for 75% adherence to 7 performance measures and 50% adherence to Arrival at First Hospital to PCI less than or equal to 120 minutes.

STEMI: Gold Referring or Silver Referring
These hospitals are recognized, in addition to their baseline gold or silver award, for 75% or higher adherence for 8 performance measures.

NSTEMI: Gold and Silver
These hospitals are recognized, in addition to their baseline gold or silver award, for 65% adherence to Dual Antiplatelet prescription at discharge and 75% or high compliance on each of the four performance measures. 75% or higher adherence for 8 performance measures.

Target: Heart Failure
These hospitals in addition to their achievement of Gold or Silver are recognized for 50% or higher performance to all relevant Target Measures.

Target: Stroke Honor Roll
These hospitals, in addition to their achievement of Gold or Silver, are recognized for 75% or higher performance in Time to IV thrombolytic therapy in 60 minutes or less.

Target: Stroke Honor Roll - Elite Plus
These hospitals, in addition to their achievement of Gold or Silver, are recognized for 75% or higher adherence for Time to IV thrombolytic therapy in 45 minutes or less and 50% or higher in Time to IV thrombolytic therapy in 30 minutes or less.

Target: Stroke Honor Roll – Elite
These hospitals, in addition to their achievement of Gold or Silver, are recognized for 75% or higher performance in Time to IV thrombolytic therapy in 60 minutes or less.

Target: Stroke Honor Roll Advanced Therapy
These hospitals, in addition to their achievement of Gold or Silver, are recognized for Door to Device times in at least 50% of applicable patients within 90 minutes for direct arriving and within 60 minutes for transfers.

Target: Type 2 Diabetes Honor Roll™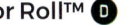
A national honor roll program for hospitals participating in Get With The Guidelines® (HF, Stroke) to reinforce evidence-based guidelines with hospitals that qualify for a Silver level or higher achievement award in the related Get With The Guidelines module. These hospitals must be able to demonstrate at least 90% compliance for 12 consecutive months (calendar year) for the "Overall Diabetes Cardiovascular Initiative Composite Score" measure in the selected module.

© 2021 American Heart Association

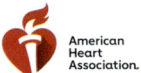

SPONSORED CONTENT

Find Your Hospital Listed Alphabetically By State

For a searchable map of hospitals by region and across the U.S., visit heart.org/myhealthcare.

ALABAMA

Hospital	Awards
Brookwood Baptist Medical Center, Birmingham	G+ E+ AT
Coosa Valley Medical Center, Sylacauga	G+ D S+
Crestwood Medical Center, Huntsville	G G+ D
Cullman Regional Medical Center, Cullman, AL, Cullman	S+ G+ E+ D
Flowers Hospital, Dothan	G+ D
Grandview Medical Center, Birmingham	G+ D
Huntsville Hospital, Huntsville	G G+ D
Medical Center Enterprise, Enterprise	G+ D
Mobile Infirmary, Mobile	G G+ E D
North Alabama Medical Center, Florence	G+
Princeton Baptist Medical Center, Birmingham	G+ E D
Riverview Regional Medical Center, Gadsden	G+ D
Shelby Baptist Medical Center, Alabaster	G+ HR
Southeast Health Medical Center, Dothan	G+
Thomas Hospital, Fairhope	G+
UAB Hospital, Birmingham	G HR G+ E D S+
USA Health University Hospital, Mobile	G+ E+ D

ALASKA

Hospital	Awards
Alaska Regional Hospital, Anchorage	G+ E D
Fairbanks Memorial Hospital, Fairbanks	G+ D
Mat-Su Regional Medical Center, Palmer	G+ D
Providence Alaska Medical Center, Anchorage	G+ E D S+

ARIZONA

Hospital	Awards
Abrazo Arrowhead Campus, Glendale	G+ E D
Abrazo Central Campus, Phoenix	G+ E AT D
Banner Baywood Medical Center, Mesa	G+ E D
Banner Boswell Medical Center, Sun City	G+ E D
Banner Del E Webb Medical Center, Sun City West	G+ E D
Banner Desert Medical Center, Mesa	G+ E AT D
Banner Estrella Medical Center, Phoenix	G+ E D
Banner Thunderbird Medical Center, Glendale	G+ HR D
Banner University Medical Center Phoenix, Phoenix	G+ E AT D
Banner University Medical Center Tucson, Tucson	G+ E D
Carondelet St. Mary's Hospital, Tucson	G+ E+
Dignity Health - Chandler Regional Medical Center, Chandler	G+ E+ D
Dignity Health - Mercy Gilbert Medical Center, Gilbert	G+ E D
HonorHealth Deer Valley Medical Center, Phoenix	G+ E+ D
HonorHealth John C. Lincoln Medical Center, Phoenix	G+ E D
HonorHealth Scottsdale Osborn Medical Center, Scottsdale	G+ E+ AT D
HonorHealth Scottsdale Shea Medical Center, Phoenix	G+ E D
HonorHealth Scottsdale Thompson Peak Medical Center, Scottsdale	G+ D
Mayo Clinic Arizona, Phoenix	S G+ E+ D
Mountain Vista Medical Center, Mesa	G+ D
Phoenix VA Healthcare System, Phoenix	G
St. Joseph's Hospital and Medical Center, Phoenix	G+ HR G+ HR D
Summit Healthcare Association, Show Low	G+ E+ D
The Neurological Institute at Carondelet St. Joseph's Hospital, Tucson	G+ E+
Tucson Medical Center, Tucson	G+ E D
Valleywise Health Medical Center, Phoenix	G * S

ARKANSAS

Hospital	Awards
Baptist Health Medical Center - Conway, Conway	G D
Baptist Health Medical Center, Little Rock	G+ D
Baptist Health-Fort Smith, Fort Smith	S+ G+ D
CHI St. Vincent Hot Springs, Hot Springs	G+ G+ S
CHI St. Vincent Infirmary, Little Rock	G+ S
CHI St. Vincent Morrilton, Morrilton	S+
Conway Regional Medical Center, Conway	G+ HR G+
Forrest City Medical Center, Forrest City	G
Johnson Regional Medical Center, Clarksville	G+ D
Mercy Hospital Fort Smith, Fort Smith	G+ E+ D
Mercy Hospital Rogers, Rogers	G+ D
NEA Baptist Memorial Hospital, Jonesboro	G+ E D
North Arkansas Regional Medical Center, Harrison	G+ E
Saint Mary's Regional Medical Center, Russellville	G+ E D
St. Bernards Five Rivers Medical Center, Pocahontas	G+ G+
St. Bernards Medical Center, Jonesboro	G+ S
UAMS Medical Center, Little Rock	G+ E
Washington Regional Medical Center, Fayetteville	G+ E AT D G+ S
White River Health System, Batesville	G+ D

CALIFORNIA

Hospital	Awards
Adventist Health + Rideout, Marysville	G+ E G
Adventist Health - Glendale, Glendale	G+ E+ D
Adventist Health Bakersfield, Bakersfield	G HR G+ E D D
Adventist Health Hanford, Hanford	G+ HR
Adventist Health Lodi Memorial, Lodi	G+ E D
Adventist Health Ukiah Valley, Ukiah	G+ D
Adventist Health White Memorial, Los Angeles	G+ E+ D
Alameda Hospital, Alameda	G+ HR D
Alvarado Hospital Medical Center, San Diego	G+ D
Antelope Valley Hospital, Lancaster	G+ HR AT
Arrowhead Regional Medical Center, Colton	G+ E D
Beverly Hospital, Montebello	G+ D
California Hospital Medical Center, Los Angeles	G+ E D
Cedars-Sinai Marina del Rey Hospital, Marina del Rey	G+ D
Cedars-Sinai Medical Center, Los Angeles	G+ E+ D
Centinela Hospital Medical Center, Inglewood	G+ D
CHA Hollywood Presbyterian Medical Center, Los Angeles	G+ D
CHOC Children's Hospital, Orange	S
Coast Plaza Hospital, Norwalk	G+ D
Community Hospital of the Monterey Peninsula, Monterey	G+ E D
Community Memorial Hospital, Ventura	G+ D
Community Regional Medical Center, Fresno	G+ HR D
Corona Regional Medical Center, Corona	G+ E D
Desert Regional Medical Center, Inc., Palm Springs	G+ E+ D
Desert Valley Hospital, Victorville	G+ HR S D D
Dignity Health Arroyo Grande Community Hospital, Arroyo Grande	G+ D
Dignity Health Bakersfield Memorial Hospital, Bakersfield	G+ E D G+ S
Dignity Health Dominican Hospital, Santa Cruz	G+ HR G+ HR D
Dignity Health Marian Regional Medical Center, Santa Maria	G+ E D
Dignity Health Mercy Hospital of Bakersfield, Bakersfield	G+ HR
Dignity Health Mercy Hospital of Folsom, Folsom	G+ HR
Dignity Health Mercy Medical Center Merced, Merced	G+ D

KEY TO THE AWARDS

GWTG - STROKE:
- G+ Gold Plus Achievement
- G Gold Achievement
- S+ Silver Plus Achievement
- S Silver Achievement

GWTG - HEART FAILURE:
- G+ Gold Plus Achievement
- G Gold Achievement
- S+ Silver Plus Achievement
- S Silver Achievement

GWTG - RESUSCITATION:
- G Gold Achievement
- S Silver Achievement

GWTG - AFIB:
- G Gold Achievement
- S Silver Achievement

© 2021 American Heart Association

*These hospitals received Get With The Guidelines-Resuscitation awards from the American Heart Association for two or more patient populations.

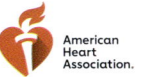

SPONSORED CONTENT

Hospital	Awards
Dignity Health Mercy Medical Center Redding, Redding	G+ E D
Dignity Health Methodist Hospital of Sacramento, Sacramento	G+ E+
Dignity Health Northridge Hospital Medical Center, Northridge	G+ E D
Dignity Health Saint Francis Memorial Hospital, San Francisco	G+
Dignity Health Sequoia Hospital, Redwood City	G+
Dignity Health Sierra Nevada Memorial Hospital, Grass Valley	G+ E+ D
Dignity Health St Bernardine Medical Center, San Bernardino	
Dignity Health St. John's Pleasant Valley Hospital, Camarillo	G+ E+
Dignity Health St. John's Regional Medical Center, Oxnard	G+ E D G+
Dignity Health St. Joseph's Medical Center, Stockton	D G+
Dignity Health St. Mary's Medical Center, San Francisco	G+ D
Dignity Health Woodland Memorial Hospital, Woodland	G+ E+
Doctors Medical Center, Modesto	G+ E D
Eisenhower Health, Rancho Mirage	G+ E D
El Camino Health, Mountain View	G+ E D
Emanate Health-Queen of the Valley Hospital, West Covina	G+ E D
Encino Hospital Medical Center, Encino	HR
Fairchild Medical Center, Yreka	S+ HR
Garden Grove Hospital Medical Center, Garden Grove	G+ HR G+ D D
Garfield Medical Center, Monterey Park	HR
Glendale Memorial Health Care Center, Glendale	S+
Good Samaritan Hospital, San Jose	S+ E
Hazel Hawkins Memorial Hospital, Hollister	S+
Henry Mayo Newhall Hospital, Valencia	
Hoag Hospital Irvine, Irvine	G+
Hoag Memorial Hospital Presbyterian, Newport Beach	G+ HR G+ E AT D
Huntington Beach Hospital, Huntington Beach	S+ HR D
Huntington Hospital, Pasadena	HR
JFK Memorial Hospital, Indio	S+
John Muir Medical Center - Concord, Concord	G+ G+ E D G+
John Muir Medical Center - Walnut Creek, Walnut Creek	G+ G+ HR AT D G
Kaiser Foundation Hospital - Antioch, Antioch	G+ E
Kaiser Foundation Hospital - Fontana Medical Center, Fontana	G+ E+ D
Kaiser Foundation Hospital - Fremont, Fremont	G+ G+ E+ D
Kaiser Foundation Hospital - Fresno, Fresno	G+ E+ D
Kaiser Foundation Hospital - Manteca, Manteca	G+ E
Kaiser Foundation Hospital - Modesto, Modesto	G+ E D
Kaiser Foundation Hospital - Oakland, Oakland	G+ E+ D
Kaiser Foundation Hospital - Ontario Medical Center, Ontario	G+ E+ D
Kaiser Foundation Hospital - Orange County, Anaheim	G+ E D
Kaiser Foundation Hospital - Orange County, Irvine	G+ E+ D
Kaiser Foundation Hospital - Redwood City, Redwood City	G+ G+ E+ AT D G
Kaiser Foundation Hospital - Richmond, Richmond	G+ E+
Kaiser Foundation Hospital - Roseville, Roseville	G+ E+
Kaiser Foundation Hospital - Sacramento, Sacramento	G+ G+ E+ AT D
Kaiser Foundation Hospital - San Diego Medical Center, San Diego	G+ E D
Kaiser Foundation Hospital - San Francisco, San Francisco	G+ HR E+ S
Kaiser Foundation Hospital - San Jose, San Jose	G+ E+ D
Kaiser Foundation Hospital - San Leandro, San Leandro	G+ E+ D
Kaiser Foundation Hospital - San Rafael, San Rafael	G+ E+ D
Kaiser Foundation Hospital - Santa Clara, Santa Clara	G+ HR G+ E+ D
Kaiser Foundation Hospital - Santa Rosa, Santa Rosa	G+ G+ E+ D
Kaiser Foundation Hospital - South Bay, Harbor City	G+ E+ D
Kaiser Foundation Hospital - South Sacramento, Sacramento	G+ G+ E+ D
Kaiser Foundation Hospital - South San Francisco, South San Francisco	G+ G+ E+ D
Kaiser Foundation Hospital - Vacaville, Vacaville	G+ E+ D
Kaiser Foundation Hospital - Vallejo, Vallejo	G+ E+ D
Kaiser Foundation Hospital - Walnut Creek, Walnut Creek	G+ E+ D
Kaiser Foundation Hospital - West Los Angeles, Los Angeles	G+ E+ D
Kaiser Foundation Hospital - Zion Medical Center, San Diego	G+ E+ D
Kaiser Foundation Hospital Woodland Hills, Woodland Hills	G+ E+ D
Kaiser Permanente - Downey Medical Center, Downey	G+ E D
Kaiser Permanente Baldwin Park Medical Center, Baldwin Park	G+ G+ E+ D D
Kaiser Permanente Los Angeles Medical Center, Los Angeles	G+ AT D
Kaiser Permanente Moreno Valley Medical Center, Moreno Valley	G+ E D
Kaiser Permanente Panorama City Medical Center, Panorama City	G+ E D
Kaiser Permanente Riverside Medical Center, Riverside	G+ E D
Kaweah Delta Health Care District, Visalia	G+ E D
Keck Hospital of USC, Los Angeles	G+ HR D
Kern Medical, Bakersfield	G+ D
La Palma Intercommunity Hospital, La Palma	G+ HR D
Lakewood Regional Medical Center, Lakewood	G+ HR D
Loma Linda University Children's Hospital, Loma Linda	G *
Loma Linda University Medical Center Murrieta, Murrieta	G+ D
Loma Linda University Medical Center, Loma Linda	G G E
Long Beach Medical Center, Long Beach	G+ HR E D D
Los Alamitos Medical Center, Los Alamitos	D
Los Robles Regional Medical Center, Thousand Oaks	G+ E+ AT D
MarinHealth Medical Center, Greenbrae	G+ E+ D
Marshall Medical Center, Placerville	G+ E D
MemorialCare - Saddleback Medical Center, Laguna Hills	G+ E D
Mercy General Hospital, Sacramento	G+ E D
Mercy San Juan Medical Center, Carmichael	G+ E D
Methodist Hospital of Southern California, Arcadia	G+ E D
Mission Hospital Regional Medical Center, Mission Viejo	G+ E+ AT D
Montclair Hospital Medical Center, MONTCLAIR	HR
NorthBay Healthcare Group, Fairfield	G+ D
O'Connor Hospital, San Jose	S+ E
Orange County Global Medical Center, Santa Ana	G+ E D
Oroville Hospital, Oroville	G+
Palmdale Regional Medical Center, Palmdale	G+ D
Paradise Valley Hospital, National City	G+ HR G+ E D
Petaluma Valley Hospital, Petaluma	G+ D
PIH Health Downey Hospital, Downey	G+ D
PIH Health Good Samaritan Hospital, Los Angeles	G+ E
PIH Health Whittier Hospital, Whittier	G+ D
Pomona Valley Hospital Medical Center, Pomona	G+ G+ E+
Providence Cedars Sinai Tarzana Medical Center, Tarzana	G+ D
Providence Holy Cross Medical Center, Mission Hills	G+ E D D
Providence Little Company of Mary Medical Center - San Pedro, San Pedro	G+ E D
Providence Little Company of Mary Medical Center - Torrance, Torrance	G+ E+ AT D
Providence Saint John's Health Center, Santa Monica	G+ E+ AT D
Providence Saint Joseph Medical Center, Burbank	G+ E D
Queen of the Valley Medical Center, Napa	G+ D
Redlands Community Hospital, Redlands	G+ HR D
Regional Medical Center of San Jose, San Jose	G+ E
Riverside Community Hospital, Riverside	G+ E AT
Riverside University Health System, Moreno Valley	G S G+ E D
Ronald Reagan UCLA Medical Center, Los Angeles	G+ HR G+ E D D
Salinas Valley Memorial Healthcare System, Salinas	G+ HR G+ E D D G+ G
San Antonio Regional Hospital, Upland	G+ D
San Dimas Community Hospital, San Dimas	
San Joaquin General Hospital, French Camp	G+ E D
San Ramon Regional Medical Center, San Ramon	G+ E D
Santa Barbara Cottage Hospital, Santa Barbara	G+ E S+
Santa Monica-UCLA Medical Center Orthopedic and Hospital, Santa Monica	S+ HR D D
Scripps Green Hospital, La Jolla	G+
Scripps Memorial Hospital Encinitas, Encinitas	G+ E+ D
Scripps Memorial Hospital La Jolla, La Jolla	G+ E+ AT D
Scripps Mercy Hospital, San Diego and Chula Vista, San Diego	G+ E+ AT D
Shasta Regional Medical Center, Redding	G+ HR E D D
Sherman Oaks Hospital, Sherman Oaks	D D

MISSION LIFELINE: STEMI:
- G+ Gold Plus Receiving
- G+ Gold Plus Referring
- G Gold Receiving
- G Gold Referring
- S+ Silver Plus Receiving
- S+ Silver Plus Referring
- S Silver Receiving
- S Silver Referring

MISSION LIFELINE: NSTEMI:
- G Gold
- S Silver

TARGET HF | TARGET STROKE:
- HR Target: Heart Failure
- HR Target: Stroke Honor Roll
- E+ Target: Stroke Honor Roll Elite Plus
- E Target: Stroke Honor Roll Elite
- AT Target: Stroke Honor Roll Advanced Therapy
- D Target: Type 2 Diabetes Honor Roll™

© 2021 American Heart Association

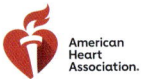

SPONSORED CONTENT

(CALIFORNIA CONTINUED)

Hospital	Awards
Sierra View Medical Center, **Porterville**	G+ D
Sierra Vista Regional Medical Center, **San Luis Obispo**	G+
Southwest Healthcare System-Inland Valley Medical Center and Rancho Springs Medical Center, **Wildomar**	G+ E D
St. Francis Medical Center, **Lynwood**	G+ D
St. Joseph Hospital, **Orange**	G+ E
St. Jude Medical Center, **Fullerton**	G+ E+ D
St. Louise Regional Hospital, **Gilroy**	G+ E D
St. Mary Medical Center, **Long Beach**	G
Stanford Childrens Health, **Menlo Park**	G *
Stanford HealthCare - ValleyCare, **Pleasanton**	G+
Stanford Healthcare, **Stanford**	G G+ HR
Temecula Valley Hospital, **Temecula**	G+ E D G+
Torrance Memorial Medical Center, **Torrance**	G+ HR G E D D
Tri-City Medical Center, **Oceanside**	G+ E D G+
Twin Cities Community Hospital, **Templeton**	G+ HR
UC San Diego Health - Jacobs Medical Center, **La Jolla**	G+ E AT D
UC San Diego Health - UC San Diego Medical Center, **San Diego**	G+ E AT D
UCI Health, **Orange**	G+ HR G+ E+ D
University of California San Francisco (UCSF), **San Francisco**	G+ E D S+
University of California, Davis Medical Center, **Sacramento**	G+ E+
USC Verdugo Hills Hospital, **Glendale**	G+ E D
VA Loma Linda Hospital, **Loma Linda**	G+
Valley Presbyterian Hospital, **Van Nuys**	G+ E D
Ventura County Medical Center/Santa Paula Hospital, **Ventura**	G+ E D
Washington Hospital Healthcare System, **Fremont**	G+
West Hills Hospital and Medical Center, **West Hills**	G+ HR

COLORADO

Hospital	Awards
Boulder Community Health Foothills Hospital, **Boulder**	G+ E D
Centura Health - Avista Adventist Hospital, **Louisville**	G+
Centura Health - Castle Rock Adventist Hospital, **Castle Rock**	G+
Centura Health - Littleton Adventist Hospital, **Littleton**	G+ E+ D
Centura Health - Longmont United Hospital, **Longmont**	G+ E D
Centura Health - Parker Adventist Hospital, **Parker**	G+ E D
Centura Health - Penrose Hospital, **Colorado Springs**	G+ E+ D
Centura Health - Porter Adventist Hospital, **Denver**	G+ HR D
Centura Health - St. Anthony Hospital, **Lakewood**	G+ HR G+ E D D G+ S
Centura Health - St. Anthony North Hospital, **Westminster**	G+ D D G
Centura Health - St. Francis Medical Center, **Colorado Springs**	G+ E D
Denver Health Medical Center, **Denver**	S+ D
Good Samaritan Medical Center, **Lafayette**	G+ E
North Colorado Medical Center, **Greeley**	G+ E D
North Suburban Medical Center, **Thornton**	E+ D
Parkview Medical Center, **Pueblo**	G+ HR G+ E D D
Platte Valley Medical Center, **Brighton**	G+
Presbyterian/St. Luke's Medical Center, **Denver**	G+ HR D S
Rose Medical Center, **Denver**	G+ E+ D
SCL Health - Lutheran Medical Center, **Wheat Ridge**	G+ E+ AT
SCL Health - Saint Joseph Hospital, **Denver**	G+ E D
SCL Health - St. Mary's Medical Center, **Grand Junction**	G+ E D
Sky Ridge Medical Center, **Lone Tree**	G+ E+ AT D
Swedish Medical Center, **Englewood**	G+ HR S+ E+ AT D
The Medical Center of Aurora, **Aurora**	G+ D
UCHealth Highlands Ranch Hospital, **Highlands Ranch**	S+ HR
UCHealth Medical Center of the Rockies, **Loveland**	G+ HR G+ E+ D D D G
UCHealth Memorial Hospital North, **Colorado Springs**	S+ HR D
UCHealth Memorial Hospital, **Colorado Springs**	G+ HR G+ E D D
UCHealth Poudre Valley Hospital, **Fort Collins**	G+ HR G+ E D
UCHealth University of Colorado Hospital, **Aurora**	G G+ HR S G+ E D

CONNECTICUT

Hospital	Awards
Connecticut Children's Medical Center, **Hartford**	G *
Danbury Hospital, part of Nuvance Health, **Danbury**	G+ HR S+ HR G+ D
Greenwich Hospital, **Greenwich**	G+ E D
Griffin Hospital, **Derby**	G+ D
Hartford HealthCare St. Vincent's Medical Center, **Bridgeport**	G+ HR G+ E+ D D D
Hartford Hospital, **Hartford**	G+ E D G+
Manchester Memorial Hospital, **Manchester**	G+
MidState Medical Center, **Meriden**	G+ E D
New Milford Hospital, part of Nuvance Health, **New Milford**	S+ HR
Norwalk Hospital, **Norwalk**	G+ E G
Saint Francis Hospital and Medical Center, **Hartford**	G+ HR S+ E S+ D
Sharon Hospital, **Sharon**	G+
Stamford Hospital, **Stamford**	G+ HR D G G
The Hospital of Central Connecticut, **New Britain**	G+ E D
The William W. Backus Hospital, **Norwich**	G+ HR
UCONN Health / John Dempsey Hospital, **Farmington**	G+ E G
Waterbury Hospital, **Waterbury**	G+ E G
Windham Hospital, **Windham**	G+ E
Yale - New Haven Hospital, **New Haven**	G+ E D

DELAWARE

Hospital	Awards
Bayhealth Medical Center - Kent General Hospital, **Dover**	S G+ E S+
Bayhealth Sussex Campus, **Milford**	G+
Beebe Healthcare, **Lewes**	G+ G G+ D D S
Christiana Care Health Services, Inc., **Newark**	G+ G+ E+ AT D G+ D
Saint Francis Inc., **Wilmington**	G+ D
TidalHealth Nanticoke, **Seaford**	G+ G+ HR D G

DISTRICT OF COLUMBIA

Hospital	Awards
Howard University Hospital, **Washington**	G+ E D
MedStar Georgetown University Hospital, **Washington**	G+ E+ D
MedStar Washington Hospital Center, **Washington**	G+ E AT D
Sibley Memorial Hospital, **Washington**	G+ D
The George Washington University Hospital, **Washington**	G+ E D

FLORIDA

Hospital	Awards
AdventHealth Altamonte Springs, **Altamonte Springs**	G+ E D
AdventHealth Apopka, **Apopka**	G+ E D
AdventHealth Celebration, **Celebration**	G+ E D
AdventHealth Dade City, **Dade City**	S+ D
AdventHealth Daytona Beach, **Daytona Beach**	G+ E D
AdventHealth DeLand, **DeLand**	G+ E D
AdventHealth East Orlando, **Orlando**	G+ E D
AdventHealth Fish Memorial, **Orange City**	G+ E D
AdventHealth Kissimmee, **Kissimmee**	G+ E D
AdventHealth New Smyrna Beach, **New Smyrna Beach**	G+ E+ D
AdventHealth North Pinellas, **Tarpon Springs**	G+ HR D
AdventHealth Ocala, **Ocala**	G+ HR D
AdventHealth Orlando, **Orlando**	G+ E+ D
AdventHealth Palm Coast, **Palm Coast**	G+ E D
AdventHealth Waterman, **Tavares**	G+ E D
AdventHealth Wesley Chapel, **Wesley Chapel**	G+ E D
AdventHealth Winter Park, **Winter Park**	G+ E D
Aventura Hospital and Medical Center, **Aventura**	G+
Baptist Hospital of Miami, **Miami**	G+ E+ AT D
Baptist Hospital, **Pensacola**	G+

KEY TO THE AWARDS

GWTG - STROKE:
- G+ Gold Plus Achievement
- G Gold Achievement
- S+ Silver Plus Achievement
- S Silver Achievement

GWTG - HEART FAILURE:
- G+ Gold Plus Achievement
- G Gold Achievement
- S+ Silver Plus Achievement
- S Silver Achievement

GWTG - RESUSCITATION:
- G Gold Achievement
- S Silver Achievement

GWTG - AFIB:
- G Gold Achievement
- S Silver Achievement

© 2021 American Heart Association

*These hospitals received Get With The Guidelines-Resuscitation awards from the American Heart Association for two or more patient populations.

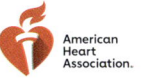

SPONSORED CONTENT

Hospital	Awards
Baptist Medical Center - Beaches (Baptist Health), **Jacksonville Beach**	G+ D
Baptist Medical Center - Jacksonville (Baptist Health), **Jacksonville**	E+ AT D
Baptist Medical Center - South (Baptist Health), **Jacksonville**	G+ D
Baptist Medical Center of Nassau, Inc., **Fernandina Beach**	E D
Bay Medical Center-Sacred Heart Health System, **Panama City**	G+ S
Bayfront Health St. Petersburg, **St. Petersburg**	G+ E D
Boca Raton Regional Hospital, **Boca Raton**	G+ E AT D
Brandon Regional Hospital, **Brandon**	G+ E+
Broward Health Coral Springs, **Coral Springs**	G+ D
Broward Health Imperial Point, **Fort Lauderdale**	G+ D
Broward Health Medical Center, **Fort Lauderdale**	G+ E AT D
Broward Health North, **Pompano Beach**	G+ E+ AT D
Cape Canaveral Hospital, **Cocoa Beach**	G+ E D
Cape Coral Hospital, **Cape Coral**	G+ E D
Capital Regional Medical Center, **Tallahassee**	G+ D
Citrus Memorial Hospital, also known as Citrus Memorial Health System, **Inverness**	S+ E D
Cleveland Clinic Florida, **Weston**	G+ E+ D
Cleveland Clinic Indian River Hospital, **Vero Beach**	G+ HR G+ E D
Cleveland Clinic Martin Health, **Stuart**	G+ E+ AT D
Delray Medical Center, **Delray Beach**	G+ E AT D
Doctors Hospital of Sarasota, **Sarasota**	E D
Dr. P. Phillips Hospital, **Orlando**	S+ HR G G+ HR E AT D
Fawcett Memorial Hospital, **Port Charlotte**	G+ E AT D
FLORIDA MEDICAL CENTER a campus of North Shore, **Fort Lauderdale**	G+ E+ AT D
Fort Walton Beach Medical Center, **Fort Walton Beach**	G+ E+ D
Good Samaritan Medical Center, **West Palm Beach**	G+ E
Gulf Breeze Hospital, **Gulf Breeze**	G+ HR
Gulf Coast Medical Center, **Fort Myers**	G+ E D
Halifax Health, **Daytona Beach**	G+ HR
Hialeah Hospital, **Hialeah**	G+ D
Holmes Regional Medical Center, **Melbourne**	G+ E+ AT D
Holy Cross Hospital, **Fort Lauderdale**	G+ HR G+ E+ AT D D
Homestead Hospital, **Homestead**	S+ HR D
Jackson Memorial Hospital, **Miami**	E+
Jackson North Medical Center, **North Miami Beach**	G+
Jackson South Medical Center, **Miami**	G+ E D
JFK Medical Center, **Atlantis**	G+ E+ D
Jupiter Medical Center, **Jupiter**	G+ HR
Kendall Regional Medical Center, **Miami**	G+ E+
Lakeland Regional Health Medical Center, **Lakeland**	G+ E
Lakewood Ranch Medical Center, **Bradenton**	G+ E
Largo Medical Center, **Largo**	G+ E+
Lower Keys Medical Center, **Key West**	S+ D
Manatee Memorial Hospital, **Bradenton**	G+ E+ G
Mayo Clinic Florida, **Jacksonville**	S+ E
Mease Countryside Hospital, **Safety Harbor**	G
Memorial Hospital Jacksonville, **Jacksonville**	G+
Memorial Hospital Miramar, **Miramar**	
Memorial Hospital Pembroke, **Pembroke Pines**	G+ E+ D
Memorial Hospital West, **Pembroke Pines**	G+ E+ AT D
Memorial Regional Hospital, **Hollywood**	G+ E+ AT D
Mercy Hospital, **Miami**	G+ E+ D
Morton Plant Hospital, **Clearwater**	S+
Mount Sinai Medical Center, **Miami Beach**	G+ HR D
NCH Healthcare System, **Naples**	G+ E
Nicklaus Children's Hospital, **Miami**	G
North Florida Regional Medical Center, **Gainesville**	G+ E AT D
Northside Hospital and Tampa Bay Heart Institute, **St. Petersburg**	G+ E D
Ocala Health, **Ocala**	G+ E D
Orange Park Medical Center, **Orange Park**	G G G+ E+ D
Orlando Health South Seminole Hospital, **Longwood**	S+
Orlando Regional Medical Center, **Orlando**	S S+ HR G+ E AT D D
Osceola Regional Medical Center, **Kissimmee**	G+ E+ AT D
Palm Bay Hospital, **Palm Bay**	G+ E D
Palm Beach Gardens Medical Center, **Palm Beach Gardens**	G+ E
Palmetto General Hospital, **Hialeah**	G+ E+ AT D
Physicians Regional Healthcare System, **Naples**	G+ HR
Regional Medical Center Bayonet Point, **Hudson**	G+ E+ D
Rockledge Regional Medical Center, **Rockledge**	G+ D
Sacred Heart Health System, **Pensacola**	G+ D
Sarasota Memorial Health Care System, **Sarasota**	G+ D
South Florida Baptist Hospital, **Plant City**	S
South Lake Hospital, **Clermont**	
South Miami Hospital, **South Miami**	G+ E+ D
St. Joseph's Hospital- North, **Lutz**	G+
St. Joseph's Hospital, **Tampa**	G+
St. Lucie Medical Center, **Port Saint Lucie**	G+ E D
St. Mary's Medical Center, **West Palm Beach**	G+ E+ AT
St. Vincent's Medical Center Southside, **Jacksonville**	G+ HR
St. Vincent's Medical Center-Clay County, **Middleburg**	S D
Tallahassee Memorial HealthCare, **Tallahassee**	G+ E D
Tampa General Hospital, **Tampa**	G+ E D
UF Health Leesburg Hospital, **Leesburg**	G+ D
UF Health Shands Hospital, **Gainesville**	G+ E AT D
UF Health The Villages Hospital, **The Villages**	G+ D
University of Miami Health System, **Miami**	G+ E D
Venice Regional Bayfront Health, **Venice**	G+ HR D
Viera Hospital, **Viera**	G+ E D
Wellington Regional Medical Center, **Wellington**	G+ D
West Boca Medical Center, **Boca Raton**	G+
West Florida Hospital, **Pensacola**	G+ E D
West Kendall Baptist Hospital, **Miami**	G+ HR D
Westside Regional Medical Center, **Plantation**	G+ E+ D

GEORGIA

Hospital	Awards
AdventHealth Gordon, **Calhoun**	G+ E+ D
Appling Healthcare System, **Baxley**	G+
AU Medical Center, **Augusta**	G G+ G+ E+ D
Cartersville Medical Center, **Cartersville**	G+ E D
Coliseum Medical Centers, **Macon**	G+ E+ D D G
Coliseum Northside Hospital, **Macon**	S+
Colquitt Regional Medical Center, **Moultrie**	G+ D
Doctors Hospital Augusta, **Augusta**	G+ E D
East Georgia Regional Medical Center, **Statesboro**	S+ HR D
Eastside Medical Center, **Snellville**	
Effingham Health System, **Springfield**	
Emory Decatur Hospital, **Decatur**	G+ D
Emory Johns Creek Hospital, **Duluth**	G S
Emory Saint Joseph's Hospital, **Atlanta**	G+ E D G D
Emory University Hospital Midtown, **Atlanta**	G+ HR D S G
Emory University Hospital, **Atlanta**	G+ E+ D D G
Floyd Medical Center, **Rome**	G+ HR D
Grady Health System, **Atlanta**	G+ HR E+ AT D D
Habersham Medical Center, **Demorest**	G G+ E D
Hamilton Medical Center, **Dalton**	G+ E+ D
Houston Healthcare, **Warner Robins**	G+ E AT D
Meadows Regional Medical Center, **Vidalia**	S+ E D
Medical Center Navicent Health, **Macon**	G G+ E+ D

MISSION LIFELINE: STEMI:
- G+ Gold Plus Receiving
- G+ Gold Plus Referring
- G Gold Receiving
- G Gold Referring
- S+ Silver Plus Receiving
- S+ Silver Plus Referring
- S Silver Receiving
- S Silver Referring

MISSION LIFELINE: NSTEMI:
- G Gold
- S Silver

TARGET HF | TARGET STROKE:
- HR Target: Heart Failure
- HR Target: Stroke Honor Roll
- E+ Target: Stroke Honor Roll Elite Plus
- E Target: Stroke Honor Roll Elite
- AT Target: Stroke Honor Roll Advanced Therapy
- D Target: Type 2 Diabetes Honor Roll™

© 2021 American Heart Association

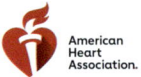

SPONSORED CONTENT

Hospital	Awards
Memorial University Medical Center, **Savannah**	G+ E D
Northeast Georgia Medical Center, Barrow, **Winder**	S+ D
Northeast Georgia Medical Center, Braselton, **Braselton**	G+ E+ D
Northeast Georgia medical Center, Gainesville, **Gainesville**	G+ E AT D
Northside Hospital Atlanta, **Atlanta**	G+ E+ D D G
Northside Hospital Cherokee, **Canton**	G+ G E+ D D G
Northside Hospital Forsyth, **Cumming**	G+ HR E+ D D G
Northside Hospital Gwinnett/Duluth, **Lawrenceville**	G+ HR E+ D G+ G
Perry Hospital, **Perry**	S+ D
Phoebe Putney Memorial Hospital, **Albany**	G S G+ E D
Piedmont Athens Regional Medical Center, **Athens**	S+ HR E D
Piedmont Columbus Midtown, **Columbus**	G+ HR D
Piedmont Fayette Hospital, **Fayetteville**	G+ G+ E D
Piedmont Henry Hospital, **Stockbridge**	G+ HR D
Piedmont Hospital, **Atlanta**	E AT D
Piedmont Mountainside Hospital, **Jasper**	S+ D
Piedmont Newnan Hospital, **Newnan**	G+ E D
Piedmont Newton Hospital, **Covington**	G+ HR D
Piedmont Rockdale Hospital, **Conyers**	G+ D
Piedmont Walton Hospital, **Monroe**	S+ D
Polk Medical Center, **Cedartown**	G+ HR D
Redmond Regional Medical Center, **Rome**	G+ HR G+ E+ D D
South Georgia Medical Center, **Valdosta**	G D
Southeast Georgia Health System, **Brunswick**	G D
Southern Regional Medical Center, **Riverdale**	G+ E D G G
St. Francis Hospital, Inc., **Columbus**	HR D
St. Joseph's Hospital, **Savannah**	G+
St. Mary's Hospital, **Athens**	G+ HR
St. Mary's Sacred Heart Hospital, **Lavonia**	S+ D
Tanner Medical Center/Carrollton, **Carrollton**	G+ E D
Tift Regional Medical Center, **Tifton**	G+ HR D
University Hospital, **Augusta**	G+ HR D
WellStar Atlanta Medical Center South, **Atlanta**	S+ D
WellStar Atlanta Medical Center, **Atlanta**	S+ D
Wellstar Cobb Hospital, **Austell**	S+ HR G+ HR D G S
Wellstar Douglas Hospital, **Douglasville**	HR S G
WellStar Kennestone Regional Hospital, **Marietta**	S+ HR G+ E+ AT D G
WellStar North Fulton Hospital, **Roswell**	HR AT D G
WellStar Paulding Hospital, **Dallas**	S+ HR D S G
WellStar West Georgia Medical Center, **LaGrange**	S+ D G

GUAM

Hospital	Awards
Guam Regional Medical City, **Dededo**	S S D

HAWAII

Hospital	Awards
Adventist Health Castle, **Kailua**	G G D
Hilo Medical Center, **Hilo**	S G+ E+ D
Kaiser Foundation Hospital Moanalua Medical Center, **Honolulu**	G+ HR G+ E D D G
Kona Community Hospital, **Kealakekua**	S HR
Kuakini Medical Center, **Honolulu**	G+
Maui Memorial Medical Center, **Wailuku**	G+ HR G+ E D D
Pali Momi Medical Center, **Aiea**	G+ E D
Straub Medical Center, **Honolulu**	G+ E D
The Queen's Medical Center Punchbowl, **Honolulu**	G G+ E+ D
The Queen's Medical Center West O'ahu, **Ewa Beach**	G+ D
Wilcox Medical Center, **Lihue**	G+ E D

IDAHO

Hospital	Awards
Eastern Idaho Regional Medical Center, **Idaho Falls**	G+ E D
Portneuf Medical Center, **Pocatello**	G AT D
St. Luke's Boise and Meridian Medical Centers, **Boise**	G+

ILLINOIS

Hospital	Awards
Advocate Christ Medical Center, **Oak Lawn**	G+ E D G
Advocate Condell Medical Center, **Libertyville**	G+ E
Advocate Good Samaritan Hospital, **Downers Grove**	G+ E D
Advocate Good Shepherd Hospital, **Barrington**	G+ D
Advocate Illinois Masonic Medical Center, **Chicago**	G+ E D
Advocate Lutheran General Hospital, **Park Ridge**	G+ E D
Advocate Sherman Hospital, **Elgin**	G+ HR G+ D D S
Advocate South Suburban Hospital, **Hazel Crest**	G+ D
Advocate Trinity Hospital, **Chicago**	G+ E+
Alton Memorial Hospital - BJC Healthcare, **Alton**	S+
AMITA Health Adventist Medical Center GlenOaks, **Glendale Heights**	G+ E
AMITA Health Adventist Medical Center, Bolingbrook, **Bolingbrook**	G+ D
AMITA Health Alexian Brothers Medical Center, **Elk Grove Village**	G+ E D
AMITA Health Resurrection Medical Center, **Chicago**	G+ D
AMITA Health Saint Francis Hospital, **Evanston**	G+ HR
AMITA Health Saint Joseph Chicago, **Chicago**	G+ D
AMITA Health St. Alexius Medical Center Hoffman Estates, **Hoffman Estates**	G+ E D
AMITA Saint Joseph Medical Center, **Joliet**	S+ D
Blessing Hospital, **Quincy**	G+ E D
Carle BroMenn Medical Center, **Normal**	G+ E D
Carle Foundation Hospital, **Urbana**	G+ E+ D
Cook County Health, **Chicago**	G+ D G
Decatur Memorial Hospital, **Decatur**	G+ HR
Edward Hospital, **Naperville**	G+ E D
Herrin Hospital, **Herrin**	G+ HR D
HSHS St. John's Hospital, **Springfield**	G+ AT D
HSHS St. Mary's Hospital, **Decatur**	G+ D
Humboldt Park Health, **Chicago**	S+
Illinois Valley Community Hospital, **Peru**	S+
Loyola University Medical Center, **Maywood**	G+ E AT D S G
MacNeal Hospital, **Berwyn**	G+ E D
Memorial Hospital of Carbondale, **Carbondale**	G+ HR D
Mercy Hospital & Medical Center, **Chicago**	G+ D S
Mount Sinai Hospital, **Chicago**	G+
Northwest Community Hospital, **Arlington Heights**	G G+ HR G+ E D
Northwestern Medicine Central DuPage Hospital, **Winfield**	G+ HR G+ E D D
Northwestern Medicine Delnor Hospital, **Geneva**	G+ HR S E D D
Northwestern Medicine Huntley, **Huntley**	G+
Northwestern Medicine Kishwaukee Hospital, **Dekalb**	G+ S+ E D D
Northwestern Medicine Lake Forest Hospital, **Lake Forest**	G+ HR E D D
Northwestern Medicine McHenry, **McHenry**	G+ HR D
Northwestern Memorial Hospital, **Chicago**	G+ E+ D D G
OSF HealthCare Saint Anthony's Health Center, **Alton**	G+ E D
OSF Saint Anthony Medical Center, **Rockford**	G+ E+ AT D
OSF Saint Francis Medical Center, **Peoria**	G+ HR D
OSF St. Joseph Medical Center, **Bloomington**	G+ E D
Presence Saint Joseph Medical Center, **Joliet**	S+ D
Riverside Medical Center, **Kankakee**	G+ HR D
Rush Copley Medical Center, **Aurora**	G+
Rush Oak Park Hospital, **Oak Park**	G+ D
Rush University Medical Center, **Chicago**	G+ E AT D G G
SwedishAmerican Hospital, A Division of UW Health, **Rockford**	G+ E D
UChicago Medicine, **Chicago**	G+ G+ E D G

KEY TO THE AWARDS

GWTG - STROKE:
- G+ Gold Plus Achievement
- G Gold Achievement
- S+ Silver Plus Achievement
- S Silver Achievement

GWTG - HEART FAILURE:
- G+ Gold Plus Achievement
- G Gold Achievement
- S+ Silver Plus Achievement
- S Silver Achievement

GWTG - RESUSCITATION:
- G Gold Achievement
- S Silver Achievement

GWTG - AFIB:
- G Gold Achievement
- S Silver Achievement

© 2021 American Heart Association

*These hospitals received Get With The Guidelines-Resuscitation awards from the American Heart Association for two or more patient populations

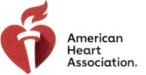

SPONSORED CONTENT

Hospital	Awards
UI Health, Chicago	G+ HR G+ E+ AT S D
UnityPoint Health - Methodist, Peoria	G+ HR G
UnityPoint Health - Proctor, Peoria	S
Vista Medical Center East, Waukegan	S+ D

INDIANA

Hospital	Awards
Ascension St. Vincent Anderson, Anderson	G D
Ascension St. Vincent Hospital, Indianapolis	S G+ E+ AT D
Baptist Health Floyd, New Albany	G+ E D
Community Heart and Vascular, Indianapolis	G+
Community Hospital - North, Indianapolis	S+ D
Community Hospital East, Indianapolis	E
Community Hospital of Anderson, Anderson	S+
Community Hospital, Community Healthcare System, Munster	G+ E AT D
Community South, Indianapolis	G+
Deaconess Gateway Hospital, Newburgh	G+ E D
Elkhart General Hospital, Elkhart	G+ D
Eskenazi Health, Indianapolis	G+ HR D
Franciscan Health - Crown Point, Crown Point	S+ E D
Franciscan Health Indianapolis, Indianapolis	G+ HR G+ E
Franciscan Health Lafayette East, Lafayette	G+ HR
Franciscan Health Michigan City, Michigan City	G+ E D
Good Samaritan, Vincennes	G+ HR
Indiana University Health Arnett, Lafayette	G+ HR
Indiana University Health Ball Memorial Hospital, Muncie	G G G+ HR D
Indiana University Health Methodist Hospital, Indianapolis	G G * HR
Indiana University Health North Hospital, Carmel	S+
IU Health Bloomington Hospital, Bloomington	G+ HR
IU Health West Hospital, Avon	G+
Lutheran Hospital, Fort Wayne	G+ HR D
Memorial Hospital, South Bend	G+ D
Memorial Hospital and Health Care Center, Jasper	G+ E D
Methodist Hospitals, Inc., Gary	G+ HR D
Parkview Health, Fort Wayne	G+ E D
Porter Regional Hospital, Valparaiso	G+ E D
Reid Health, Richmond	G+ D
St. Catherine Hospital, Inc., East Chicago	G+ D
St. Mary Medical Center, Hobart	G+ E D
St. Vincent Evansville, Evansville	G+ HR
Terre Haute Regional Hospital, Terre Haute	S+
Union Hospital, Terre Haute	G+ E

IOWA

Hospital	Awards
Allen Hospital, Waterloo	D
CHI Health Mercy Hospital Council Bluffs, Council Bluffs	G+ E D
Genesis Health System- Davenport, Davenport	G+ E
Mercy Iowa City an affiliate of MercyOne, Iowa City	G+
Mercy Medical Center-Cedar Rapids, Cedar Rapids	G+
MercyOne Clinton Medical Center, Clinton	G
MercyOne Des Moines Medical Center, Des Moines	G+ AT
MercyOne Dubuque Medical Center, Dubuque	G+ D G+ G
MercyOne North Iowa Medical Center, Mason City	G+
MercyOne, Sioux City	G+ HR G+ G D
Methodist Jennie Edmundson Hospital, Council Bluffs	G+ G
Montgomery County Memorial Hospital, Red Oak	G+
Myrtue Medical Center, Harlan	G+
Southeast Iowa Regional Medical Center, West Burlington	G+
Trinity Bettendorf, Bettendorf	G+
UnityPoint Health - St. Luke's Hospital, Cedar Rapids	G+ HR D
UnityPoint Health -St. Luke's, Sioux City	G+ HR G D
UnityPoint Health Trinity Regional Medical Center, Fort Dodge	G+
University of Iowa Hospitals and Clinics, Iowa City	S *

KANSAS

Hospital	Awards
AdventHealth Shawnee Mission, Shawnee Mission	G+ HR S G+ S
Ascension Via Christi St. Francis, Wichita	G+ E D
Centura Health- St. Catherine Hospital, Garden City	G+
HaysMed. part of The University of Kansas Health, Hays	G+ E D
Hutchinson Regional Medical Center, Hutchinson	S+ E D G+
Lawrence Memorial Hospital, Lawrence	S
Olathe Medical Center, Olathe	G+ E D
Providence Medical Center, Kansas City	G+ E D
Saint Luke's South Hospital, Overland Park	G+ E D
Salina Regional Health Center, Salina	G+ E+ D
Stormont-Vail HealthCare, Topeka	G+ HR E D
The University of Kansas Health System St. Francis Campus, Topeka	G+
The University of Kansas Health System, Kansas City	HR G+ E+ AT D D
Wesley Medical Center, Wichita	G+ E D

KENTUCKY

Hospital	Awards
Baptist Health Hardin, Elizabethtown	G+ E+ D
Baptist Health LaGrange, LaGrange	G+ HR
Baptist Health Lexington Hospital, Lexington	G+ HR G+ E+ AT D
Baptist Health Louisville, Louisville	S+ D
Baptist Health Madisonville, Madisonville	G+ D
Baptist Health Paducah, Paducah	G+ E D
Frankfort Regional Medical Center, Frankfort	G+ E
King's Daughters Medical Center, Ashland	G+
Mercy Health Lourdes Hospital, Paducah	S+ D
Norton Audubon Hospital, Louisville	G+ D G+
Norton Brownsboro Hospital, Louisville	G+ E AT D G+
Norton Hospital, Louisville	HR D G+
Owensboro Health Regional Hospital, Owensboro	
Pikeville Medical Center, Inc., Pikeville	
Saint Joseph Hospital, Lexington	HR
St. Elizabeth Edgewood, Edgewood	G G+ HR E D
St. Elizabeth Florence, Florence	G G+ HR G+ HR D D
St. Elizabeth Ft. Thomas, Fort Thomas	G G+ HR G+ E D D
The Medical Center at Bowling Green, Bowling Green	G+ HR E D
TJ Samson Community Hospital, Glasgow	S D
University of Kentucky Hospital, Lexington	G+ E+ D
University of Louisville Hospital, Louisville	E+
UofL Health - Mary & Elizabeth, Louisville	G+ E
UofL Health Jewish Hospital, Louisville	E E G+

LOUISIANA

Hospital	Awards
Children's Hospital, New Orleans	G
East Jefferson General Hospital, Metairie	G+ HR G+ HR
Glenwood Regional Medical Center, West Monroe	G+ E D
Lakeview Regional Medical Center, a campus of Tulane Medical Center, Covington	G G+ HR D
New Orleans East Hospital, New Orleans	G+ E D
Ochsner LSU Health System, Shreveport	G+
Ochsner Medical Center - Kenner, Kenner	G+
Ochsner Medical Center - New Orleans, New Orleans	S
Ochsner Medical Center - Northshore, Slidell	E
Ochsner Medical Center Baton Rouge, Baton Rouge	G+ HR
Our Lady of Lourdes Regional Medical Center, Lafayette	G+ E D
Our Lady of the Lake Regional Medical Center, Baton Rouge	G+ E D

MISSION LIFELINE: STEMI:
- G+ Gold Plus Receiving
- G+ Gold Plus Referring
- G Gold Receiving
- G Gold Referring
- S+ Silver Plus Receiving
- S+ Silver Plus Referring
- S Silver Receiving
- S Silver Referring

MISSION LIFELINE: NSTEMI:
- G Gold
- S Silver

TARGET HF | TARGET STROKE:
- HR Target: Heart Failure
- HR Target: Stroke Honor Roll
- E+ Target: Stroke Honor Roll Elite Plus
- E Target: Stroke Honor Roll Elite
- AT Target: Stroke Honor Roll Advanced Therapy
- D Target: Type 2 Diabetes Honor Roll™

© 2021 American Heart Association

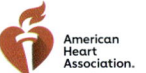

SPONSORED CONTENT

(KENTUCKY CONTINUED)

Hospital	Awards
Rapides Regional Medical Center, Alexandria	S G+ E D
St. Charles Parish Hospital, Luling	G+
St. Frances Cabrini Hospital, Alexandria	S+ HR D
St. Tammany Parish Hospital, Covington	G+ E
Touro Infirmary, New Orleans	G+ E D
Tulane Medical Center, New Orleans	G+ E+ D
University Medical Center New Orleans (UMCNO), New Orleans	G+ HR D
West Jefferson Medical Center, Marrero	G+ E D
Willis-Knighton Health System, Shreveport	G+ E D

MAINE

Hospital	Awards
Central Maine Medical Center, Lewiston	G+ HR D
Eastern Maine Medical Center, Bangor	S G+ HR D
Maine Medical Center, Portland	G
Mercy Hospital, EMHS member, Portland	G+ S D
Pen Bay Medical Center, Rockport	G G+ E
York Hospital, York	G+

MARYLAND

Hospital	Awards
Adventist HealthCare Shady Grove Medical Center, Rockville	G+ E D G
Adventist HealthCare White Oak Medical Center, Silver Spring	G+ E D G G
Anne Arundel Medical Center, Annapolis	G+ E D G+
Ascension Saint Agnes Hospital, Baltimore	G+ E D
Atlantic General Hospital, Berlin	G+ D
CalvertHealth Medical Center, Prince Frederick	G+ D
Carroll Hospital Center, Westminster	G+ E D
ChristianaCare - Union Hospital, Elkton	G+ E D
Doctors Community Medical Center, Lanham	G+ E D
Frederick Health Hospital, Frederick	G+ E D G G
Garrett Regional Medical Center, Oakland	S+
Greater Baltimore Medical Center, Baltimore	G+ E D
Holy Cross Germantown Hospital, Germantown	G+ E D
Holy Cross Hospital, Silver Spring	G+ E D
Howard County General Hospital, Columbia	G+ D S S
Johns Hopkins Bayview Medical Center, Baltimore	G+ E D S G
MedStar Franklin Square Medical Center, Baltimore	G+ E D G
MedStar Good Samaritan Hospital, Baltimore	S+ D
MedStar Harbor Hospital, Baltimore	G+ E D
MedStar Montgomery Medical Center, Olney	G+ HR D
MedStar Southern Maryland Hospital Center, Clinton	G+ HR D
MedStar St. Mary's Hospital, Leonardtown	S+
MedStar Union Memorial Hospital, Baltimore	G+ E D G
Mercy Medical Center, Baltimore	G+ D
Meritus Medical Center, Hagerstown	G+ E D
Northwest Hospital, Randallstown	G+ E D
Peninsula Regional Medical Center, Salisbury	G+ HR
Sinai Hospital of Baltimore, Baltimore	G+ E+ AT D G+ G
Suburban Hospital Johns Hopkins Medicine, Bethesda	G+ HR D G G
The Johns Hopkins Hospital, Baltimore	G* S G+ D G G
University of Maryland Baltimore Washington Medical Center, Glen Burnie	G+ E D G S
University of Maryland Charles Regional Medical Center, La Plata	G+ E D
University of Maryland Harford Memorial Hospital, Havre De Grace	G+ HR D
University of Maryland Medical Center, Baltimore	G+ E D
University of Maryland Prince George's Hospital Center, Cheverly	E D G
University of Maryland Shore Medical Center at Easton, Easton	G+ D
University of Maryland St. Joseph Medical Center, Towson	G+ D G
University of Maryland Upper Chesapeake Medical Center, Bel Air	G+ HR D
UPMC Western Maryland, Cumberland	G+ HR D G G

MASSACHUSETTS

Hospital	Awards
Addison Gilbert Hospital, Gloucester	G+ E D
Baystate Franklin Medical Center, Greenfield	G+ D
Baystate Medical Center, Springfield	G+ HR D G+
Baystate Noble Hospital, Westfield	G+ E D
Baystate Wing Hospital, Palmer	S+ D
Berkshire Medical Center, Pittsfield	G+ HR D G
Beth Israel Deaconess Hospital - Milton, Milton	D
Beth Israel Deaconess Hospital - Needham, Needham	G+ E D
Beth Israel Deaconess Hospital-Plymouth, Plymouth	G+ E D
Beth Israel Deaconess Medical Center, Boston	G+ HR G G+ E+ AT
Beverly Hospital, Beverly	D
Boston Children's Hospital, Boston	G *
Boston Medical Center, Boston	G+ E+ AT D
Brigham and Women's Faulkner Hospital, Boston	G+ S D
Brigham and Women's Hospital, Boston	G+ HR D HR
Cape Cod Hospital, Hyannis	G+ HR D
Cooley Dickinson Hospital, Northampton	G+ D
Emerson Hospital, Concord	G+
Falmouth Hospital, member Cape Cod Healthcare, Falmouth	G+ E D
Holy Family Hospital - Haverhill, Haverhill	S+
Holy Family Hospital - Methuen, Methuen	S+
Holyoke Medical Center, Holyoke	G+ E+ D D
Lahey Hospital & Medical Center, Burlington, Burlington	G+ E AT D
Lawrence General Hospital, Lawrence	S
Lowell General Hospital - Main Campus, Lowell	D
Massachusetts General Hospital, Boston	G+ E AT D
Mercy Medical Center, Springfield	G+ E
MetroWest Medical Center - Framingham Union Hospital, Framingham	G
Milford Regional Medical Center, Milford	G+ D
Mount Auburn Hospital, Cambridge	G+ E D
Newton-Wellesley Hospital, Newton	G G+ HR G+ HR D D
Norwood Hospital, A Steward Family Hospital, Norwood	G+
Saint Vincent Hospital, Worcester	G+ E D
Signature Healthcare Brockton Hospital, Brockton	S
South Shore Hospital, South Weymouth	G
Southcoast Health St. Luke's Hospital, New Bedford	G+ E D
Southcoast Health Tobey Hospital, Wareham	G+ E D
Steward St. Elizabeth's Medical Center, Brighton	G+ D
Sturdy Memorial Hospital, Attleboro	G+ E D
Tufts Medical Center, Boston	G+ E AT D
UMASS Memorial HealthAlliance-Clinton Hospital, Leominster	G+ D
UMass Memorial Medical Center, Worcester	G G+ E D

MICHIGAN

Hospital	Awards
Ascension Borgess Hospital, Kalamazoo	S+ D
Ascension Providence Hospital-Novi Campus, Novi	G+ E D
Ascension Providence Hospital-Southfield Campus, Southfield	G+ E D
Ascension Providence Rochester Hospital, Rochester	G+ D
Ascension St. John Hospital and Medical Center, Detroit	G+ E AT D
Ascension St. Mary's Hospital, Saginaw	G+ E AT D
Bronson Methodist Hospital, Kalamazoo	G+ E
Covenant HealthCare, Saginaw	G+ E+
Garden City Hospital, Garden City	G+ E D D D
Genesys Regional Medical Center, Grand Blanc	G+ E D
Henry Ford Allegiance Health, Jackson	G+ E D
Henry Ford Hospital and Health Network, Detroit	G+ HR D
Henry Ford Macomb Hospital, Clinton Township	G+ E D
Henry Ford West Bloomfield Hospital, West Bloomfield	G+ E D
Henry Ford Wyandotte Hospital, Wyandotte	G+ HR D

KEY TO THE AWARDS

GWTG - STROKE:
- G+ Gold Plus Achievement
- G Gold Achievement
- S+ Silver Plus Achievement
- S Silver Achievement

GWTG - HEART FAILURE:
- G+ Gold Plus Achievement
- G Gold Achievement
- S+ Silver Plus Achievement
- S Silver Achievement

GWTG - RESUSCITATION:
- G Gold Achievement
- S Silver Achievement

GWTG - AFIB:
- G Gold Achievement
- S Silver Achievement

© 2021 American Heart Association

*These hospitals received Get With The Guidelines-Resuscitation awards from the American Heart Association for two or more patient populations.

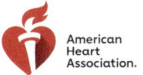

SPONSORED CONTENT

Hospital	Awards
Hurley Medical Center, Flint	G+ E D
McLaren Bay Region, Bay City	G+ E D
McLaren Flint, Flint	G+ E+ AT D
McLaren Greater Lansing, Lansing	G+
McLaren Lapeer Region, Lapeer	S+ E+ D
McLaren Macomb, Mount Clemens	G+ E D
McLaren Northern Michigan, Petoskey	G+ E+ D
McLaren Port Huron Hospital, Port Huron	G+ HR D
Mercy Health Saint Mary's, Grand Rapids	G+ E+ AT
Metro Health – University of Michigan Health, Wyoming	G+ E+
MidMichigan Medical Center-Midland an affiliate of MidMichigan Health System, Midland	S+ D
Munson Medical Center, Traverse City	G+ E
ProMedica Charles and Virginia Hickman Hospital, Adrian	G+
ProMedica Monroe Regional Hospital, Monroe	
Sparrow Hospital, Lansing	G+ E D
Spectrum Health Blodgett Hospital, Grand Rapids	S+ HR
Spectrum Health Butterworth, Grand Rapids	S+ HR G+ AT E D
Spectrum Health Lakeland, Saint Joseph	G+ HR D
St. Joseph Mercy Oakland, Pontiac	G+ E D
St. Mary Mercy Hospital, Livonia	G+ E D
University of Michigan Health System, Ann Arbor	G* G+ E AT

MINNESOTA

Hospital	Awards
Abbott Northwestern Hospital, Minneapolis	G+ E AT D
CentraCare St. Cloud Hospital, Saint Cloud	G+ HR G* G+ E D D
Essentia Health East. St. Mary's Medical Center, Duluth	G+ HR E AT D
Hennepin Healthcare System, Inc., Minneapolis	G+ E
M Health Fairview University of Minnesota Medical Center, Minneapolis	G+ HR
Mayo Clinic Hospital, Saint Marys Campus, Rochester	G+ HR
Mercy Hospital, Coon Rapids	G G+
North Memorial Health Hospital, Robbinsdale	G+ E D
Park Nicollet Methodist Hospital, Saint Louis Park	G+ E G
Regions Hospital, Saint Paul	E
St. Luke's, Duluth	D D
United Hospital, Saint Paul	G+ E+ AT D

MISSISSIPPI

Hospital	Awards
Baptist Memorial Hospital - DeSoto, Southaven	G+ E D
Baptist Memorial Hospital - Golden Triangle, Columbus	S+
Baptist Memorial Hospital - North Mississippi, Oxford	G+ D
Forrest General Hospital, Hattiesburg	G+ HR D G+ G
Greenwood Leflore Hospital, Greenwood	E D
Magnolia Regional Health Center, Corinth	G+ HR
Memorial Hospital at Gulfport, Gulfport	G+ HR
Merit Health Wesley, Hattiesburg	S+ HR
Methodist Healthcare, Olive Branch, Olive Branch	
Mississippi Baptist Medical Center, Jackson	G+ HR E D D
North Mississippi Medical Center, Tupelo	G+ E
Ocean Springs Hospital, Ocean Springs	G D G+
Singing River Hospital, Pascagoula	D
St. Dominic Memorial Hospital, Jackson	G+ E AT
University of Mississippi Health Care, Jackson	G+ E

MISSOURI

Hospital	Awards
Barnes-Jewish Hospital, Saint Louis	S HR G+ E+ D D G S
Boone Hospital Center, Columbia	G+ E G+ G
Capital Region Medical Center, Jefferson City	G+
Centerpoint Medical Center, Independence	G+ HR G+ E D
Cox Medical Center Branson, Branson	
Cox Medical Center South, Springfield	
Freeman Health System, Joplin	G+ HR D S+ G
Lake Regional Health System, Osage Beach	G+ E D
Lee's Summit Medical Center, Lees Summit	G+ E D
Liberty Hospital, Liberty	G+ HR D
Mercy Hospital Jefferson, Crystal City	G+ E D
Mercy Hospital Joplin, Joplin	G+ E+ D S+ G
Mercy Hospital Lincoln, Troy	S+
Mercy Hospital South, Saint Louis	G+ HR S G+ E+ AT
Mercy Hospital Springfield, Springfield	G+ E D
Mercy Hospital St. Louis, Saint Louis	S E D
Mercy Hospital Washington, Washington	G+ D
Missouri Baptist Medical Center, Saint Louis	G+ E+ D
Mosaic Life Care, Saint Joseph	S+ E D
North Kansas City Hospital, North Kansas City	S+ E D
Phelps Health, Rolla	S+ G+
Research Medical Center, Kansas City	G+ HR G+ E D
Saint Francis Medical Center, Cape Girardeau	G+
Saint Luke's East Hospital, Lees Summit	G+ HR D S
Saint Luke's Hospital of Kansas City, Kansas City	G+ HR G+ E+ AT D D G+ G
Saint Luke's North Hospital, Kansas City	G+ E D S
Southeast Health, Cape Girardeau	G+ HR S+ D D S
SSM Health DePaul Hospital, Bridgeton	G+ E AT D
SSM Health Saint Louis University Hospital, Saint Louis	G+ E+ D
SSM Health St. Mary's Hospital, St. Louis	G+ E+ D
St. Joseph Medical Center, Kansas City	S+ G+ D
St. Mary's Health Center, Jefferson City	S+ HR D
St. Mary's Medical Center, Blue Springs	G+ HR G+ E D G G
University of Missouri Health Care, Columbia	S+ HR D

MONTANA

Hospital	Awards
Benefis Health System, Great Falls	G+ HR G+
Billings Clinic, Billings	
Bozeman Health Deaconess Hospital, Bozeman	G+ E D D
Community Medical Center, Missoula	S
Logan Health, Kalispell	G+ HR E D D G+ G
Providence St. Patrick Hospital, Missoula	G G+ E D G
St. Peter's Hospital, Helena	G
St. Vincent Healthcare, Billings	G+ E+ D

NEBRASKA

Hospital	Awards
Bryan Medical Center, Lincoln	G+ E D
CHI Health Creighton University Medical Center Bergan Mercy, Omaha	G+ E D
CHI Health Good Samaritan Hospital, Kearney	G+ D
CHI Health Immanuel Medical Center, Omaha	G+ E+ D
CHI Health Lakeside Hospital, Omaha	G+ E D
CHI Health St. Elizabeth, Lincoln	G
CHI Health St. Francis Medical Center, Grand Island	G+ E D
Faith Regional Health Services, Norfolk	G+ E D
Great Plains Health, North Platte	G+ E D G G
Kearney Regional Medical Center, Kearney	G+ D
Mary Lanning Healthcare, Hastings	G+ D
Nebraska Medicine – Bellevue, Bellevue	G+ D
Nebraska Medicine, Omaha	G+ E AT D
Regional West Medical Center, Scottsbluff	S+ E

MISSION LIFELINE: STEMI:
- G+ Gold Plus Receiving
- G+ Gold Plus Referring
- G Gold Receiving
- G Gold Referring
- S+ Silver Plus Receiving
- S+ Silver Plus Referring
- S Silver Receiving
- S Silver Referring

MISSION LIFELINE: NSTEMI:
- G Gold
- S Silver

TARGET HF | TARGET STROKE:
- HR Target: Heart Failure
- HR Target: Stroke Honor Roll
- E+ Target: Stroke Honor Roll Elite Plus
- E Target: Stroke Honor Roll Elite
- AT Target: Stroke Honor Roll Advanced Therapy
- D Target: Type 2 Diabetes Honor Roll™

© 2021 American Heart Association

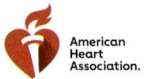

SPONSORED CONTENT

NEVADA

Hospital	Awards
Carson Tahoe Regional Medical Center, **Carson City**	S+ D
Centennial Hills Hospital Medical Center, **Las Vegas**	G+ HR D G+
Desert Springs Hospital Medical Center, **Las Vegas**	G G+ E D G S
Dignity Health St. Rose Dominican Hospital - San Martin Campus, **Las Vegas**	G+ E D
Dignity Health St. Rose Dominican Hospital - Siena Campus, **Henderson**	G+ HR D
Henderson Hospital, **Henderson**	G+
MountainView Hospital, **Las Vegas**	G+ E D
Northern Nevada Medical Center, **Sparks**	G+ E+ D G
Renown Regional Medical Center, **Reno**	G+ HR G+ D G+ S
Saint Mary's Regional Medical Center, **Reno**	G+ HR D D
Southern Hills Hospital & Medical Center, **Las Vegas**	G+ D
Spring Valley Hospital Medical Center, **Las Vegas**	G+ E AT G+ S
Summerlin Hospital Medical Center, **Las Vegas**	G+ D
Sunrise Hospital & Medical Center, **Las Vegas**	G+ E+ AT D
UMC Hospital, **Las Vegas**	G+ D
Valley Hospital Medical Center, **Las Vegas**	G+ E AT

NEW HAMPSHIRE

Hospital	Awards
Catholic Medical Center, **Manchester**	G+ HR D
Dartmouth-Hitchcock Medical Center, **Lebanon**	G S G+ E D
Exeter Hospital, **Exeter**	S+ HR D
Parkland Medical Center, **Derry**	G+ E
Portsmouth Regional Hospital, **Portsmouth**	G+ D
St. Joseph Hospital, **Nashua**	G+ E D
Wentworth-Douglass Hospital, **Dover**	S+ HR G+ D

NEW JERSEY

Hospital	Awards
AtlantiCare Regional Medical Center, **Pomona**	S+
Capital Health Medical Center- Hopewell, **Pennington**	G+ E D
Capital Health Regional Medical Center, **Trenton**	G+ E AT D
CarePoint Health - Bayonne Medical Center, **Bayonne**	G+ D
CarePoint Health - Christ Hospital, **Jersey City**	G+ HR G+ D
CarePoint Health - Hoboken University Medical Center, **Hoboken**	G+
CentraState Medical Center, **Freehold**	G+ HR G+ E D
Chilton Medical Center, **Pompton Plains**	G+ E+ D
Cooper University Health Care, **Camden**	G+ HR AT D
Deborah Heart and Lung Center, **Browns Mills**	G
Hackensack Meridian Health Bayshore Medical Center, **Holmdel**	G+ G+ E D
Hackensack Meridian Health Hackensack University Medical Center, **Hackensack**	G+ E D
Hackensack Meridian Health Jersey Shore University Medical Center, **Neptune**	G+ G+ E D
Hackensack Meridian Health JFK Medical Center, **Edison**	G+ E D
Hackensack Meridian Health Mountainside Medical Center, **Montclair**	G+ HR D
Hackensack Meridian Health Ocean Medical Center, **Brick**	S+ E D D
Hackensack Meridian Health Palisades Medical Center, **North Bergen**	G+ G+ HR
Hackensack Meridian Health Pascack Valley Medical Center, **Westwood**	G+ D
Hackensack Meridian Health Riverview Medical Center, **Red Bank**	G+ HR G+ E D
Hackensack Meridian Health Southern Ocean Medical Center, **Manahawkin**	G+ E D
Hackensack Meridian Raritan Bay Medical Center, **Perth Amboy**	G+ D
Hackettstown Medical Center, **Hackettstown**	G+ E+ D
Holy Name Medical Center, **Teaneck**	G+ E D
Hunterdon Healthcare, **Flemington**	G+ E
Inspira Medical Center Elmer, **Elmer**	G+
Inspira Medical Center Mullica Hill, **Mullica Hill**	G
Inspira Medical Center Vineland, **Vineland**	G+ D

Hospital	Awards
Jefferson Cherry Hill Hospital, **Cherry Hill**	G+ D
Jefferson Stratford Hospital, **Stratford**	G+ D
Jefferson Washington Township Hospital, **Turnersville**	G+ D
Jersey City Medical Center-a RWJBarnabas Health Facility, **Jersey City**	G+ HR
Monmouth Medical Center, **Long Branch**	G+ HR
Morristown Medical Center, **Morristown**	G+ E+ D
Newark Beth Israel Medical Center, **Newark**	G+ D
Newton Medical Center, **Newton**	G+ E+ D
Overlook Medical Center, **Summit**	G+ E+ AT
Penn Medicine Princeton Medical Center, **Plainsboro**	S+ HR G+ D
Robert Wood Johnson University Hospital Somerset, **Somerville**	G+ HR D
Robert Wood Johnson University Hospital, **New Brunswick**	G+ E+ AT
Saint Clare's Denville Hospital, **Denville**	G+ HR G+ D G+
Saint Peter's University Hospital, **New Brunswick**	G+ HR
St. Francis Medical Center, **Trenton**	
St. Joseph's University Medical Center, **Paterson**	S+ E D D
St. Joseph's Wayne Medical Center, **Wayne**	G+ E D
St. Luke's Warren Hospital, **Phillipsburg**	G+ E D
St. Mary's General Hospital, **Passaic**	G+ D
The Valley Hospital, **Ridgewood**	G+ HR
Trinitas Regional Medical Center, **Elizabeth**	G
University Hospital, **Newark**	G+ HR G+ E D S
Virtua Our Lady of Lourdes Hospital, **Camden**	G+ D D
Virtua West Jersey, **Marlton**	G+

NEW MEXICO

Hospital	Awards
Eastern New Mexico Medical Center, **Roswell**	S+ E+
Lovelace Medical Center, **Albuquerque**	G+ HR G+ E+ D D
Lovelace Westside Hospital, **Albuquerque**	G+ D
MountainView Regional Medical Center, **Las Cruces**	G+
New Mexico VA Health Care System, **Albuquerque**	S
Presbyterian Healthcare Services, **Albuquerque**	G+
University of New Mexico Hospitals, **Albuquerque**	G+ HR G+ E+ D D G

NEW YORK

Hospital	Awards
Albany Med, **Albany**	G+ HR D G+
Arnot Ogden Medical Center, **Elmira**	G+ E D
Auburn Community Hospital, **Auburn**	G+ E D
Bassett Medical Center, **Cooperstown**	G+ E D
BronxCare Health System, **Bronx**	G G+ HR G+ D D G G
Catholic Health - Kenmore Mercy Hospital, **Buffalo**	G+ D
Catholic Health - Mercy Hospital of Buffalo, **Buffalo**	G+ E D D
Catholic Health - Mount St. Mary's Hospital, **Lewiston**	G+ D
Catholic Health- Sisters of Charity Hospital, **Buffalo**	G+ D
Cayuga Medical Center, **Ithaca**	G+ E D
Cohen Children's Medical Center, **New Hyde Park**	G
Columbia Memorial Hospital, **Hudson**	G+ D
Crouse Hospital, **Syracuse**	G+ HR G+ E+ AT D
Ellis Medicine, **Schenectady**	G+ E D S+
F.F. Thompson Hospital, **Canandaigua**	G+ E D
Faxton St. Luke's Healthcare, an affiliation of Mohawk Valley Health System, **Utica**	G+ HR D
Flushing Hospital Medical Center, **Flushing**	G+ HR D
Garnet Health Medical Center - Catskills, **Harris**	G+
Garnet Health Medical Center, **Middletown**	G+ D
Gates Vascular Institute / Buffalo General Medical Center, **Buffalo**	G+ D D
Geneva General Hospital, **Geneva**	G+ HR D
Glen Cove Hospital, **Glen Cove**	S D
Glens Falls Hospital, **Glens Falls**	G+ D
Good Samaritan Hospital Medical Center, **West Islip**	G+ E D

KEY TO THE AWARDS

GWTG - STROKE:
- G+ Gold Plus Achievement
- G Gold Achievement
- S+ Silver Plus Achievement
- S Silver Achievement

GWTG - HEART FAILURE:
- G+ Gold Plus Achievement
- G Gold Achievement
- S+ Silver Plus Achievement
- S Silver Achievement

GWTG - RESUSCITATION:
- G Gold Achievement
- S Silver Achievement

GWTG - AFIB:
- G Gold Achievement
- S Silver Achievement

© 2021 American Heart Association

*These hospitals received Get With The Guidelines-Resuscitation awards from the American Heart Association for two or more patient populations.

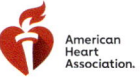

SPONSORED CONTENT

Good Samaritan Hospital, a member of WMC Health, **Suffern** ..... G+ E D
Guthrie Corning Hospital, **Corning** ..... G+ D
HealthAlliance: Broadway Campus a Member of the WMC Health Network, **Kingston** ..... G+
Highland Hospital, **Rochester** ..... G+ HR G+ HR
Huntington Hospital, **Huntington** ..... G+ E D G+
Jamaica Hospital Medical Center, **Richmond Hill** ..... G+ G+ E AT D S
John T. Mather Memorial Hospital, **Port Jefferson** ..... G+ E D
Lenox Hill Hospital, **New York** ..... G+ E+
LIJ Medical Center at Forest Hills, **Forest Hills** ..... G+ D
LIJ Valley Stream, **Valley Stream** ..... G+ HR
Long Island Community Hospital, **Patchogue** ..... G+ E D
Long Island Jewish Medical Center, **New Hyde Park** ..... G+ HR
Maimonides Medical Center, **Brooklyn** ..... G+ E D
Mercy Medical Center, **Rockville Centre** ..... G+ E D
MidHudson Regional Hospital of WMC Health, **Poughkeepsie** ..... G+ D
Millard Fillmore Suburban Hospital, **Williamsville** ..... G+
Montefiore Medical Center - Moses Campus, **Bronx** ..... G+ E
Montefiore Medical Center - Weiler Campus, **Bronx** ..... S+ HR
Montefiore Mount Vernon Hospital, **Mount Vernon** ..... G+ E
Montefiore New Rochelle Hospital, **New Rochelle** ..... G+ E D
Montefiore Nyack Hospital, **Nyack** ..... G+ E
Montefiore St. Luke's Cornwall, **Newburgh** ..... G+ E D G
Mount Sinai Beth Israel, **New York** ..... G G+ E AT D G
Mount Sinai Brooklyn, **Brooklyn** ..... G+ E
Mount Sinai Morningside, **New York** ..... G+ D D G+ S
Mount Sinai Queens, **Astoria** ..... G+ E D
Mount Sinai South Nassau, **Oceanside** ..... G+ HR G+ E D
Mount Sinai West, **New York** ..... HR AT D
Nassau University Medical Center, **East Meadow** ..... G+ HR G+ E D D
Newark–Wayne Community Hospital, **Newark** ..... HR
NewYork-Presbyterian Brooklyn Methodist Hospital, **Brooklyn** ..... G+ E+ D
NewYork-Presbyterian Hudson Valley Hospital, **Cortlandt Manor** ..... G+ E D
NewYork-Presbyterian Queens, **Flushing** ..... G+ E D G
NewYork-Presbyterian/Columbia University Medical Center, **New York** ..... G+ E+ AT
NewYork-Presbyterian/Lawrence Hospital, **Bronxville** ..... G+ E D G
NewYork-Presbyterian/Lower Manhattan Hospital, **New York** ..... G+ E D
NewYork-Presbyterian/The Allen Hospital, **New York** ..... G+ E D
NewYork-Presbyterian/Weill Cornell Medical Center, **New York** ..... G+ E D
North Shore University Hospital, **Manhasset** ..... S+
Northern Dutchess Hospital, **Rhinebeck** ..... S+
Northern Westchester Hospital, **Mount Kisco** ..... G+ HR
NYC Health + Hospitals/Bellevue, **New York** ..... G+ HR G G+ E D D G G
NYC Health + Hospitals/Coney Island, **Brooklyn** ..... S G+ HR D
NYC Health + Hospitals/Elmhurst, **Elmhurst** ..... G G G E+ D
NYC Health + Hospitals/Harlem, **New York** ..... S+ D
NYC Health + Hospitals/Jacobi, **Bronx** ..... G+ HR G G+ E D D
NYC Health + Hospitals/Kings County, **Brooklyn** ..... G G G E D
NYC Health + Hospitals/Lincoln, **Bronx** ..... G+ E D D
NYC Health + Hospitals/Metropolitan, **New York** ..... S+ G+
NYC Health + Hospitals/North Central Bronx, **Bronx** ..... G+
NYC Health + Hospitals/Queens, **Jamaica** ..... G
NYC Health + Hospitals/Woodhull, **Brooklyn** ..... G G D
NYU Langone Hospital - Brooklyn, **Brooklyn** ..... G+ E+ AT D S
NYU Langone Hospital – Long Island, **Mineola** ..... S G E+ AT
NYU Langone Hospitals, **New York** ..... G+ E+ AT D G
Our Lady of Lourdes Memorial Hospital, **Binghamton** ..... G+ D
Peconic Bay Medical Center, **Riverhead** ..... G+ E D
Phelps Hospital, Northwell Health, **Sleepy Hollow** ..... G+ E AT
Plainview Hospital, **Plainview** ..... G+ D

Putnam Hospital Center, **Carmel** ..... G+
Richmond University Medical Center, **Staten Island** ..... G+
Rochester General Hospital, **Rochester** ..... S+ G+ E D
Rochester Regional Health United Memorial Medical Center, **Batavia** ..... G+ D
Rome Memorial Hospital, **Rome** ..... G+
Saint Joseph's Medical Center, **Yonkers** ..... D
Samaritan Hospital, **Troy** ..... D
Saratoga Hospital, **Saratoga Springs** ..... S+ G
SBH Health System, **Bronx** ..... S+ G+ E D D
Soldiers & Sailors Memorial Hospital, **Penn Yan** ..... S
South Shore University Hospital, **Bay Shore** ..... G+ E+ D G+
Southampton Hospital, **Southampton** ..... G+ E D
St. Catherine of Siena Medical Center, **Smithtown** ..... G+ E D
St. Charles Hospital, **Port Jefferson** ..... D
St. Francis Hospital, The Heart Center, **Roslyn** ..... G+ HR E D D
St. John's Episcopal Hospital, **Far Rockaway** ..... G+ HR D
St. John's Riverside Hospital, **Yonkers** ..... D
St. Joseph Hospital, **Bethpage** ..... G+ E D
St. Peter's Hospital, **Albany** ..... G+ D
Staten Island University Hospital South Campus / Northwell Health, **Staten Island** ..... G+ E D
Staten Island University Hospital, **Staten Island** ..... G+ E D
Stony Brook University Hospital, **Stony Brook** ..... G+ G E+ D
Syosset Hospital, **Syosset** ..... G+
The Brooklyn Hospital Center, **Brooklyn** ..... G+ HR E D D
The Mount Sinai Hospital, **New York** ..... G+ HR E AT D D
UHS Wilson Medical Center, **Johnson City** ..... G+ HR HR
Unity Hospital, **Rochester** .....
University Hospital of Brooklyn - SUNY Downstate Medical Center, **Brooklyn** ..... G+ D
University of Vermont Healthnetwork-Champlain Valley Physician's Hospital, **Plattsburgh** ..... S D
Upstate University Hospital, **Syracuse** ..... G+ HR G G+ E+ D D
UR Medicine / Noyes Health, **Dansville** ..... G+
UR Medicine Strong Memorial Hospital, **Rochester** ..... S G+ HR G E AT G+
Vassar Brothers Medical Center, **Poughkeepsie** ..... D G+
White Plains Hospital, **White Plains** ..... S+ HR E D D G
Wyckoff Heights Medical Center, **Brooklyn** ..... G+ HR

NORTH CAROLINA

Angel Medical Center, **Franklin** ..... G+ E+
Annie Penn Hospital, **Reidsville** ..... G+ HR D
Atrium Health Cabarrus, **Concord** ..... G+ E AT D G+ G
Atrium Health Cleveland, **Shelby** ..... G+ E D
Atrium Health Kings Mountain, **Kings Mountain** ..... G+
Atrium Health Lincoln, **Lincolnton** ..... G+ E D
Atrium Health Mercy, **Charlotte** ..... G+ D
Atrium Health Pineville, **Charlotte** ..... E D G+ G
Atrium Health Stanly, **Albemarle** .....
Atrium Health Union, **Monroe** ..... G+ E D
Atrium Health University City, **Charlotte** .....
Atrium Health's Carolinas Medical Center, **Charlotte** ..... G+ E+ AT D G+
Blue Ridge Regional Hospital, **Sprice Pine** ..... G+
Cape Fear Valley Medical Center, **Fayetteville** ..... G G+ HR G G+ E D G+ G
CarolinaEast Medical Center, **New Bern** ..... S
Carolinas HealthCare System Blue Ridge-Morganton, **Morganton** ..... G+ E D
CaroMont Regional Medical Center, **Gastonia** ..... G+ HR
Carteret Health Care Medical Center, **Morehead City** ..... G G+ HR G D D S
Central Carolina Hospital, **Sanford** ..... S+ D
Cone Health - Alamance Regional, **Burlington** ..... G+ E D
Cone Health, **Greensboro** ..... G G+ E+ D

MISSION LIFELINE: STEMI:
G+ Gold Plus Receiving
G+ Gold Plus Referring
G Gold Receiving
G Gold Referring
S+ Silver Plus Receiving
S+ Silver Plus Referring
S Silver Receiving
S Silver Referring

MISSION LIFELINE: NSTEMI:
G Gold
S Silver

TARGET HF | TARGET STROKE:
HR Target: Heart Failure
HR Target: Stroke Honor Roll
E+ Target: Stroke Honor Roll Elite Plus
E Target: Stroke Honor Roll Elite
AT Target: Stroke Honor Roll Advanced Therapy
D Target: Type 2 Diabetes Honor Roll™

© 2021 American Heart Association

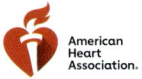

SPONSORED CONTENT

Hospital	Awards
Duke Raleigh Hospital, Raleigh	G+ E D
Duke University Hospital, Durham	G+ HR G+ E D D D G
Durham VA HealthCare System, Durham	G D S
FirstHealth Moore Regional Hospital - Hoke, Raeford	
FirstHealth Moore Regional Hospital, Pinehurst	G+ HR
Frye Regional Medical Center, Hickory	G+ HR G+ E D G+ D
Hugh Chatham Memorial Hospital, Elkin	S+ E D
Iredell Memorial Hospital, Statesville	HR G+
Johnston Health, Smithfield	S+ D
Lake Norman Regional Medical Center, Mooresville	S+ E D
Mission Hospital McDowell, Marion	G+ E D
Mission Hospitals, Inc., Asheville	E+ D
Nash UNC Health Care, Rocky Mount	G+ HR G D
New Hanover Regional Medical Center, Wilmington	G+ G+ E+ AT D
Northern Regional Hospital, Mount Airy	S+ HR
Novant Health Brunswick Medical Center, Bolivia	G+
Novant Health Forsyth Medical Center, Winston-Salem	G+ HR G+ E+ AT D D G+ G
Novant Health Huntersville Medical Center, Huntersville	G+ HR G+ E D
Novant Health Kernersville Medical Center, Kernersville	S+
Novant Health Matthews Medical Center, Matthews	G+ HR G+ E D
Novant Health Mint Hill Medical Center, Charlotte	G+ HR G+ E S S
Novant Health Presbyterian Medical Center, Charlotte	G+ HR G+ E+ AT D D
Novant Health Rowan Medical Center, Salisbury	G+ HR HR G+ D
Novant Health Thomasville Medical Center, Thomasville	G+ G+
Onslow Memorial Hospital, Jacksonville	G G+ D
Pardee UNC Health Care, Hendersonville	G+ E D
Sentara Albemarle Medical Center, Elizabeth City	G+ E D
The Outer Banks Hospital, Nags Head	G+ E
Transylvania Regional Hospital, Brevard	G+ E D
UNC Hospitals, Chapel Hill	G+ E AT D G+ G
UNC Lenoir Health Care, Kinston	G+ D
UNC REX Healthcare, Raleigh	G+ E+ D
Vidant Beaufort Hospital, Washington	G+ D
Vidant Chowan Hospital, Edenton	G+ D
Vidant Duplin Hospital, Kenansville	G+ D
Vidant Edgecombe Hospital, Tarboro	G+ D
Vidant Medical Center, Greenville	G+ E+ D G G
Vidant North Hospital, Roanoke Rapids	G+ D
Vidant Roanoke-Chowan Hospital, Ahoskie	G+ HR
Wake Forest Baptist Health High Point Medical Center, High Point	G+
Wake Forest Baptist Health Lexington Medical Center, Lexington	G+ D
Wake Forest Baptist Medical Center, Winston-Salem	G+ E D
WakeMed Cary Hospital, Cary	G+ HR G+ HR D D
WakeMed Health & Hospitals - Raleigh Campus, Raleigh	G+ HR G+ HR D D
Watauga Medical Center, Boone	G+ HR

NORTH DAKOTA

Hospital	Awards
Altru Health System, Grand Forks	G+ E D
CHI St. Alexius Health Bismarck, Bismarck	G+ E D G G
Essentia Health, Fargo	G+ E D
Jamestown Regional Medical Center, Jamestown	S+
Sanford Bismarck Medical Center, Bismarck	G+ E D
Sanford Medical Center Fargo, Fargo	G+ E AT D
Trinity Health, Minot	G+ E

OHIO

Hospital	Awards
Adena Regional Medical Center, Chillicothe	G+ HR S
Ashtabula County Medical Center, Ashtabula	G+ D
Atrium Medical Center, Middletown	G
Aultman Alliance Community Hospital, Alliance	S+
Aultman Hospital, Canton	G+
Blanchard Valley Health System, Findlay	G+ E
Cincinnati Children's, Cincinnati	
Cleveland Clinic Akron General Medical Center, Akron	G+ E D
Cleveland Clinic Avon Hospital, Avon	G G+ E D
Cleveland Clinic Euclid Hospital, Euclid	S G+ HR
Cleveland Clinic Fairview Hospital, Cleveland	G G+ E D
Cleveland Clinic Hillcrest Hospital, Mayfield Heights	G+ E D
Cleveland Clinic Marymount Hospital, Garfield Heights	G+ E D
Cleveland Clinic Medina Hospital, Medina	S G+ E D
Cleveland Clinic Mercy Hospital, Canton	G HR G+ E D D D
Cleveland Clinic South Pointe Hospital, Warrensville Heights	G+ E D
Cleveland Clinic Union Hospital, Dover	G+ E D
Cleveland Clinic, Cleveland	G+ HR G * E AT D D
Coshocton Regional Medical Center, Coshocton	G+
Fairfield Medical Center, Lancaster	G+ E
Firelands Regional Medical Center, Sandusky	S+ G+ S
Fort Hamilton Hospital, Hamilton	G+ E D
Genesis Healthcare System, Zanesville	G+ D
Grandview Medical Center System, Dayton	G+ D
Greene Memorial Hospital, Xenia	G+ E D
Kettering Health Network Troy Hospital, Troy	S+
Kettering Medical Center, Dayton	G+ HR D
Licking Memorial Hospital, Newark	G G
Lima Memorial Health System, Lima	S+ D
Louis Stokes Cleveland VA Medical Center, Cleveland	G+ HR D
McLaren St. Luke's, Maumee	D
Mercy Health - Anderson Hospital, Cincinnati	G+ HR D
Mercy Health - Fairfield Hospital, Fairfield	G+ HR G+ HR D D
Mercy Health - St. Elizabeth Boardman Hospital, Boardman	S+ D
Mercy Health - St. Elizabeth Youngstown Hospital, Youngstown	G HR G+ E D D
Mercy Health Clermont Hospital, Batavia	G+
Mercy Health West Hospital, Cincinnati	G+ HR G+ HR D
Miami Valley Hospital, Dayton	G+ HR D
Mount Carmel Health System, Columbus	G+ D
Mount Carmel St. Ann's, Westerville	G+ E
Ohio State University Wexner Medical Center, Columbus	G+ E+ D
OhioHealth Doctors Hospital, Columbus	S+ HR D
OhioHealth Grant Medical Center, Columbus	G+ E D
OhioHealth Mansfield Hospital, Mansfield	G+ E
OhioHealth Marion General Hospital, Marion	G+ HR D
OhioHealth Riverside Methodist Hospital, Columbus	G+ E+ D
Pomerene Hospital, Millersburg	S+ G+
ProMedica Flower Hospital, Sylvania	G+ HR D
ProMedica Toledo Hospital, Toledo	G+ HR AT D
Soin Medical Center, Beavercreek	G+ D
Southwest General Health Center, Middleburg Heights	G G+ D G G
Springfield Regional Medical Center, Springfield	G+ HR S+ D
St. Rita's Medical Center, Lima	G+ D
Summa Akron City Hospital, Akron	G+ E+ D
Sycamore Medical Center, Miamisburg	G+ D
The Christ Hospital, Cincinnati	G
The Jewish Hospital Mercy Health, Cincinnati	G+ D
The MetroHealth System, Cleveland	G G+ HR G+ E D D
The Ohio State University Wexner Medical Center East Hospital, Columbus	S+ D
The University of Toledo Medical Center, Toledo	G+ HR D
TriHealth Bethesda North Hospital, Cincinnati	G+ D
UH Regional Hospitals, Bedford Medical Center and Richmond Medical Center, Richmond Heights	G+ D
University Hospitals Ahuja Medical Center, Beachwood	G+ E D

KEY TO THE AWARDS

GWTG - STROKE:
- G+ Gold Plus Achievement
- G Gold Achievement
- S+ Silver Plus Achievement
- S Silver Achievement

GWTG - HEART FAILURE:
- G+ Gold Plus Achievement
- G Gold Achievement
- S+ Silver Plus Achievement
- S Silver Achievement

GWTG - RESUSCITATION:
- G Gold Achievement
- S Silver Achievement

GWTG - AFIB:
- G Gold Achievement
- S Silver Achievement

© 2021 American Heart Association

*These hospitals received Get With The Guidelines-Resuscitation awards from the American Heart Association for two or more patient populations.

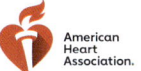

SPONSORED CONTENT

Hospital	Awards
University Hospitals Cleveland Medical Center, Cleveland	G+ E+ AT D
University Hospitals Conneaut Medical Center, Conneaut	S+
University Hospitals Elyria Medical Center, Elyria	G+ E D
University Hospitals Geauga Medical Center, Chardon	G+ E+ D
University Hospitals Geneva Medical Center, Geneva	G+ D
University Hospitals Parma Medical Center, Parma	G+ E D
University Hospitals Portage Medical Center, Ravenna	G+ E D
University Hospitals Samaritan Medical Center, Ashland	S
University Hospitals St. John Medical Center, Cleveland	G+ E D
University of Cincinnati Medical Center, Cincinnati	G+ HR G+ AT
Upper Valley Medical Center, Troy	G+
West Chester Hospital, West Chester	G+ HR D
Western Reserve Hospital, LLC, Cuyahoga Falls	G+ HR D
Wooster Community Hospital, Wooster	G+ E D

OKLAHOMA

Hospital	Awards
Ascension St. John Medical Center, Tulsa	G+ E D
Comanche County Memorial Hospital, Lawton	G+ HR D
Hillcrest Hospital South, Tulsa	G+ E
Hillcrest Medical Center, Tulsa	G+ HR E D
INTEGRIS Baptist Medical Center, Oklahoma City	G+ E D
INTEGRIS Southwest Medical Center, Oklahoma City	G+
Jane Phillips Medical Center, Bartlesville	S+ G
McAlester Regional Health Center, McAlester	G+ D
Mercy Hospital Oklahoma City Comprehensive Stroke Center, Oklahoma City	G+ E
Norman Regional Health System, Norman	G+ E D D
Northeastern Health System, Tahlequah	S+ HR D
OU Medical Center, Oklahoma City	G+ E D
Saint Francis Hospital, Tulsa	S G+ E D
St. Anthony Hospital, Oklahoma City	G+ E D
St. Mary's Regional Medical Center, Enid	G+ D
Stillwater Medical Center, Stillwater	G+ HR

OREGON

Hospital	Awards
Asante Rogue Regional Medical Center, Medford	G+ G+ G
Bay Area Hospital, Coos Bay	S
Good Samaritan Regional Medical Center, Corvallis	S S+ D
Kaiser Sunnyside Medical Center, Clackamas	G+ E+ D
Kaiser Westside Medical Center, Hillsboro	G+ E D
Legacy Emanuel Medical Center, Portland	G+ E
Legacy Good Samaritan Medical Center, Portland	G+ HR D
Legacy Meridian Park Medical Center, Tualatin	G+ E
Legacy Mount Hood Medical Center, Gresham	G+ E D
OHSU Health Hillsboro Medical Center, Hillsboro	G+ D
OHSU, Portland	G+ HR S S+ D
PeaceHealth Sacred Heart Medical Center RiverBend, Springfield	E AT D
Providence Hood River Memorial Hospital, Hood River	G+ D
Providence Medford Medical Center, Medford	G+ D
Providence Milwaukie Hospital, Milwaukie	G+ HR D
Providence Newberg Medical Center, Newberg	G+ HR D
Providence Portland Medical Center, Portland	G+ E D G+ S
Providence Seaside Hospital, Seaside	G+
Providence St. Vincent Medical Center, Portland	G+ E D G+ S
Providence Willamette Falls Medical Center, Oregon City	G+ D
Samaritan Albany General Hospital, Albany	G+ E D
Samaritan Lebanon Community Hospital, Lebanon	G+ E D
Samaritan Pacific Communities Hospital, Newport	G+ E D
Sky Lakes Medical Center, Klamath Falls	G+ D
St. Charles Medical Center, Bend	G+ HR D
Tillamook Regional Medical Center, Tillamook	S+

PENNSYLVANIA

Hospital	Awards
Abington-Lansdale Hospital, Lansdale	G+ HR
ACMH Hospital, Kittanning	S+ D
Allegheny General Hospital, Pittsburgh	S G+ HR G+ E D
Allegheny Valley Hospital, Natrona Heights	G+ HR G+ D
Aria Jefferson Health Systems Bucks, Langhorne	G
Brandywine Hospital, Coatesville	G+ HR
Bryn Mawr Hospital, Bryn Mawr	G+ E AT D G+
Butler Memorial Hospital, Butler	G+ D
Canonsburg Hospital, Canonsburg	S+
Chester County Hospital, West Chester	S G+ HR D D D
Chestnut Hill Hospital, Philadelphia	G+ E D
Conemaugh Memorial Medical Center, Johnstown	G+ E D
Crozer-Chester Medical Center, Upland	G+ E+ AT D
Delaware County Memorial Hospital, Drexel Hill	G+ D
Doylestown Hospital, Doylestown	G+ HR G G+ E G G
Einstein Medical Center - Philadelphia, Philadelphia	G+ E AT D
Einstein Medical Center Montgomery, East Norriton	G+ E
Evangelical Community Hospital, Lewisburg	G+ D
Excela Health Frick Hospital, Mount Pleasant	G+
Excela Health Latrobe, Latrobe	G+
Excela Health Westmoreland Hospital, Greensburg	G+
Forbes Hospital, Monroeville	G+ HR HR D
Geisinger Community Medical Center, Scranton	G+ D G
Geisinger Jersey Shore Hospital, Jersey Shore	
Geisinger Lewistown Hospital, Lewistown	S+ D
Geisinger Medical Center, Danville	S+ HR G+ HR D D D
Geisinger St. Luke's Hospital, Orwigsburg	S+ E D
Geisinger Wyoming Valley, Wilkes Barre	G+ E D G+
Grand View Health, Sellersville	G G+ HR S+ D D
Heritage Valley Beaver, Beaver	G+ HR D
Holy Redeemer Hospital, Meadowbrook	G+ E
Jeanes Hospital - Temple University Health System, Philadelphia	G+ D
Jefferson Abington Hospital, Abington	G+ E D G+
Jefferson Hospital, Clairton	G+ HR D
Jefferson Torresdale Hospital, Philadelphia	G+ HR D
Lankenau Medical Center, Wynnewood	G+ E D
Lehigh Valley Health Network Cedar Crest, Allentown	G+ E AT D
Lehigh Valley Hospital - Hazleton, Hazleton	G+ HR G+ E D D
Lehigh Valley Hospital - Schuylkill, Pottsville	G+ E D
Lehigh Valley Pocono, East Stroudsburg	G+
Lower Bucks Hospital, Bristol	G+
Meadville Medical Center, Meadville	G+ HR D
Mercy Fitzgerald Hospital, Darby	G G+
Monongahela Valley Hospital, Monongahela	G G+ HR G+ E D D G
Moses Taylor Hospital, Scranton	G+
Mount Nittany Medical Center, State College	G+ E D
Nazareth Hospital, Philadelphia	G+ D
Paoli Hospital, Paoli	D D
Penn Highlands DuBois, DuBois	G+ E
Penn Highlands Elk, Saint Marys	G+ E D
Penn Medicine Lancaster General Hospital, Lancaster	S+ HR G+ E D
Penn Presbyterian Medical Center, Philadelphia	S G+ HR G+ E D D S+
Penn State Health Holy Spirit Medical Center, Camp Hill	G G+ HR D D
Penn State Hershey Medical Center, Hershey	G+ HR G+ E AT D
Pennsylvania Hospital, Philadelphia	G+ G+ D D
Phoenixville Hospital, Phoenixville	G+ HR D
Pinnacle Health System - West Shore Hospital, Mechanicsburg	G+ G

MISSION LIFELINE: STEMI:
- G+ Gold Plus Receiving
- G+ Gold Plus Referring
- G Gold Receiving
- G Gold Referring
- S+ Silver Plus Receiving
- S+ Silver Plus Referring
- S Silver Receiving
- S Silver Referring

MISSION LIFELINE: NSTEMI:
- G Gold
- S Silver

TARGET HF | TARGET STROKE:
- HR Target: Heart Failure
- HR Target: Stroke Honor Roll
- E+ Target: Stroke Honor Roll Elite Plus
- E Target: Stroke Honor Roll Elite
- AT Target: Stroke Honor Roll Advanced Therapy
- D Target: Type 2 Diabetes Honor Roll™

© 2021 American Heart Association

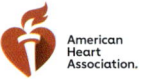

SPONSORED CONTENT

(PENNSYLVANIA CONTINUED)

- Pottstown Hospital, **Pottstown** — G+ E D
- Reading Hospital-Tower Health, **West Reading** — G+ HR G+ E+ AT D G+
- Regional Hospital of Scranton, **Scranton** — G+ E D
- Riddle Hospital, **Media** — G+ D G
- Robert Packer Hospital, **Sayre** — G+ HR
- Roxborough Memorial Hospital, **Philadelphia** — G+ D
- Saint Vincent Health System, **Erie** — G+ HR E D
- St. Clair Hospital, **Pittsburgh** — G+ D
- St. Joseph Regional Health Network, **Reading** — G+ HR
- St. Luke's Allentown Campus, **Allentown** — G+ E D
- St. Luke's Hospital - Anderson Campus, **Easton** — G+ E D
- St. Luke's Hospital - Miners Campus, **Coaldale** — G+ D
- St. Luke's Hospital Quakertown Campus, **Quakertown** — G+ E D
- St. Luke's Lehighton Campus, **Lehighton** — G+ E D
- St. Luke's Monroe Campus, **Stroudsburg** — G+ E D
- St. Luke's University Hospital, **Bethlehem** — G+ E AT D
- St. Mary Medical Center, **Langhorne** — G G+ E
- Steward Sharon Regional Medical Center, **Sharon** — G+ E D
- Suburban Community Hospital, **Norristown** — G+ E D
- Temple University Hospital, **Philadelphia** — G+ E D
- The Children's Hospital of Philadelphia, **Philadelphia** — G *
- The Hospital of the University of Pennsylvania, **Philadelphia** — S G+ HR G+ E D D D
- Thomas Jefferson University Hospital, **Philadelphia** — G+ E AT D
- UPMC Altoona, **Altoona** — G+ AT D
- UPMC Carlisle, **Carlisle** — G+ HR G+ D D G+ S
- UPMC East, **Monroeville** — G+ E
- UPMC Hamot, **Erie** — G+ HR G+ E+ AT D
- UPMC Jameson, **New Castle** — S+
- UPMC McKeesport, **McKeesport** — G+
- UPMC Mercy Pittsburgh, **Pittsburgh** — G+ E AT
- UPMC Northwest, **Seneca** — G+
- UPMC Passavant, **Pittsburgh** — G+
- UPMC Pinnacle Hanover Hospital, **Hanover** — S
- UPMC Pinnacle Harrisburg, Community and West Shore Campuses, **Harrisburg** — G+ HR G+ HR D D G+ G
- UPMC Pinnacle Lititz Hospital, **Lititz** — G+ E D
- UPMC Pinnacle Memorial Hospital, **York** — G+ D S S
- UPMC Presbyterian, **Pittsburgh** — G+ E AT
- UPMC Shadyside, **Pittsburgh** — S+ HR
- UPMC Somerset, **Somerset** — G+ HR D
- UPMC St. Margaret, **Pittsburgh** — G+
- UPMC Williamsport, **Williamsport** — G+
- Washington Health System, **Washington** — G+ D
- Wayne Memorial Hospital, **Honesdale** — G+ HR
- WellSpan Chambersburg Hospital, **Chambersburg** — G+ HR E
- WellSpan Ephrata Community Hospital, **Ephrata** — G+ HR G+ E+
- WellSpan Gettysburg Hospital, **Gettysburg** — S+ HR G+ E
- WellSpan Good Samaritan Hospital, **Lebanon** — G+ HR G+ E
- WellSpan Health - York Hospital, **York** — G G+ HR G E+ AT
- WellSpan Waynesboro Hospital, **Waynesboro** — G+
- West Penn Hospital, **Pittsburgh** — G+ HR G+ D
- Wilkes Barre General Hospital, **Wilkes Barre** — G+ E D
- WVU Medicine Uniontown Hospital, **Uniontown** — G+ E D

PUERTO RICO

- Hospital HIMA - San Pablo - Caguas, **Caguas** — G+ HR G+ HR D

RHODE ISLAND

- Kent Hospital, **Warwick** — G+ HR D
- Landmark Medical Center, **Woonsocket** — G+ E D
- Newport Hospital, **Newport** — G+ D
- Our Lady of Fatima Hospital, **North Providence** — G
- Rhode Island Hospital, **Providence** — G+ E AT D
- South County Hospital, **Wakefield** — G+
- The Miriam Hospital, **Providence** — G+ E D

SOUTH CAROLINA

- Aiken Regional Medical Center, **Aiken** — S+ G+ HR
- AnMed Health, **Anderson** — G+ D
- Beaufort Memorial Hospital, **Beaufort** — G+ E D G
- Bon Secours St. Francis Eastside, **Greenville** — D
- Bon Secours St. Francis Hospital, **Charleston** — G+ E D
- Bon Secours St. Francis-Downtown, **Greenville** — G+ HR G+ HR AT D D
- Carolina Pines Regional Medical Center, **Hartsville** — S+ HR
- Conway Medical Center, **Conway** — G+ E D
- Grand Strand Medical Center, **Myrtle Beach** — G+ E+ AT D
- Hampton Regional Medical Center, **Varnville** — S+ E D
- Hilton Head Hospital, **Hilton Head** — G+ E D
- Lexington Medical Center, **West Columbia** — G+ G+ E+ D D G+ G
- McLeod Health Loris, **Loris** — G+ D
- McLeod Health Seacoast, **Little River** — G+ HR D
- McLeod Regional Medical Center, **Florence** — G+ D
- Mount Pleasant Hospital, **Mount Pleasant** — G+ D
- MUSC Health - Lancaster Medical Center, **Lancaster** — G+ D
- MUSC Health, **Charleston** — G+ HR D
- Pelham Medical Center, **Greer** — S HR
- Piedmont Medical Center, **Rock Hill** — G+ E
- Prisma Health Baptist Hospital, **Columbia** — G
- Prisma Health Baptist Parkridge Hospital, **Columbia** — S
- Prisma Health Greenville Memorial Hospital, **Greenville** — G+ E+ AT D
- Prisma Health Greer Memorial Hospital, **Greer** — G+ HR D
- Prisma Health Hillcrest Memorial Hospital, **Simpsonville** — G+ D
- Prisma Health Richland Hospital, **Columbia** — S G G S G+ E D G+
- Ralph H. Johnson VA Medical Center, **Charleston** — G G+ E+ D
- Regional Medical Center of Orangeburg & Calhoun Counties, **Orangeburg** — S G+ E D
- Roper Hospital, **Charleston** — G+ E D
- Roper St. Francis Berkeley Hospital, **Summerville** — S+ E D
- Self Regional Healthcare, **Greenwood** — G+ HR G+
- Spartanburg Medical Center - Church Street Campus, **Spartanburg** — G HR G+ HR D D
- Tidelands Waccamaw Community Hospital, **Murrells Inlet** — G+ HR D
- Trident Medical Center, **Charleston** — G E+ D

SOUTH DAKOTA

- Sanford USD Medical Center, **Sioux Falls** — G HR
- Monument Health Rapid City Hospital, **Rapid City** — S+

TENNESSEE

- Baptist Memorial Hospital Memphis, **Memphis** — G+ E AT D
- Blount Memorial Hospital, **Maryville** — G+ E+ D
- CHI Memorial, **Chattanooga** — G+ E D
- Erlanger Health System, **Chattanooga** — G+ E+ AT D
- Fort Sanders Regional Medical Center, **Knoxville** — G+ E+ AT D G G
- Holston Valley Medical Center, **Kingsport** — G+ D D G+

KEY TO THE AWARDS

GWTG - STROKE:
- G+ Gold Plus Achievement
- G Gold Achievement
- S+ Silver Plus Achievement
- S Silver Achievement

GWTG - HEART FAILURE:
- G+ Gold Plus Achievement
- G Gold Achievement
- S+ Silver Plus Achievement
- S Silver Achievement

GWTG - RESUSCITATION:
- G Gold Achievement
- S Silver Achievement

GWTG - AFIB:
- G Gold Achievement
- S Silver Achievement

© 2021 American Heart Association

*These hospitals received Get With The Guidelines-Resuscitation awards from the American Heart Association for two or more patient populations.

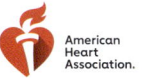

SPONSORED CONTENT

Hospital	Awards
LeConte Medical Center, Sevierville	G+ D
Methodist Healthcare, North, Memphis	G+ HR D
Methodist Healthcare, South, Memphis	G+ E D
Methodist LeBonheur Healthcare, Germantown	S+ HR D
Methodist Medical Center, Oak Ridge	G+ E+ D G
Methodist University Hospital, Memphis	G+ HR D
North Knoxville Medical Center, Powell	G+ D
NorthCrest Medical Center, Springfield	S+
Parkwest Medical Center, Knoxville	G+ E+ D G+
Roane Medical Center, Harriman	G+
Saint Thomas Midtown Hospital, Nashville	G G+ E D
Saint Thomas Rutherford Hospital, Murfreesboro	G+ E D
Saint Thomas West Hospital, Nashville	G G+ E AT
St. Francis Hospital - Bartlett, Bartlett	G+ E D
Sumner Regional Medical Center, Gallatin	G+ D
The University of Tennessee Medical Center, Knoxville	G+ E+ AT
TriStar Centennial Medical Center, Brentwood	G+ E D
TriStar Hendersonville Medical Center, Hendersonville	G+ E+ D
TriStar Skyline Medical Center, Nashville	G+ E D
TriStar Stonecrest Medical Center, Smyrna	S+ HR D
TriStar Summit Medical Center, Hermitage	G+ E D
Vanderbilt University Medical Center, Nashville	G+ E D
Williamson Medical Center, Franklin	S

TEXAS

Hospital	Awards
AdventHealth - Central Texas, Killeen	G+ HR D G+ G
Ascension Providence, Waco	G+ D
Ascension Seton Hays, Kyle	S+ E D
Ascension Seton Medical Center Austin, Austin	G+ HR D
Ascension Seton Williamson, Round Rock	G+ E D
Baptist Health System, San Antonio	G+ HR D
Baptist Hospitals of Southeast Texas, Beaumont	S+ E D
Baylor Scott & White All Saints Medical Center - Fort Worth, Fort Worth	G+ E D
Baylor Scott & White Heart and Vascular Hospital, Dallas	G+ G
Baylor Scott & White Medical Center - Brenham, Brenham	S+ E
Baylor Scott & White Medical Center - Centennial, Frisco	S+ D
Baylor Scott & White Medical Center - College Station, College Station	G+ E
Baylor Scott & White Medical Center - Grapevine, Grapevine	G+ E D
Baylor Scott & White Medical Center - Hillcrest, Waco	G+ E D
Baylor Scott & White Medical Center - Irving, Irving	S+ E D
Baylor Scott & White Medical Center - Lake Pointe, Rowlett	G+ HR D
Baylor Scott & White Medical Center - Lakeway, Lakeway	G+ E D
Baylor Scott & White Medical Center - Marble Falls, Marble Falls	G+ E
Baylor Scott & White Medical Center - McKinney, McKinney	G+ E D
Baylor Scott & White Medical Center - Plano, Plano	G+ E+ D
Baylor Scott & White Medical Center - Round Rock, Round Rock	G+ E D G+
Baylor Scott & White Medical Center - Temple, Temple	G+ E D G
Baylor Scott & White The Heart Hospital - Plano, Plano	G+ HR D
Baylor University Medical Center at Dallas, Dallas	G+ E+ AT
Ben Taub Hospital, Houston	G+ HR G+ E D D G+ G
Brazosport Regional Health System, Lake Jackson	S+ E
BSA Health System, Amarillo	G+
Carrollton Regional Medical Center, Carrollton	S S
Cedar Park Regional Medical Center, Cedar Park	
CHI St. Joseph Health College Station Hospital, College Station	S+ D S+
CHI St. Joseph Health Regional, Bryan	G+ E+ G+ D
CHI St. Luke's Health – Baylor St. Luke's Medical Center, Houston	G G+ D
Children's Medical Center Dallas, Dallas	G S
CHRISTUS Good Shepherd Health System - Longview, Longview	G+ E+ D
CHRISTUS Good Shepherd Health System - Marshall, Marshall	G+ E D
CHRISTUS Santa Rosa Health, San Antonio	G
CHRISTUS Spohn Hospital Corpus Christi - Shoreline, Corpus Christi	G+ E D
CHRISTUS Spohn Hospital Corpus Christi - South, Corpus Christi	G+ E D
CHRISTUS St. Michael Health System, Texarkana	G+ D
CHRISTUS St. Michael Hospital - Atlanta, Atlanta	G+ E
Citizens Medical Center, Victoria	G+ E D D
Corpus Christi Medical Center, Corpus Christi	G+ HR
Covenant Medical Center, Lubbock	HR D
Cuero Regional Hospital, Cuero	
Dallas Regional Medical Center, Mesquite	G+ E D G S
Del Sol Medical Center, El Paso	G+ E D
Dell Seton Medical Center at The University of Texas, Austin	G+ HR D
DeTar Healthcare System, Victoria	G D G
Doctors Hospital at Renaissance, Edinburg	G+ HR G+ E D D G+
Doctors Hospital of Laredo, Laredo	G+ E D
Harlingen Medical Center, Harlingen	G+ D
HCA Houston Healthcare - Clear Lake, Webster	G+ E D
HCA Houston Healthcare - Kingwood, Kingwood	G+ D
HCA Houston Healthcare - Northwest, Houston	G+ E D
HCA Houston Healthcare - Southeast, Pasadena	G
HCA Houston Healthcare - Tomball, Tomball	G+ D
HCA Houston Healthcare - West, Houston	G+ E D
Heart Hospital of Austin, Austin	S+ D
Hendrick Medical Center South, Abilene	S+
Hendrick Medical Center, Abilene	G+ E D G
Houston Methodist Baytown Hospital, Baytown	G+ E D
Houston Methodist Clear Lake Hosptial, Nassau Bay	G+ E D
Houston Methodist Hospital, Houston	S+ HR G G+ E D
Houston Methodist Sugar Land Hospital, Sugar Land	G+ E+ D
Houston Methodist The Woodlands Hospital, The Woodlands	G+ E D
Houston Methodist West Hospital, Houston	G+ E D
Houston Methodist Willowbrook Hospital, Houston	G+ E D
JPS Health Network, Fort Worth	G G+ E+ D D
Knapp Medical Center, Weslaco	G+ E D
Medical Center Hospital, Odessa	G+ G+ E D D
Medical City Dallas, Dallas	G S *
Medical City Plano, Plano	G+ HR
Methodist Charlton Medical Center, Dallas	G+ HR D
Methodist Dallas Medical Center, Dallas	G+ E D
Methodist Hospital	Metropolitan, San Antonio	G+ E D
Methodist Hospital	Northeast, San Antonio	G+ E D
Methodist Hospital	Stone Oak, San Antonio	G+ E D
Methodist Hospital, San Antonio	G+ E+ D
Methodist Mansfield Medical Center, Mansfield	G+ D G+
Methodist Richardson Medical Center, Richardson	G+ HR D
Midland Memorial Hospital, Midland	G+ D
Mission Regional Medical Center, Mission	S+ D
Northwest Texas Healthcare System, Amarillo	G+ E D
OakBend Medical Center Williams Way Campus, Richmond	G+
OakBend Medical Center, Richmond	G+ D
Odessa Regional Medical Center, Odessa	G+ D
Parkland Health & Hospital System, Dallas	G+ E D
Rio Grande Regional Hospital, McAllen	
Shannon Medical Center, San Angelo	G+ HR G+ HR D G+ G
South Texas Health System, Edinburg	G+ E AT D
Southwest General Hospital, San Antonio	G+ D
St. David's Georgetown Hospital, Georgetown	S+ HR D S
St. David's Medical Center, Austin	G+ E D S+ G
St. David's North Austin Medical Center, Austin	G+ E G G
St. David's Round Rock Medical Center, Round Rock	G+ E D D
St. David's South Austin Medical Center, Austin	G+ E D G+ G
St. Joseph Medical Center, Houston	G+ D
St. Luke's Health - Memorial Lufkin, Lufkin	G G+ E D D

MISSION LIFELINE: STEMI:
- G+ Gold Plus Receiving
- G+ Gold Plus Referring
- G Gold Receiving
- G Gold Referring
- S+ Silver Plus Receiving
- S+ Silver Plus Referring
- S Silver Receiving
- S Silver Referring

MISSION LIFELINE: NSTEMI:
- G Gold
- S Silver

TARGET HF | TARGET STROKE:
- HR Target: Heart Failure
- HR Target: Stroke Honor Roll
- E+ Target: Stroke Honor Roll Elite Plus
- E Target: Stroke Honor Roll Elite
- AT Target: Stroke Honor Roll Advanced Therapy
- D Target: Type 2 Diabetes Honor Roll™

© 2021 American Heart Association

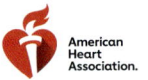

SPONSORED CONTENT

(TEXAS CONTINUED)

- St. Luke's Health - The Woodlands Hospital, **The Woodlands** — G+ E D G+ G
- Texas Health Arlington Memorial Hospital, **Arlington** — G+ E S
- Texas Health Harris Methodist Hospital Fort Worth, **Fort Worth** — G+ E S
- Texas Health Harris Methodist Hospital Hurst-Euless-Bedford, **Bedford** — S+ D G+
- Texas Health Harris Methodist Hospital Southwest Fort Worth, **Fort Worth** — S
- Texas Health Heart & Vascular Hospital Arlington, **Arlington** — G+ HR S
- Texas Health Huguley Hospital Fort Worth South, **Burleson** — G S
- Texas Health Presbyterian Hospital Dallas, **Dallas** — G+ E D G+
- Texas Health Presbyterian Hospital Denton, **Denton** — G+ HR D G+ S
- Texas Health Presbyterian Hospital Plano, **Plano** — G+ E S
- Texoma Medical Center, **Denison** — G+ E+ AT D
- The Hospitals of Providence East Campus, **El Paso** — S+
- The Hospitals of Providence Sierra Campus, **El Paso** — G+ D
- The Hospitals of Providence Transmountain Campus, **El Paso**
- Titus Regional Medical Center, **MT Pleasant** — G+ E D G G
- United Regional Healthcare System, **Wichita Falls** — D
- University Health System, **San Antonio** — S
- University Medical Center of El Paso, **El Paso** — G+ E+ D
- UT Health East Texas, **Tyler** — G+ HR
- UT Southwestern Medical Center, **Dallas** — G+ HR AT D S
- UTMB Health Clear Lake Hospital, **Webster** — S+ D
- UTMB Health Galveston, **Galveston** — G+ E D
- Valley Baptist Medical Center-Brownsville, **Brownsville** — G+
- Valley Baptist Medical Center-Harlingen, **Harlingen** — G+ E+ D
- Valley Regional Medical Center, **Brownsville** — D
- Wadley Regional Medical Center, **Texarkana** — D
- Woodland Heights Medical Center, **Lufkin** — G+

UTAH

- Davis Hospital and Medical Center, **Layton** — S G+ HR
- Intermountain Medical Center, **Murray** — G+ E+ AT D
- Intermountain St. George Regional Hospital, **Saint George** — S G+ E+ D
- Jordan Valley Medical Center/JVMC-West Valley Campus/Mountain Point Medical Center, a Campus of JVMC, **West Jordan** — G+ HR
- Lakeview Hospital, **Bountiful** — G+ E D
- McKay-Dee Hospital, **Ogden** — G+ E+ AT D
- Mountain View Hospital - Payson, **Payson** — D
- Ogden Regional Medical Center, **Ogden** — D
- St. Mark's Hospital, **Salt Lake City** — G+ E+ D
- Timpanogos Regional Hospital, **Orem** — D
- University of Utah Health, **Salt Lake City** — G G+ E HR
- Utah Valley Hospital, **Provo** — G+ E+ AT D

VERMONT

- The University of Vermont Medical Center, **Burlington** — G G+ E D

VIRGINIA

- Augusta Health, **Fishersville** — G+ E D
- Bon Secours Mary Immaculate Hospital, **Newport News** — D
- Bon Secours Maryview Medical Center, **Portsmouth** — G+ HR D
- Bon Secours Memorial Regional Medical Center, **Mechanicsville** — G+ E S+
- Bon Secours Rappahannock General Hospital, **Kilmarnock** — G+ E
- Bon Secours Richmond Community Hospital, **Richmond** — G+
- Bon Secours St. Francis Medical Center, **Midlothian** — G+ E D
- Bon Secours St. Mary's Hospital, **Richmond** — G+ HR E D G+
- Carilion Roanoke Memorial Hospital, **Roanoke** — G+ E AT D S
- Centra Lynchburg General Hospital, **Lynchburg** — G+ HR D
- Chesapeake Regional Medical Center, **Chesapeake** — G+ E
- Fauquier Hospital, **Warrenton** — S+ D
- Inova Alexandria Hospital, **Alexandria** — G+ E+ AT D
- Inova Fair Oaks Hospital, **Fairfax** — G+ E D
- Inova Fairfax Hospital, **Falls Church** — G+ E D
- Inova Loudoun Hospital, **Leesburg** — G+ E D
- Inova Mount Vernon Hospital, **Alexandria** — G+ E D
- Martha Jefferson Hospital, **Charlottesville** — G+ E AT D
- Mary Washington Hospital, **Fredericksburg** — G+
- Novant Health UVA Health System Haymarket Medical Center, **Haymarket** — S+
- Novant Health UVA Health System Prince William Medical Center, **Manassas** — G+ G+ HR
- Reston Hospital Center, **Reston** — G+ E
- Riverside Regional Medical Center, **Newport News** — G+ E+ AT D
- Riverside Shore Memorial Hospital, **Nassawadox** — S+ D
- Riverside Walter Reed Hospital, **Gloucester** — S+ D
- Sentara CarePlex Hospital, **Hampton** — G+ HR D
- Sentara Leigh Hospital, **Norfolk** — G+ D
- Sentara Louise Obici Memorial Hospital, **Suffolk** — G+ D
- Sentara Norfolk General Hospital/Sentara Heart Hospital, **Norfolk** — G+ E AT D S S
- Sentara Northern Virginia Medical Center, **Woodbridge** — G+ E D
- Sentara Princess Anne Hospital, **Virginia Beach** — G+ E+ D
- Sentara RMH Medical Center, **Harrisonburg** — G+ E D
- Sentara Virginia Beach General Hospital, **Virginia Beach** — G+ E D
- Sentara Williamsburg Regional Medical Center, **Williamsburg** — S+ E D
- Southside Regional Medical Center, **Petersburg** — G+ D G+
- StoneSprings Hospital Center, **Dulles** — G+ D
- The University of Virginia Health System, **Charlottesville** — G+ HR G+ E D
- Twin County Regional Healthcare, **Galax** — D
- VCU Health/Community Memorial Hospital, **South Hill** — G+ D
- Virginia Commonwealth University Medical Center, **Richmond** — G+ E+ D
- Virginia Hospital Center, **Arlington** — G+ HR D
- Winchester Medical Center, **Winchester** — S G+

WASHINGTON

- Capital Medical Center, **Olympia** — S
- Confluence Health-Central Washington Hospital, **Wenatchee** — G+ E D S+ G
- EvergreenHealth Medical Center, **Kirkland** — G+ E D
- EvergreenHealth Monroe, **Monroe** — G+
- Harbor Regional Health, **Aberdeen** — D
- Harborview Medical Center, **Seattle** — G+ E D G+
- Jefferson Healthcare, **Port Townsend** — S G+ HR G+
- Kadlec Regional Medical Center, **Richland** — G+ E D
- Kittitas Valley Healthcare, **Ellensburg** — S
- Legacy Salmon Creek Medical Center, **Vancouver** — G+ E D
- MultiCare Allenmore Hospital, **Tacoma** — S+ D
- MultiCare Auburn Medical Center, **Auburn** — G+ HR D
- MultiCare Covington Medical Center, **Covington** — S+ D
- MultiCare Deaconess Hospital, **Spokane** — G+ E+ D
- MultiCare Good Samaritan Hospital, **Puyallup** — G+ E D
- MultiCare Tacoma General Hospital, **Tacoma** — G+ HR D
- MultiCare Valley Hospital, **Spokane Valley** — S D
- Overlake Medical Center & Clinics, **Bellevue** — S+ HR E D D
- PeaceHealth Southwest Medical Center, **Vancouver** — G+ E D
- PeaceHealth St. John Medical Center, **Longview** — G+ HR D
- PeaceHealth St. Joseph Medical Center, **Bellingham** — G+ E D
- PeaceHealth United General Medical Center, **Sedro Woolley** — S
- Providence Centralia Hospital, **Centralia** — G+ S D
- Providence Holy Family Hospital, **Spokane** — G+ D

KEY TO THE AWARDS

GWTG - STROKE:
- G+ Gold Plus Achievement
- G Gold Achievement
- S+ Silver Plus Achievement
- S Silver Achievement

GWTG - HEART FAILURE:
- G+ Gold Plus Achievement
- G Gold Achievement
- S+ Silver Plus Achievement
- S Silver Achievement

GWTG - RESUSCITATION:
- G Gold Achievement
- S Silver Achievement

GWTG - AFIB:
- G Gold Achievement
- S Silver Achievement

© 2021 American Heart Association

*These hospitals received Get With The Guidelines-Resuscitation awards from the American Heart Association for two or more patient populations

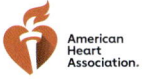

SPONSORED CONTENT

Hospital	Awards
Providence Regional Medical Center Everett, Everett	G+ E D
Providence Sacred Heart Medical Center & Children's Hospital, Spokane	E+ D
Providence St. Mary Medical Center, Walla Walla	G+ D
Providence St. Peter Hospital, Olympia	G+ G+ E D
Saint Joseph Medical Center, Tacoma	G+ HR G+ E AT D D
Saint Michael Medical Center, Bremerton	G+ HR G+ E D D
Seattle Children's Hospital, Seattle	G
St. Elizabeth Hospital, Enumclaw	S+ D
St. Francis Hospital, Federal Way	S+ HR G+ HR D
Swedish Edmonds, Edmonds	G+ E D
Swedish Medical Center - Cherry Hill Campus, Seattle	G+ E+ D
Swedish Medical Center - First Hill Campus, Seattle	G+ E D
Swedish Medical Center - Issaquah Campus, Issaquah	G+ E D
Trios Health, Kennewick	G+ E D
University of Washington Medical Center, Seattle	HR
UW Medicine	Valley Medical Center, Renton	G+ E+ D
VA Puget Sound Health Care System, Seattle Campus, Seattle	G+ D
Virginia Mason Medical Center - Seattle, Seattle	G+ E AT D D S
Yakima Valley Memorial, Yakima	G

WEST VIRGINIA

Hospital	Awards
Berkeley Medical Center, Martinsburg	S G+ D
Cabell Huntington Hospital, Huntington	G G+ HR
CAMC General Hospital, Charleston	G+ E
Camden Clark Medical Center, Parkersburg	G S+ E
Davis Medical Center, Elkins	G S
Mon Health Medical Center, Morgantown	G+ G+ D
Raleigh General Hospital, Beckley	G+ D
St. Mary's Medical Center, Huntington	G+ HR G D D
United Hospital Center, Bridgeport	G+ HR G G+ E D D
West Virginia University Hospital, Inc., Morgantown	G+ HR G+ E+ D D
Wheeling Hospital, Wheeling	S G+ D G+

WISCONSIN

Hospital	Awards
Ascension All Saints Hospital, Racine	G+ G+ E D D
Ascension Columbia St. Mary's Hospital Milwaukee, Milwaukee	G+ D
Ascension Columbia St. Mary's Hospital Ozaukee, Mequon	G+ D
Ascension St. Joseph Hospital, Milwaukee	G+ D
Aspirus Wausau Hospital, Wausau	G+ HR
Aurora BayCare Medical Center, Green Bay	G+ HR E
Aurora Lakeland Medical Center, Elkhorn	G+ HR S+
Aurora Medical Center - Grafton, Grafton	G+ E D
Aurora Medical Center - Kenosha, Kenosha	G+ HR G+ E+ D D
Aurora Medical Center - Oshkosh, Oshkosh	G+ E D
Aurora Medical Center Burlington, Burlington	G+ HR G+
Aurora Medical Center Manitowoc County, Two Rivers	G+ HR E D
Aurora Medical Center Summit, Summit	G+ G+ HR
Aurora Medical Center Washington County, Hartford	S+
Aurora Sheboygan Memorial Medical Center, Sheboygan	G G+ E
Aurora Sinai Medical Center, Milwaukee	G+ G+ D
Aurora St. Luke's Medical Center, Milwaukee	G+ HR G+ E+ D D
Aurora St. Luke's South Shore, Cudahy	G+ G+ D
Aurora West Allis Medical Center, West Allis	G+ E D
Bellin Memorial Hospital, Green Bay	D
Beloit Memorial Hospital, Beloit	S+ E
Froedtert Hospital, Milwaukee	G+ HR G G+ E+ D D
Froedtert Menomonee Falls Hospital, Menomonee Falls	G+ HR S+ E D
Froedtert West Bend Hospital, West Bend	S+ E+ D
Gundersen Lutheran Medical Center, La Crosse	G+
HSHS Sacred Heart Hospital, Eau Claire	S+
Marshfield Medical Center, Marshfield	G+ E D
Mayo Clinic Health System LaCrosse, La Crosse	G+
Mayo Clinic Health System- Eau Claire, Eau Claire	G+ D
Mercy Hospital and Trauma Center, Janesville	G+ HR
Oconomowoc Memorial Hospital, Oconomowoc	S+ D
Richland Hospital, Richland Center	S+
SSM Health St. Clare Hospital, Baraboo	G+ HR D
SSM Health St. Mary's Hospital - Madison, Madison	G+ E+ AT
St. Agnes Hospital, Fond Du Lac	G+
St. Mary's Janesville Hospital, Janesville	
ThedaCare Regional Medical Center, Appleton	S D
ThedaCare Regional Medical Center-Neenah, Neenah	G+ HR AT D
UnityPoint Health -Meriter, Madison	G+ E D
University of Wisconsin Hospital and Clinics, Madison	G+ E+ D G+ G
Upland Hills Health, Dodgeville	S+
Waukesha Memorial Hospital, Waukesha	G+ HR

WYOMING

Hospital	Awards
Cheyenne Regional Medical Center, Cheyenne	G+ G+ HR D D
Wyoming Medical Center, Casper	G+ E+ AT D

This content is available online at
https://usnewsbrandfuse.com/AmericanHeartAssociation/

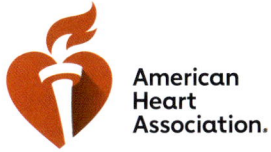

MISSION LIFELINE: STEMI:
- **G+** Gold Plus Receiving
- **G+** Gold Plus Referring
- **G** Gold Receiving
- **G** Gold Referring
- **S+** Silver Plus Receiving
- **S+** Silver Plus Referring
- **S** Silver Receiving
- **S** Silver Referring

MISSION LIFELINE: NSTEMI:
- **G** Gold
- **S** Silver

TARGET HF | TARGET STROKE:
- **HF** Target: Heart Failure
- **HR** Target: Stroke Honor Roll
- **E+** Target: Stroke Honor Roll Elite Plus
- **E** Target: Stroke Honor Roll Elite
- **AT** Target: Stroke Honor Roll Advanced Therapy
- **D** Target: Type 2 Diabetes Honor Roll™

© 2021 American Heart Association

ON MEDICINE'S FRONT LINES

Searching for Ways to Close Gaps

Providers are getting more serious about tackling health disparities

by **Joseph P. Williams**

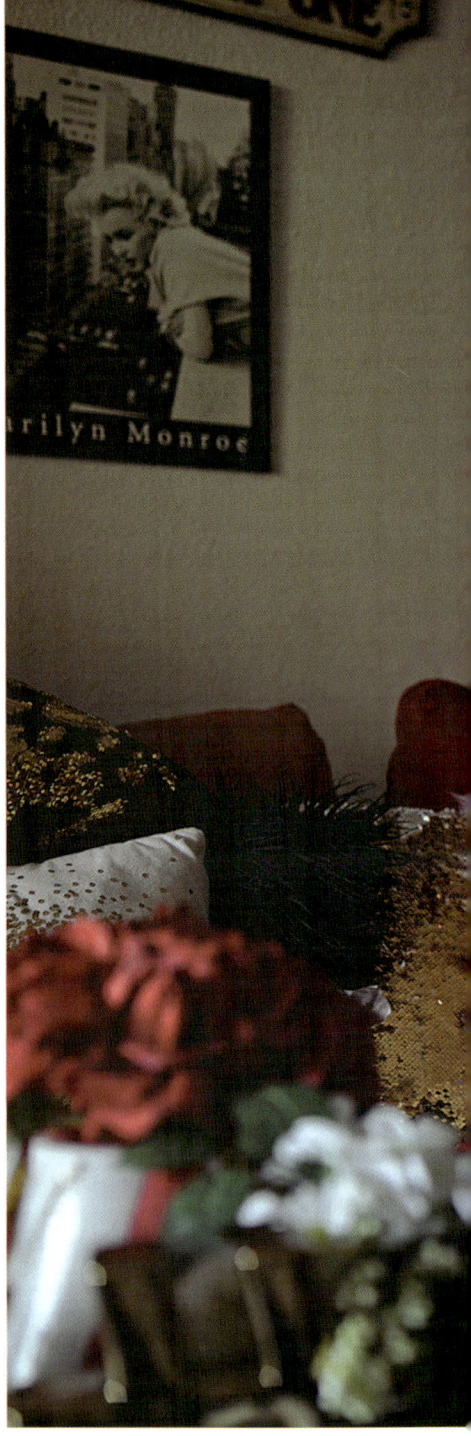

A WAKE AT 4 A.M. one morning last November, Felicia Silva of Albuquerque, New Mexico, assumed the dull ache in her left shoulder was a cramp – or maybe she'd slept on it wrong. She pushed through the pain and went to work, but her colleagues, seeing her disorientation and hearing her stutter, urged her to get medical help. Hours later, Silva found herself at Presbyterian Rust Medical Center in nearby Rio Rancho, diagnosed with a minor stroke and admitted for treatment.

Then, about a week after she was sent home, Silva got a surprising call from an administrator at Presbyterian, and it wasn't about her hospital bill. "She just reached out to me: 'I got your number from our system and I just want to know if you needed anything,'" Silva recalls. "At that time I was just out of the hospital. And I said, 'No, I'm okay.'" The agent, Amy, said she'd call back in a few weeks.

By then, Silva was dealing with a chain reaction triggered by her stroke. Forced to take short-term disability to recover, she'd seen her take-home pay plunge; food for Silva and her two school-age sons had run low, and her utility company was about to shut off the lights over a $800 past-due bill. So when Amy called again, Silva acknowledged that she was in trouble. "I said, 'Actually, I haven't gotten paid this month at all. My rent is paid, but I'm worried about groceries. All I care about is like feeding my boys and they have a roof over their head.'"

Within minutes, Amy had connected Silva to state and federal resources to help her pay her bill, and a local food pantry so she and her children could eat. "That was a huge weight lifted off my shoulders – huge," says Silva, who has fully recovered and is back at her job at a pharmaceutical company.

Social health. She didn't realize it at the time, but Silva had benefited from a growing movement in medical care that considers patients' access to healthy food and stable housing and relief from financial stress to be as important to address as their blood pressure, heart rate and

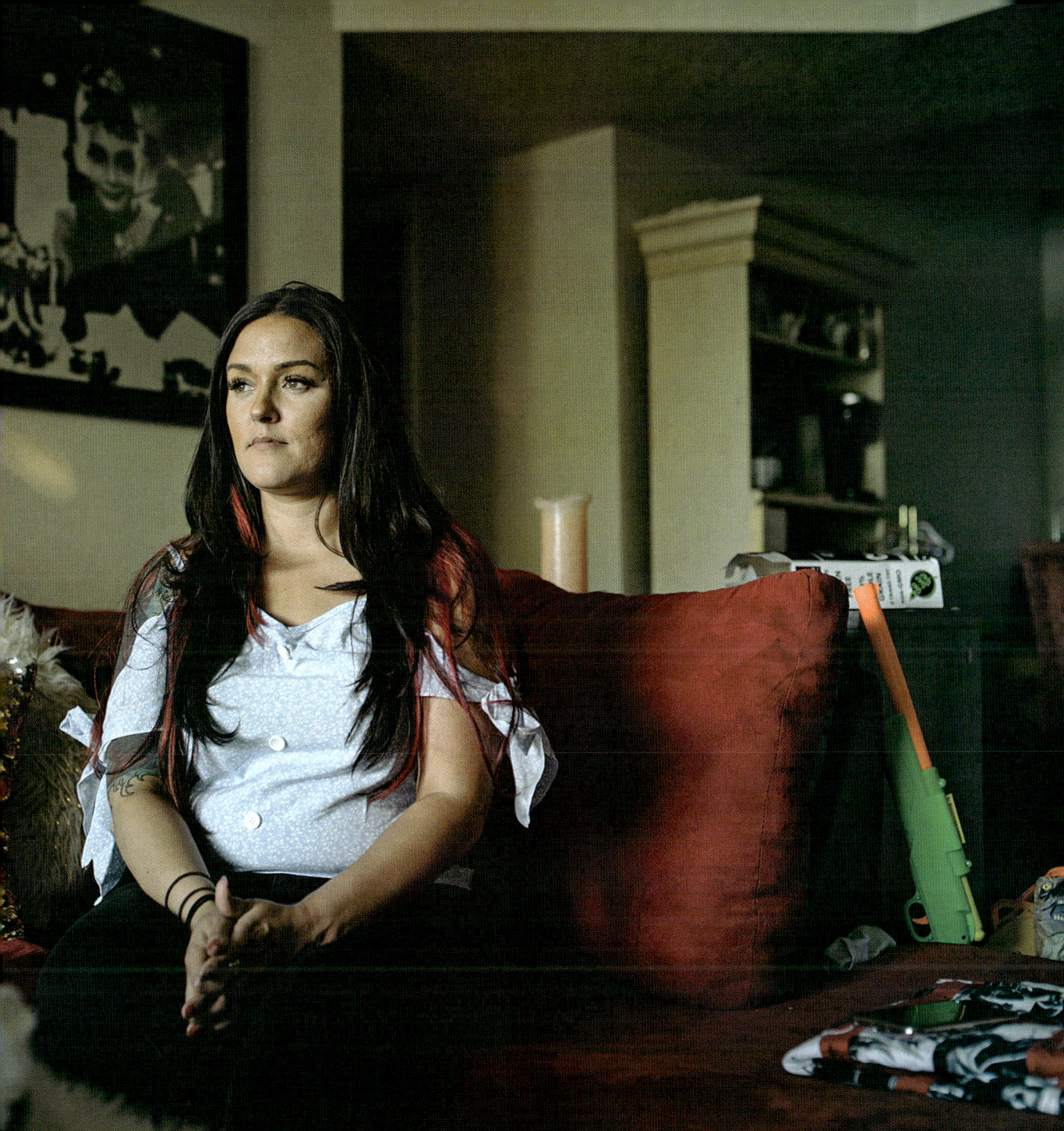

the images from an MRI. Hospitals, health systems and federally subsidized clinics are increasingly focused on the "social health" of patients – external factors, called social determinants of health, that have short- and long-term impacts on their physical wellbeing.

"Trying to help patients address their social needs is really an important emerging issue for health care managers," says Amanda Brewster, assistant professor of health policy and management at the University of California–Berkeley. "We've really seen increased atten-

FELICIA SILVA'S RETURN TO NORMALCY AFTER A STROKE WAS AIDED BY THE HOSPITAL'S ATTENTION TO HER FINANCIAL NEEDS.

tion to this topic for the past five or 10 years. And there's quite a lot of research going on across the U.S. to try to figure out what are the best ways of doing this."

The issue catapulted to the top of the national agenda last year, when headlines about the disproportionate effect of the coronavirus pandemic on Black and brown neighborhoods collided with dramatic images of protests condemning the police killings of George Floyd in Minneapolis and Breonna Taylor in Louisville, Kentucky. Experts said the same social forces that contributed to the deaths of Floyd and Taylor were helping to intensify the deadliness of the contagion in communities of color. The Centers for Disease Control and Prevention,

ON MEDICINE'S FRONT LINES

which in April declared racism a serious public health threat, attributes the higher mortality rate among African Americans – twice that of whites – in part to profound inequalities commonly found in underserved communities. Harvard researchers studying socioeconomic data on COVID fatalities found that, even on an individual level, people with markers for poor socioeconomic status – racial minorities, poor people and the undereducated, in particular – were significantly more likely to bear a "disproportionate burden" of COVID-19 mortality.

That finding was yet another data point adding to the evidence that solving longstanding health differentials between populations requires systemic solutions. Food deserts in the neighborhoods where impoverished people live, lack of quality affordable housing, employment insecurity and financial stress are among the root causes of chronic diseases like obesity and diabetes, which are particularly endemic among African Americans and Latinos. Those diseases, in turn, increase the likelihood of critical, potentially life-threatening illnesses like heart disease and kidney failure.

Meanwhile, reduced or lost income like Silva experienced can make it more difficult to buy prescriptions and keep

> **'Gun violence is an area gaining caregiver focus.'**

follow-up or physical therapy appointments, impeding a patient's recovery from an illness.

Epidemiologists also blame poor health outcomes on lack of access to the health care system: For too many people, quality primary – preventive – care and the latest advances in medicine are out of reach. That helps explain why African Americans have for decades had the highest overall cancer mortality rate of any racial or ethnic group in the country (story, Page 92).

Health disparities between African Americans and whites have "been around for forever," says Dr. Alisahah Cole, system vice president of population health innovation and policy at CommonSpirit Health. And until recently there hadn't been much effort to address them. Now, says Cole, she sees "a very intentional interest" in working toward health equity. Indeed, an increasing number of health systems are offering access to or information on food pantries, housing assistance, employment, substance abuse and financial assistance.

New leadership. At the same time, more systems are creating C-suite positions focused on achieving health equity. Rush University Medical Center, Mass General Brigham, CommonSpirit Health and Nationwide Children's Hospital, among others, have all added equity officers. The 174-year-old American Medical Association hired its first chief health equity officer in 2019: Dr. Aletha Maybank, who previously directed the Center for Health Equity within New York City's public health department.

According to a 2020 report published in Health Affairs, 57 health systems nationwide had spent some $2.5 billion on programs addressing social determinants of health. While the lion's share of that sum has gone to affordable housing, other programs address issues ranging from food insecurity to transportation and job training.

Types of support. In Toledo, Ohio, for example, ProMedica chipped in $11.5 million to Ebeid Neighborhood Promise, a $50 million neighborhood development project focused in part on health, education, jobs, family stability and social and educational services.

In Detroit, the Henry Ford Health System joined forces with the ridesharing giant Lyft to create a system aimed at getting patients who need transportation to and from appointments. Kaiser Permanente spent more than $100 million in 2020 in support of housing and food security, economic opportunity, health in schools and equity. Some has gone toward providing entrepreneurs of color with access to capital, some to grants that will give a few hundred high-school students a chance to go to college, and some to support an affordable housing nonprofit engaged in California's effort to provide interim housing and services to people experiencing homelessness.

"I do think leaders, especially health care system leaders, are being really thoughtful about this work now" and are including it in long-term strategic plans, Cole says. "I really base my work on one of my favorite Arthur Ashe quotes: 'Start where you are, use what you have, and do what you can.'"

Still, most hospitals that get tax breaks caring for indigent patients continue to spend more on unreimbursed care than they do investing to improve the health of a community, possibly because the skills and infrastructure required are so different from what's involved in delivering care.

Gun violence, which kills more than 100 people and wounds more than 230 people every day – many of whom are boys and men of color – is one factor contributing to wide disparities in life expectancy in some communities, and

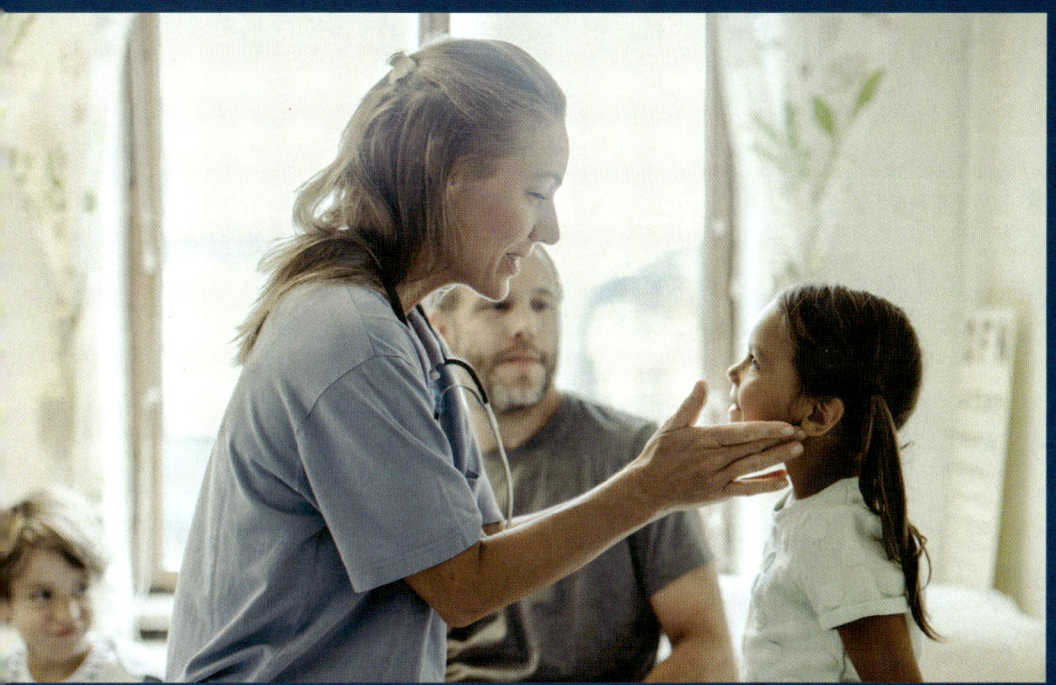

60 years and going strong.

We have proudly served Santa Clara County for six decades with unparalleled healthcare.

The American Nurses Credentialing Center awarded us the prestigious Magnet designation four consecutive times.

The Centers for Medicare & Medicaid Services (CMS) have given us a 5-star rating.

Our doctors and nurses deliver a standard of excellence in care using compassion and innovation.

Because that is what our community deserves.

Learn more at **elcaminohealth.org**

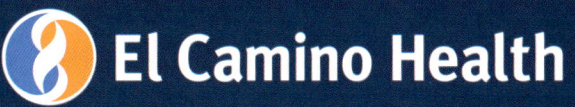

ON MEDICINE'S FRONT LINES

"Now there's 'a very intentional interest' in health equity."

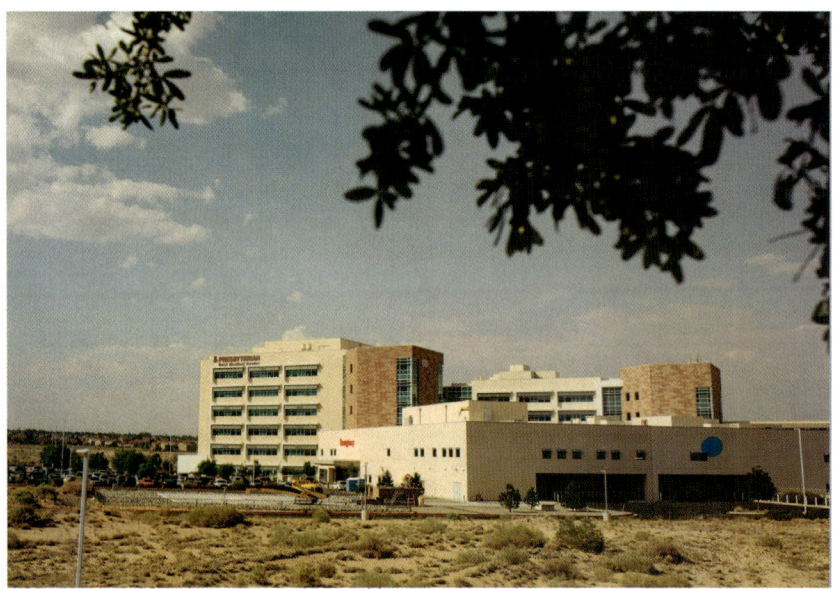

PRESBYTERIAN RUST MEDICAL CENTER IN NEW MEXICO, WHERE FELICIA SILVA WAS TREATED.

is an area gaining caregiver focus. People experiencing interpersonal violence, experts say, are at elevated risk for re-injury and violence perpetration, creating a "revolving door" of victims and offenders cycling through emergency rooms.

To close that door, hospitals are turning to hospital-based violence intervention programs, or HB-VIPs, to convince those involved to get help and choose another path. "I can have a patient come in, shot at age 18, shot again at 22, in a recovery bed at 23," says Dr. Charity Evans, an associate surgery professor at the University of Nebraska Medical Center. "Our feeling is, when these individuals come in with their first and second gunshot wounds, that that was our opportunity to intervene."

Redirection. Using a "credible messenger" to make a bedside visit – "someone from their community, that's gone through what they've gone through, who's been injured before, been in that bed," Evans says – the hospital looks to redirect the patient away from violence, offering a range of services to help with everything from battling the effects of poverty to education and job training.

Partnerships with other organizations are key to hospitals' ability to improve patients' situations, Brewster says; the medical community can't solve the problem alone. "It does take a village, if you will," agrees Barbara Petee, chief advocacy and government relations officer at ProMedica and executive director of the Root Cause Coalition, a nonprofit organization that links the health care industry with community groups to share ideas and best practices and partner to address socially-driven health disparities. "It takes hospitals, health systems and insurance companies working with social service organizations, faith-based groups and foundations" as well as federal, state and local government, Petee says.

Amen, says Andrea Norberg, executive director of the Francois-Xavier Bagnoud Center, a Rutgers University-affiliated community clinic in Newark, New Jersey. Formed in 1987 as part of the School of Nursing, the clinic was an early adopter of caregiver-community partnerships, largely because of its mission: providing family-centered care for HIV/AIDS patients as well as adults and children with other infectious diseases and immunologic disorders.

Because employers, landlords, families and even doctors often ostracized or shunned them, it wasn't unusual for AIDS patients to suffer, and often die, impoverished, with next to no financial or emotional support. The staff included specialists who connected patients to social-service resources.

Over time, the clinic's prime directive has evolved to include eliminating "barriers to interdisciplinary, client-centered, equitable, high-quality health care for those at the greatest risk for socially determined health vulnerabilities," according to its mission statement. That includes helping people gain access to job training, child care, education and behavioral-health services. "You can't really achieve your health goals unless your social situation is also addressed," explains Norberg.

Consider patients who have severe hypertension, putting them at risk for a stroke or kidney failure. Generally, Norberg says, they are sent home with blood pressure monitoring equipment. That's not possible when a patient lives on the street. "If you're homeless, it's very difficult for you to prioritize your blood pressure," she says. The focus becomes "thinking about all of the needs that a person has," she says. "Trying to help them to navigate the complexities of systems and trying to help them get to a better place."

For Felicia Silva, the offer from Presbyterian Rust Medical Center to help with getting the bills paid and putting food on the table accomplished that mission. Without that phone call from the hospital, she says, "I would have never even known, you know, that there was actually this much help out there. And there was so much help." •

Even the best can Get Better.

Ranked among the Best Hospitals in the nation once again. From cardiology to gastroenterology, there's nothing we love better than caring for you. Get to know the team that's consistently ranked among the best in Texas. Make an appointment today by scanning the QR code to download MyBSWHealth.

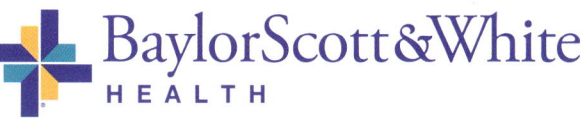

Changing Healthcare For The Better

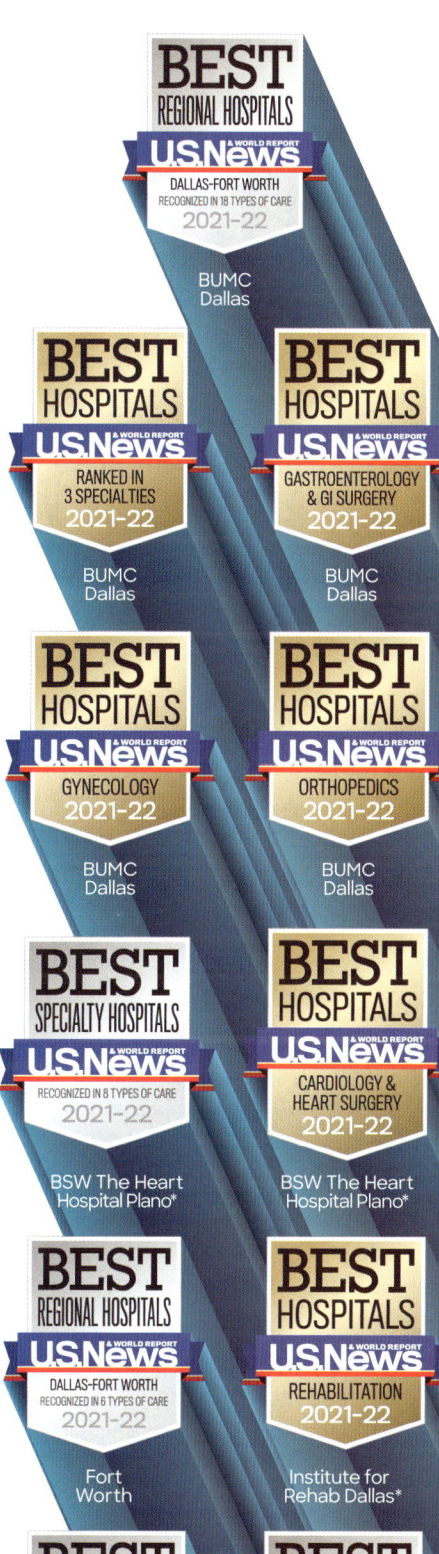

Scan to download MyBSWHealth

*Joint ownership with physicians. Not all hospitals recognized in all specialties. See USNews.com/BestHospitals for complete listings. Physicians provide clinical services as members of the medical staff at one of Baylor Scott & White Health's subsidiary, community or affiliated medical centers and do not provide clinical services as employees or agents of those medical centers or Baylor Scott & White Health. ©2021 Baylor Scott & White Health. 99-ALL-243908 L/GD

ON MEDICINE'S FRONT LINES

On the Cutting Edge of Cancer Care

Four leading experts discuss the latest advances in immunotherapy – and offer their vision of the future

LATE LAST YEAR, U.S. News hosted a webinar about the promise of cutting-edge developments in cancer care, particularly in the field of immunotherapy. Four preeminent researchers joined the discussion: **James P. Allison, Ph.D.,** chair of the department of immunology and executive director of the immunotherapy platform at The University of Texas MD Anderson Cancer Center and a recipient of the 2018 Nobel Prize in Physiology or Medicine; **Dr. Michael A. Caligiuri,** president of City of Hope National Medical Center; **Dr. Laurie H. Glimcher,** president and chief executive officer of Dana-Farber Cancer Institute; and **Dr. Carl H. June,** director of the Center for Cellular Immunotherapies in the University of Pennsylvania's Perelman School of Medicine. Edited excerpts of the conversation:

If you look back at the past 18 months, how has COVID-19 affected cancer care?

Laurie Glimcher: This has been a critical time for cancer patients, who are particularly susceptible to infection because their immune systems have been weakened. Early in the pandemic, we implemented a very robust telemedicine system; we were doing 10 to 15 telemedicine visits per week before the pandemic and quickly got up to 3,000 telemedicine visits a week within two to three weeks so that we could continue to care for our patients. And we were able to offer some patients oral medications that were as good as what they were getting in person so they didn't have to come to the hospital to be treated. So we saw a very significant drop of patients coming into Dana-Farber in the first few months of the pandemic.

Importantly, routine screenings such as mammograms, colonoscopies and pap smears dropped by as much as 96%, and cancer diagnosis dropped by nearly 50%. Ned Sharpless, director of the National Cancer Institute, predicts that we'll have a 10% increase in cancer mortality because of that. We're working hard now to tell people that they've got to resume routine screenings and seek care if it's needed.

Michael Caligiuri: One thing about a cancer hospital is that what we do is with immunosuppressed patients. The nature of infection itself is something that each of us is dealing with every day. So our preparedness was probably a bit more advanced than, say, at a more general hospital where the immunosuppressed patient is rarer.

Carl, you had your own experience with COVID-19. Tell us about that.

Carl June: It was when we had no testing in place. My internist basically said, unless you have to come to the hospital, don't. I had my own pulse oximeter to measure my oxygen. So I stayed home and fortunately didn't have any complications. But it led me to look at a lot of the issues. We've opened a trial at the University of Pennsylvania to look at whether, if we mildly suppress the immune

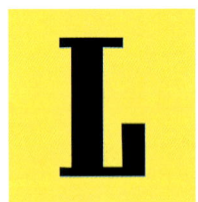

NOBEL LAUREATE JAMES P. ALLISON ARRIVES AT THE 2018 CELEBRATION WITH HIS WIFE AND COLLABORATOR, DR. PADMANEE SHARMA.

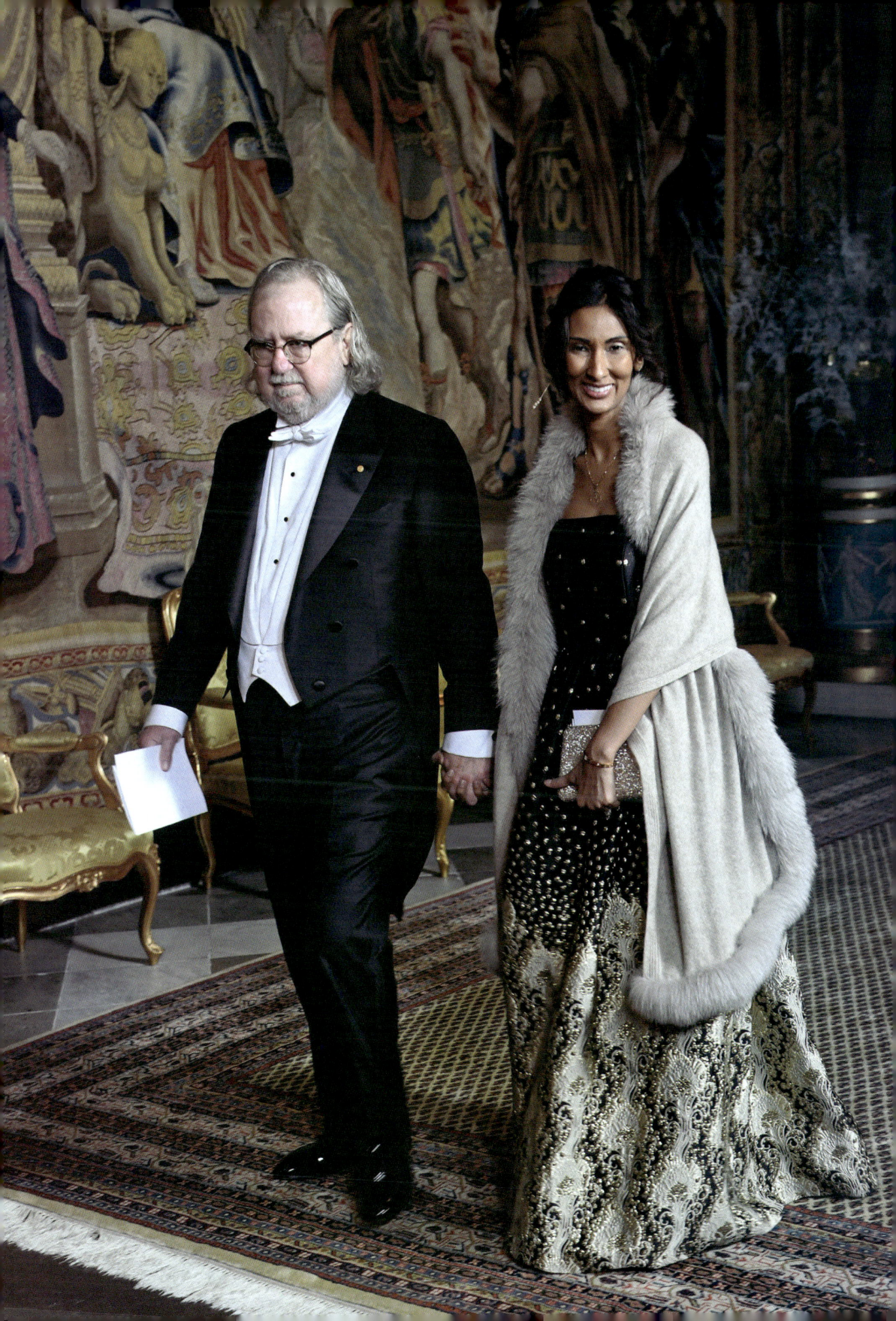

ON MEDICINE'S FRONT LINES

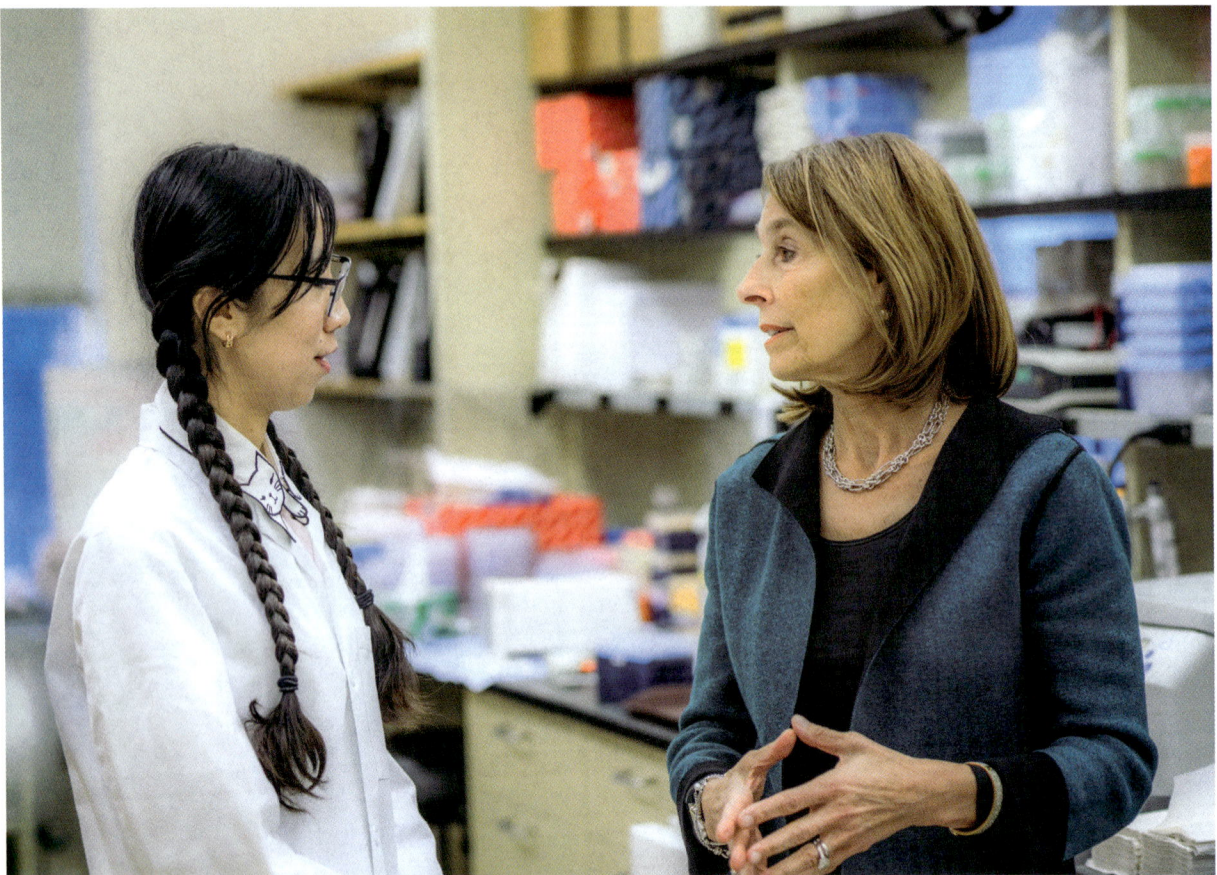

DANA-FARBER'S PRESIDENT AND CEO, DR. LAURIE H. GLIMCHER, TALKS WITH RESEARCHER HAN DONG IN THE GLIMCHER LAB.

system, we can prevent the overactivity that in a subset of people leads to increased damage.

Have your clinical trials been interrupted?
LG: The good thing – about the only good thing – about cancer is that clinical trials at Dana-Farber continued, which may have been a different experience at hospitals with trials for cardiovascular disease or any other disease.
MC: I would add that patients who go on clinical trials get superb care. They're mandated for routine follow-up and when it can't be in person, it's through telemedicine. You have patients who understand the importance of clinical trials, and they're very aggressive in pursuing the latest, greatest innovative care that they can get.
LG: For our patients, the truth is that the best option for 15% to 20% of them is to be on a clinical trial, because it's the best treatment available at the time.

There is so much promise in cancer care. Jim, can you talk about developments in immunotherapy and in particular the checkpoint inhibitors you pioneered?
James Allison: The idea of immunotherapy has been around for a long time. The first mention of it that I'm aware of was in 1906 by Paul Ehrlich, who suggested making antibodies to cancer. In the 1970s and '80s, we began to recognize that there were molecules on tumor cells that are detected by the immune system. There were a lot of trials of therapeutic vaccines for cancer that failed. But regulation of immune responses – T cell responses in particular – is more complicated than we thought. What we and others found in the early '90s was that there are active signaling pathways that shut [the immune response] down. They're there to protect you [from an] overshoot – from the immune system becoming too strong. It was those pathways that we were running into in trying to treat cancer. And so the thing that really opened up checkpoint blockade was to realize that we could block those molecules that were limiting an immune response to keep the normal immune response going and eliminate cancer. And that worked.

One of the things that's become apparent is that immune therapy has some things others don't, memory being the most notable. Once you've alerted the immune system, for a long time, perhaps the rest of your life, you've got T cells that can recognize that tumor and make sure that if it comes back, they attack it.

Will immunotherapy potentially replace other standard treatments?
JA: What we're realizing now is that if you can get radiation therapies and chemotherapies done in a way that they don't inactivate the immune system, they can be very, very, very good vaccines, if

you will. And I think we're beginning to see that come to fruition as people in those fields realize they don't have to kill every last tumor cell, and in so doing cause a lot of adverse events. You can turn, for example, a drug that targets one molecule in a tumor cell into an immune response that will target many other things. Some people say, oh, immunotherapy is going to replace chemo or radiation or surgery. I really don't think so. Certainly not across the board. I think the cancer therapy of the future will contain an element of immunotherapy to give it the ability to eliminate that last cancer cell and to provide the long-lived memory of that.

Where are you seeing the greatest success so far?

JA: With melanoma, with a strictly immunological approach [using one combination therapy], the five-year survival is over 50% in a cohort of patients who were in a phase 3 trial six years ago now. There's no reason why that can't keep going on. [The first approved checkpoint inhibitor] ipilimumab has a much lower response rate, but it's lasted for 10 years and more in a little over 20% of patients. And that's a pretty remarkable achievement, since when all this work started the median survival after diagnosis with late stage melanoma was seven months. There are a couple of patients who are almost 19 years out. After a single dose. No retreatment ever. Other cancers aren't quite so responsive yet.

The key now is to find ways of targeting additional checkpoints. At Penn there's an approach that looks promising for pancreatic cancer, which has frustrated oncologists for decades.

LG: Jim, I will never forget the story you told me about when you first met a patient whose life you had saved. You went in to see a young woman who had had stage 4 melanoma and was essentially at death's door, and who was now melanoma-free. You said you met her and started crying. I just want to thank you again for being so persevering about pushing this forward.

JA: Well, thank you for that. She was diagnosed when she was 22 years old, and now she has two teenage kids and has become a friend.

Carl, describe your pioneering work with CAR-T cells.

CJ: First I want to mention the trial that Jim referred to of pancreatic cancer. It's early data. But pancreatic cancer really hasn't changed in 50 years. If you can't cut it out, you ultimately fail. So while what Jim developed takes the brakes off the immune system, what's being tested in the trial started at Penn is pushing on the accelerator at the same time. It's a combination. I think we're going to look at all these other cancers as using combinations of therapies.

CAR-T cells are a way to step on the gas. They're made of the patient's own immune system. We take cells from the patient's blood and then rewire them in a laboratory. Those cells are genetically modified and given back to the patient.

Our first patients were treated in 2010. Last summer, the first patient came back in and still has no leukemia. So, most likely, he's cured.

Mike, tell us about the work you've been doing at City of Hope in this arena.

MC: I've spent about 35 years working on a different cell, maybe a cousin to T cells, called natural killer cells. Very similarly to T cells, they can kill a tumor, and sometimes a bit quicker. They don't have memory, which is a key

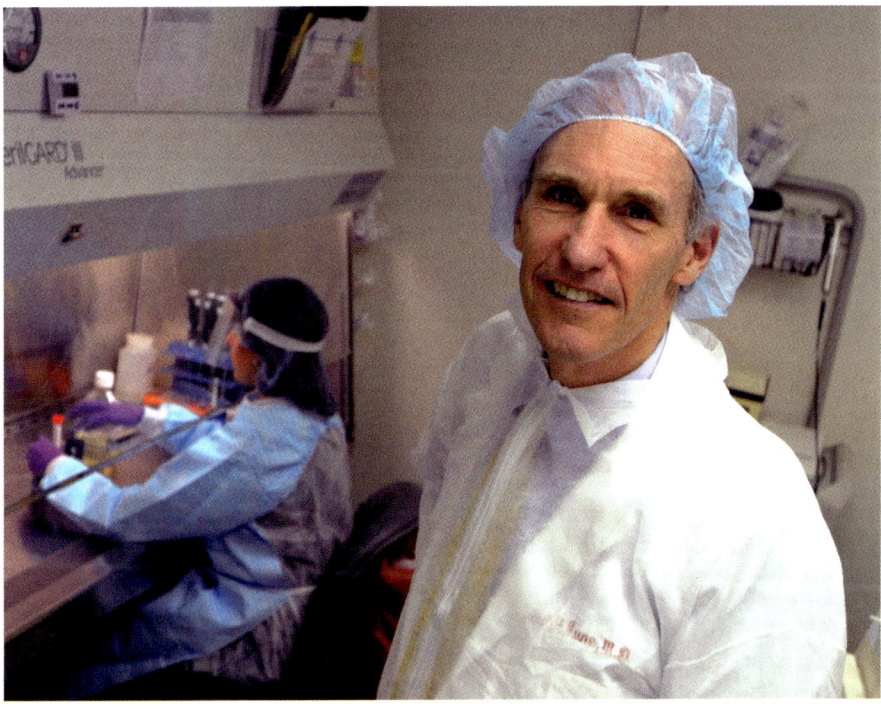

CAR-T CELL PIONEER DR. CARL H. JUNE HEADS THE CENTER FOR CELLULAR IMMUNOTHERAPIES AT PENN'S PERELMAN SCHOOL OF MEDICINE.

to T cell success. But on the other hand they're less likely to cause some of the toxicities that can result from memory. The work is about 10 years behind the work in T cells, but they're rapidly coming to the clinic now.

A study that's going to be opening at City of Hope in lung cancer combines such cells with a checkpoint inhibitor. We're finding it works to actually activate the NK cells, turning on the gas of NK cells. And importantly, they can be made from blood or out of cord blood, and can be frozen and distributed. So if they proved to be as effective as CAR-T cell therapy, or maybe in certain tumors as effective, the production and distribution should be a lot easier – what's called "off the shelf." That could hopefully drive the price down.

ON MEDICINE'S FRONT LINES

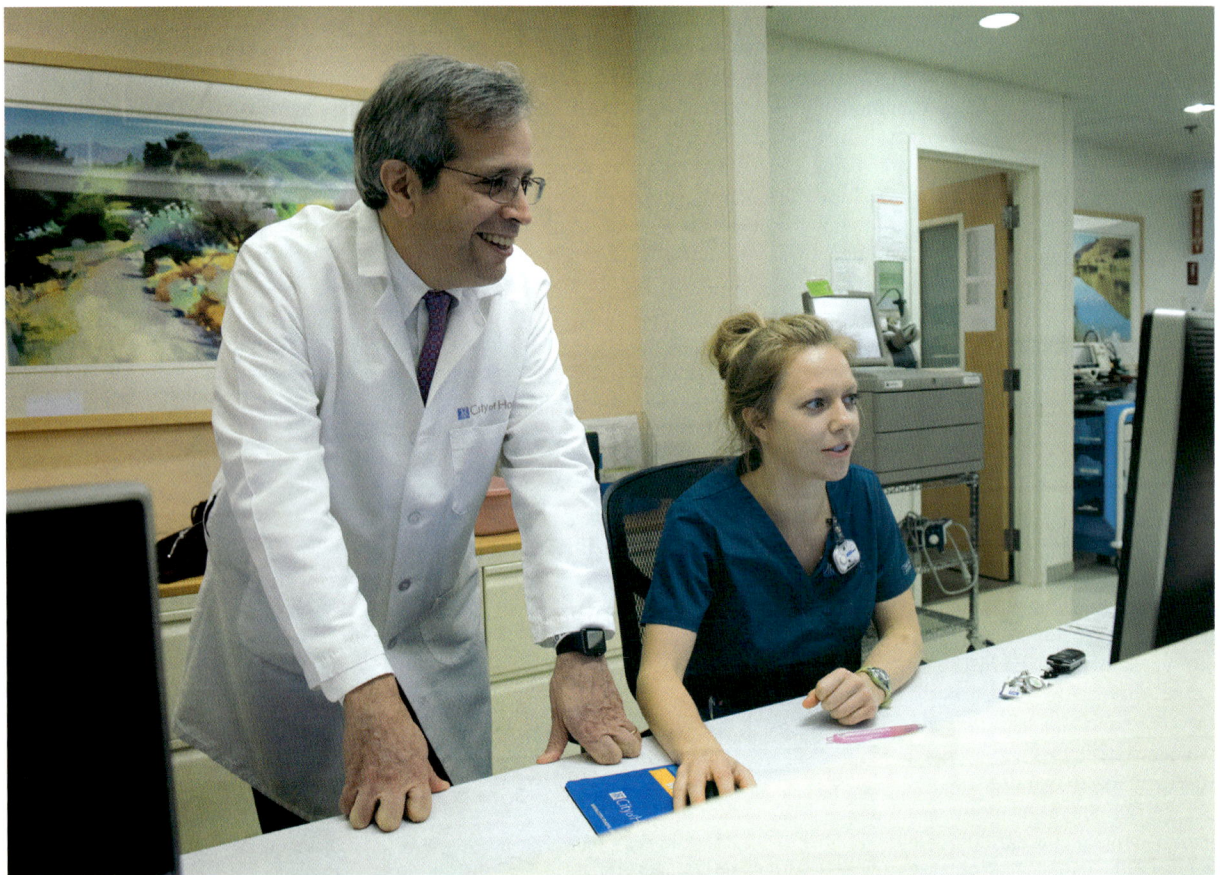

How can these very expensive treatments be made available to people who can't get to major cities?

JA: One thing with checkpoint blockade is, there are troublesome adverse events that can become very dangerous if they're not properly controlled in the big cancer centers. A lot of community doctors are afraid of these therapies, because while the adverse events are fewer and probably less severe than with most chemotherapy, the chemotherapy is very stereotypical, and the algorithm is easily taught. It's very hard to predict with these checkpoints.

So a number of people are working now on developing software programs on cell phones where patients can report how they're feeling and any events they have. That goes into a program that you can take a look at and say, well, according to what we know, we would recommend this to the community doctor. With this daily monitoring, the doctor could learn really early what's going on and get advice as to how to treat it.

LG: I think all of us would say that every patient, no matter what their zip code is, should be getting the highest quality cancer care. One way we're doing this at Dana-Farber is through a platform called Pathways, a tool to help oncologists everywhere quickly identify the best treatment for an individual patient by providing a very clear map with key factors that we use to make clinical decisions at Dana-Farber.

CITY OF HOPE PRESIDENT DR. MICHAEL A. CALIGIURI HAS SPENT 35 YEARS STUDYING NATURAL KILLER CELLS.

Cancer is an incredibly complex set of diseases, and cancer medicines change rapidly, which is a good thing. But the rapid changes force physicians and patients who don't have any oncologists nearby to interpret massive amounts of new information from publications and from clinical trials. Pathways helps physicians sort through deep and complex sets of information and shows how Dana-Farber would treat a patient with say, a rare sarcoma, or even a more common disease like breast cancer. When treating a patient, you must integrate radiology, pathology, genomics, immunoprofile and, very importantly, electronic health record data. Pathways is a roadmap based on data, so physicians can come up with the best possible treatment for their patient. And it's backed by the power of the entire cancer community.

MC: There's this huge gap between all that we're able to do as "super specialists" focused on one cancer versus what a community physician dealing with a dozen different cancers from 7:00 a.m. to 7:00 p.m. could possibly have the time to do. Pathways is a wonderful example of filling that gap. One of the things that we've initiated is called Access Hope. Employers care deeply about the care that their employees get, and we now have almost 2 million employees who are covered by Access Hope. No matter where they are in the country, they can talk to an expert in their particular cancer and get an opinion over the phone about the acuity of their situation and the next steps, and then we point them to a comprehensive cancer center: You can go here for this and you can go here for that. And that doctor in Access Hope will work with the community physician to see that they're guided if they can't get to one of our centers.

Carl, do you want to add anything?
CJ: You know, when people graduate from medical school, their training gets dated. What Laurie and Michael just described are ways to try to accelerate the generation of knowledge. The National Cancer Institute calls this translational research Type 2, which is the spread of it from our specialized centers to the community.

Bone marrow transplantation is the kind of therapy most related to CAR-T cells. When that happened back in the 1980s, people said it could never become generalized. But all the cancer centers now can do bone marrow transplants. So it's going to be really important that we learn how to train physicians.

Let's talk about the problem of disparities in care affecting communities of color. How do we tackle that?
LG: It's a multipronged answer. There's an absence of good primary care in these communities, and because of that, diagnoses are missed. So only 25% of our patients present with stage 1 cancer. For the others, the cancer has already spread and therefore is much harder to treat. [Many people] don't have access to healthy food, or time to exercise and do all the things that we know can help prevent cancer. So that's an issue we need to address.

Also, patients like to come to a place where they see people who look like themselves. When you go into a cancer center, you're afraid, and you want to see somebody you can trust. I think for many reasons there is a lack of trust in some of these communities, and justifiably so. Forty percent of the patients we see are referred to us for second or even third opinions, and of those patients, at least 20% have either been misdiagnosed or put on the wrong treatments.
MC: The onus is on us to do something about it. All of our organizations are putting in huge efforts, I believe, to educate the next generation, and also to recruit those physicians, sustain them, and bring them into the academic fold and nurture them in a way that years ago never happened.
LG: I think one real positive about the COVID-19 vaccine trials is that they worked very hard to have adequate representation of diversity. How can you approve a vaccine or a drug if you haven't tested it in multiple diverse populations?

Can the new therapies be tailored to children?
JA: I think there's a lot of attention being paid to that issue, particularly with immunotherapy of the checkpoint block type, which unleashes cells in your body. Kids are going through a lot of changes as they're developing through puberty, and T cells might recognize things that weren't there before but are beginning to be expressed. So people are proceeding to go younger and younger, but at a very, very slow rate.
CJ: There are now trials in kids with our CAR-T cells asking if, instead of being given after they've failed all kinds of chemotherapy and radiation, can these be given frontline? Can it be done safely, and spare kids the effects of chemotherapy and radiation?

Tell us about your first pediatric patient.
CJ: She had very advanced refractory leukemia, and when we treated her in 2012 she had a very violent reaction. Her temperature went to 106 degrees for three days. This was – we learned later – due to the cancer being killed by her CAR-T cells. Usually when a leukemia patient gets a fever, it's due to infection. She was on life support, with a ventilator and multiorgan failure. We found she had very high levels of a cytokine, interleukin 6, and we were able to treat that with a drug for arthritis that had a virtually miraculous effect. She's now eight years cancer-free. This was, I think, the first example where a therapy, in this case CAR-T cells, was first approved for a pediatric indication. It was approved in 2017 for ages 3 to 25.
LG: If you were to ask what is the most alarming thing in cancer nowadays, I would say it's the incidence of cancer in young people. I've seen so many patients now who are otherwise healthy who are developing metastatic colorectal cancer in their 30s or 40s. [One recent study] showed that the incidence of cancer in adolescents and young adults has increased by nearly 30% since 1973. That to me is a very scary development.

Is there anything you would particularly like people diagnosed with cancer today to know?
JA: I'd say cancer is no longer a death sentence. With melanoma, it was almost a certain death sentence a decade ago. Now the majority of those patients are going to make it five to 10 years. If we're able to extend life by a year, two years, there may be another finding that would add to that. We've got a long way to go, but we can cure a significant number of people with certain kinds of cancer now. And by cure, I mean they'll be alive 10 years after their therapy stops. ●

> '**I'd say cancer is no longer a death sentence.**'

AMERICAN OSTEOPATHIC FOUNDATION

WWW.AOF.ORG

CONGRATULATIONS!

TO OUR NATION'S TOP RISING OSTEOPATHIC PHYSICIANS AS NOMINATED BY STATE PEERS

KENDRA M. GRAY, DO
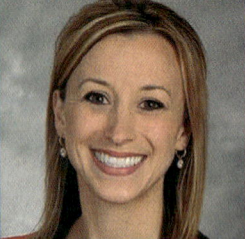
OBSTETRICS AND GYNECOLOGY
Arizona

MAJ. REGAN A. STIEGMANN, DO
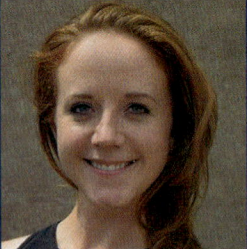
FAMILY MEDICINE
Colorado

SEAN MCCANN, DO
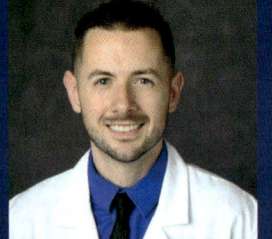
FAMILY MEDICINE
Florida

MEHRDOD EHTESHAMI, DO
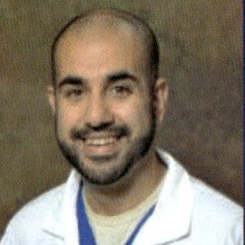
EMERGENCY MEDICINE
Georgia

MITCHELL W. SMITH, DO
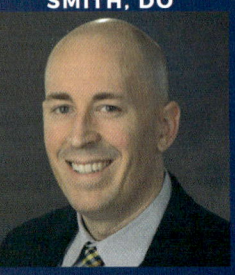
ALLERGY AND IMMUNOLOGY
Indiana

RICHARD CHARLES CALDERONE, DO
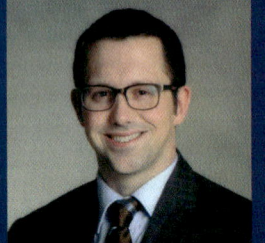
INTERNAL MEDICINE
Mississippi

CHELSEA A. NICKOLSON, DO
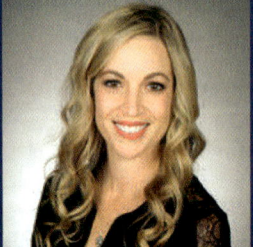
INTERNAL MEDICINE
Ohio

SARAH JULANE WOLFF, DO
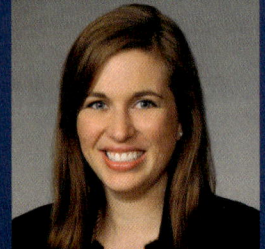
FAMILY MEDICINE
Oregon

TRAVIS JOHN GROTH, DO
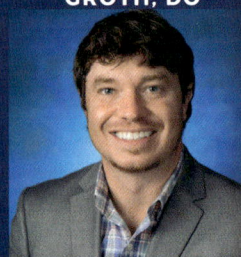
FAMILY MEDICINE
Tennessee

The American Osteopathic Foundation is pleased to celebrate the

2021 STATE EMERGING LEADERS

who are honored as new physicians in practice within the Osteopathic profession.

These exceptional individuals provide service to others through Osteopathic Medicine's tenants and principles, advocacy efforts, community service, and philanthropic spirit.

We salute their ongoing commitment to enhancing patient-centered care.

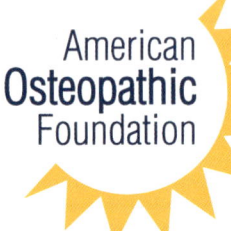

CHAPTER 2

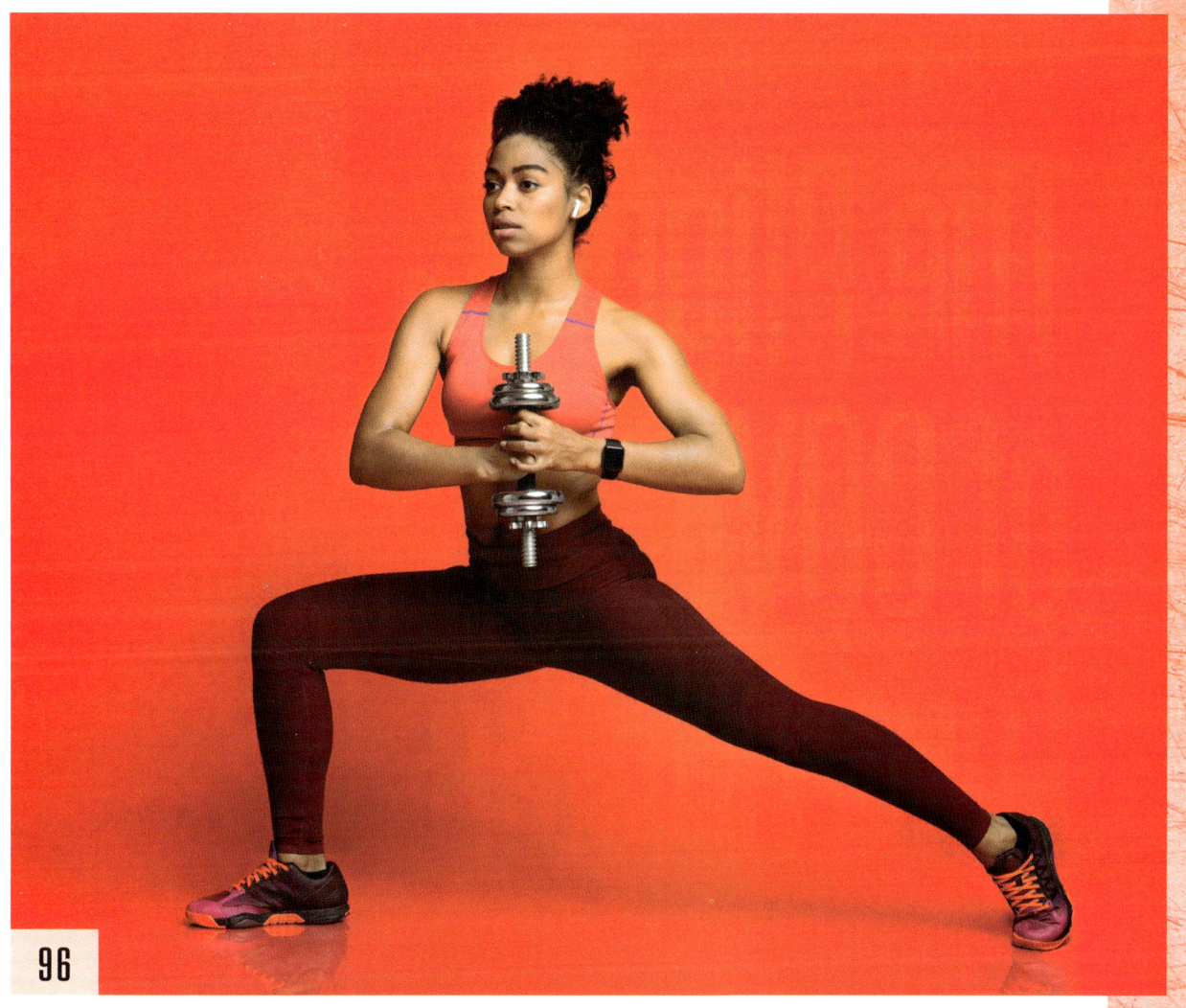

96

Patient Power

The Plight of the COVID Long Haulers **66**	Strength Training With a Purpose **96**
How to Boost Your Immune System **89**	Best Diets: Which Ones Work? **100**
Making Cancer Care Equitable **92**	Eating the Mediterranean Way **103**

PATIENT POWER

The Plight of COVID Long Haulers

There's much still to learn about the serious, lasting symptoms

by **Beth Howard**

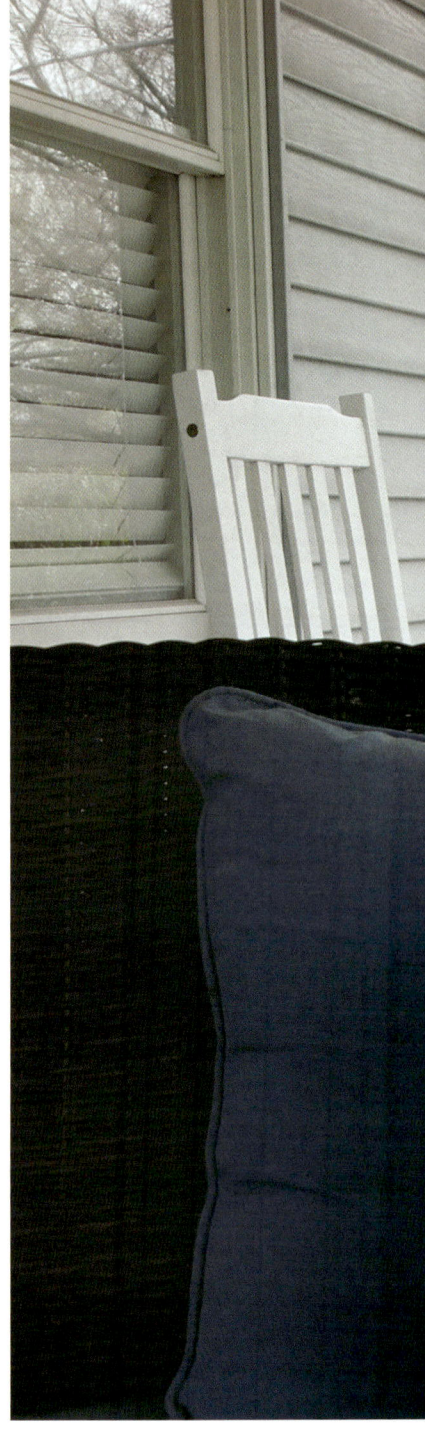

MARIA MANFREDINI, 36, was supposed to get married in Italy in June of 2020. But when the pandemic hit, the Chicago project manager and her fiancé scuttled their dream wedding and flew to Arizona for the weekend. They would come to regret that decision. Sometime during the trip – on the plane, eating at a restaurant or somewhere else – Manfredini contracted COVID-19.

After about a week of relatively mild symptoms, she seemed to get better. Then, a week or two later, she fell sick all over again. Months later, she was still feeling ill, with "chills, flu aches, pain in my ears, pain in my chest," says Manfredini, who was also bothered by burning sensations throughout her body. "Imagine having the worst flu of your life and feeling like that every day." By this past summer, she was finally hopeful about making a full recovery.

Experiences like this have become alarmingly common. As the total number of COVID cases has surged into the tens of millions, doctors and hospitals have been seeing more people with complaints that persist weeks and even months after they've recovered from the initial illness. These "long haulers" often drift from doctor to doctor with a perplexing array of symptoms that clinicians are clueless about how to treat.

Lack of experience. "It's like discovering a new disease, except you have a ton of people who need treatment now," says Dr. Zijian Chen, director of the Center for Post-COVID Care at Mount Sinai Health System in New York, one of a handful of clinics popping up around the country to address the long-term fallout. "Our experience is so limited. We're struggling to catch

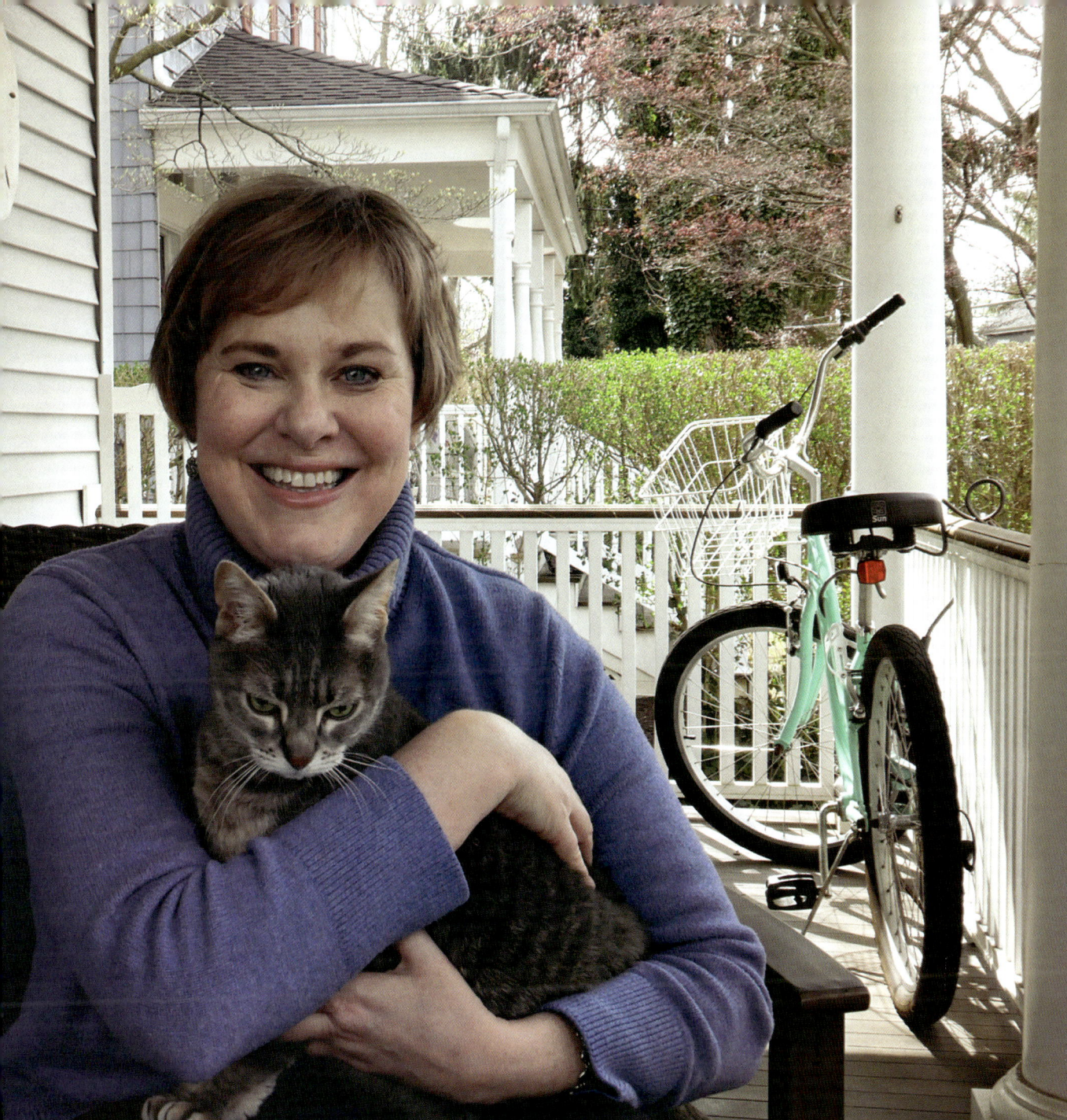

"NOW I WILL ALWAYS HAVE HEART FAILURE," SAYS SURVIVOR JEN SINGER, AT HOME IN NEW JERSEY (WITH HER CAT, BENNY).

up, to see what's working, what's not working, and looking for things that might help."

Research suggests that 10 to 35 percent of COVID patients have one or more symptoms of long COVID, the syndrome's official name. In one Chinese study, researchers found that 63 percent of more than 1,700 patients hospitalized for the disease still had fatigue or muscle weakness six months after the initial infection. Sleep problems and anxiety or depression each plagued about a quarter of the patients. Other studies have found that people struggle from post-traumatic stress disorder, stabbing chest pains, lung scarring, rashes and neurological symptoms like confusion, cognitive impairment and brain fog. In April, researchers at Washington University School of Medicine in St. Louis published a study of the impacts on more than 87,000 COVID survivors using Veterans Health Administration data. They confirmed not only the vast array of complications still affecting people six months out but also a significantly heightened risk of death in that six-month period.

"Just about every system in the body can be affected, anything from the skin to the nervous system, the kidneys and the liver,"

PATIENT POWER

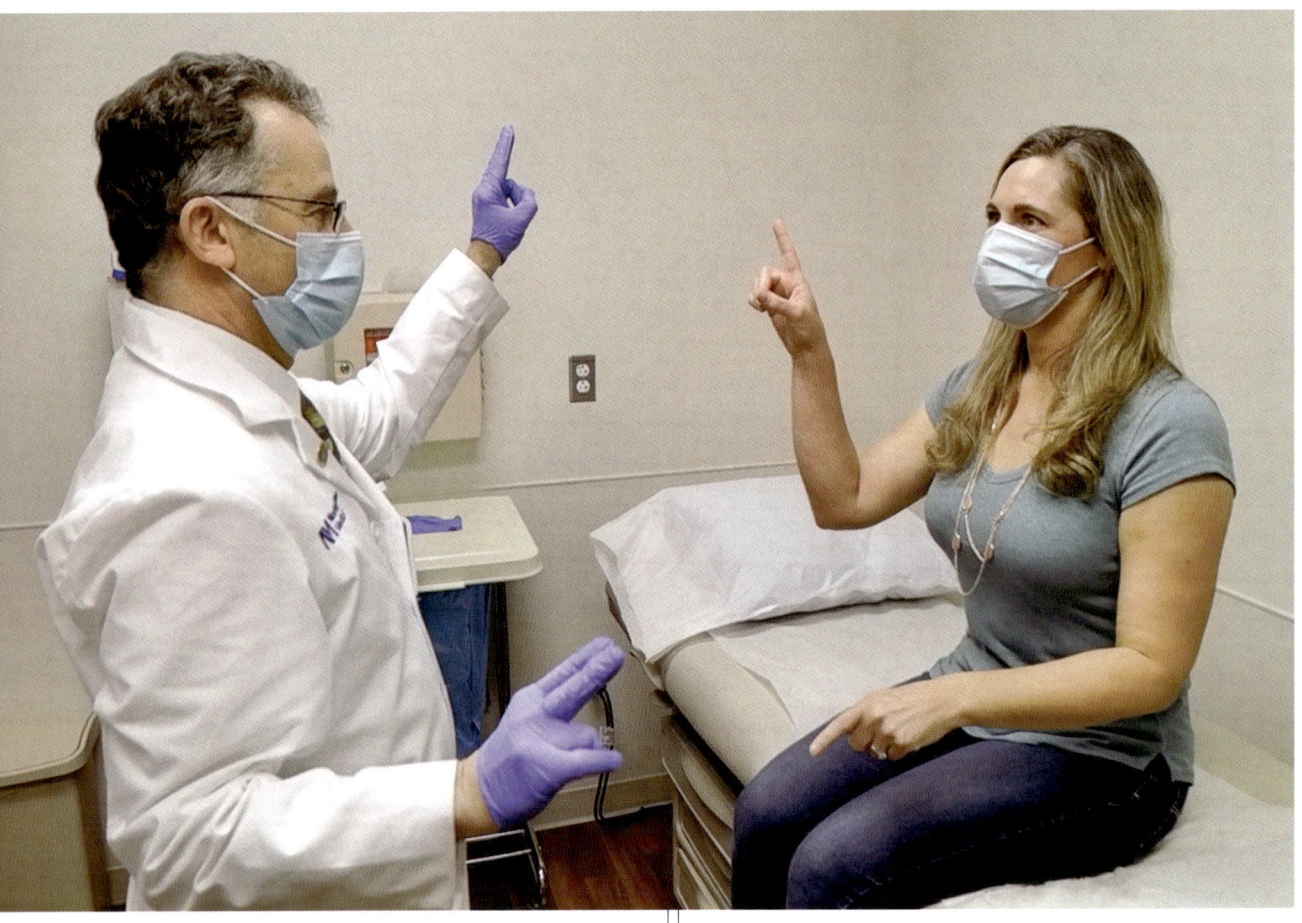

DR. IGOR KORALNIK GIVES PATIENT BETH MOORE A NEUROLOGICAL EXAM AT NORTHWESTERN'S COMPREHENSIVE COVID-19 CENTER.

says Dr. Neil Schachter, a professor of pulmonary and community medicine specializing in respiratory problems at Mount Sinai Hospital. "All of them have been implicated in the disease, either directly as a result of the infection itself or due to some of the consequences of the body's reaction to the virus."

Ground zero for COVID infection, the lungs, may take the hardest hit. In the worst case, "this virus can chew away the lungs," says Schachter. "When we look at some of the X-rays, we see pictures of the lung looking like Swiss cheese, big black holes in the middle of healthy tissue." It can also cause scarring, called fibrosis, that makes it harder to breathe. These patients may continue to feel weak and short of breath – unable to resume normal activities without getting winded – long after COVID struck. In a small study of survivors in China, 70 percent had abnormal lung CT scans and 25 percent had reduced lung function three months after discharge.

When COVID infects heart muscle, it can cause myocarditis, or inflammation in the heart wall, says Dr. Dara Lee Lewis, a cardiologist and associate physician at Brigham and Women's Hospital and an instructor in medicine at Harvard Medical School. Although some people are asymptomatic, severe cases can weaken the heart, leading to chest pain, abnormal heartbeat, shortness of breath and heart failure.

That was the outcome of Jen Singer's bout with COVID-19. The 54-year-old freelance writer in Red Bank, New Jersey, believes she was infected with the virus on a train trip on Valentine's Day 2020, before Americans were advised to take precautions. As the country went under lockdown, Singer, a non-Hodgkin's lymphoma survivor, found she could no longer bound up the stairs without stopping to catch her breath. When she developed sharp pain under her ribs, she sought help. An electrocardiogram revealed that her heart's electrical system was malfunctioning. She was later diagnosed with cardiac sarcoidosis and had to have a pacemaker inserted. "Not even two months before all this happened, I took my kids hiking in Sedona," she says. "Despite having had cancer, I was in good shape. Now I will always have heart failure."

Complex complications. Blood clot complications, some leading to heart attacks, strokes and other cardiac problems, have been reported, as have potentially dangerous heart rhythm abnormalities. Lewis suspects that many COVID survi-

EXPERTS WORK TOGETHER TO TREAT PATIENTS WITH MIS-C

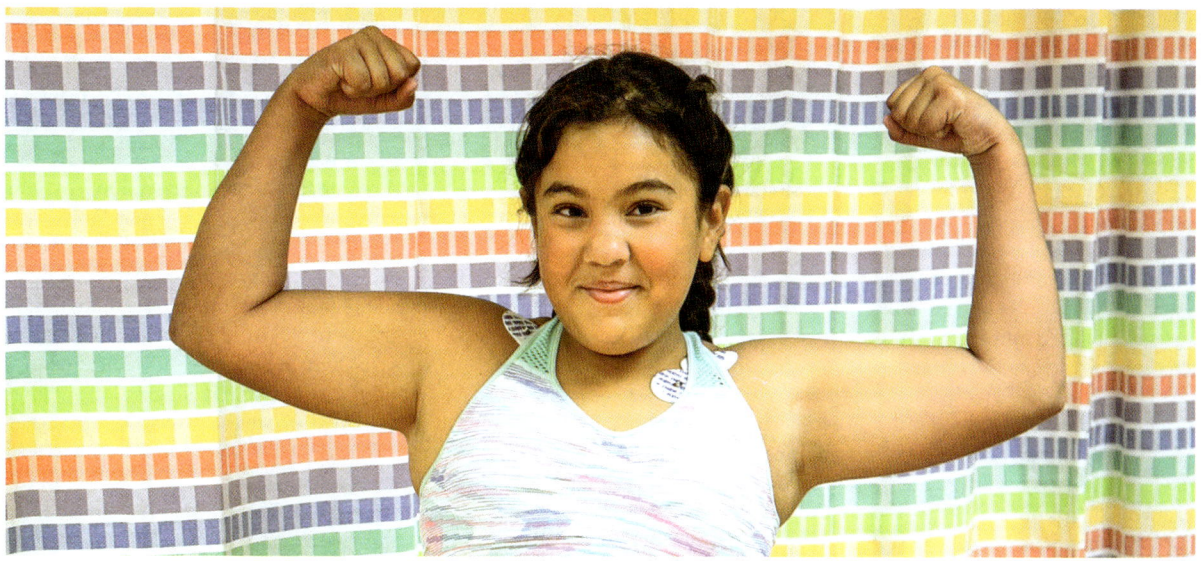

When Xitlali arrived at Children's Hospital Los Angeles during the height of the pandemic, she had a high fever, red eyes and a swollen tongue. She'd been vomiting and hallucinating. Doctors diagnosed the 8 year old with multisystem inflammatory syndrome in children (MIS-C), a condition striking kids who previously contracted COVID-19.

In the Pediatric Intensive Care Unit, specialists from cardiology, infectious diseases, endocrinology, hematology and other disciplines around the hospital used their expertise to treat Xitlali's heart, lungs and other impacted organs.

The team's collaborative efforts paid off. On her 11th day at the hospital, Xitlali went home—her heart function restored. Today, experts at Children's Hospital Los Angeles are closely monitoring her and other patients diagnosed with MIS-C, through regular cardiology appointments, evaluations in our Exercise Stress Lab and more.

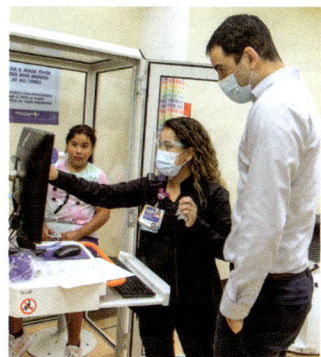

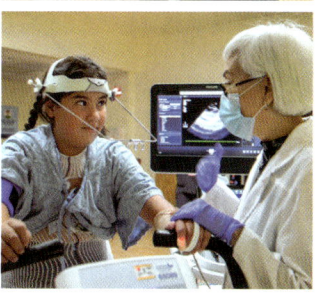

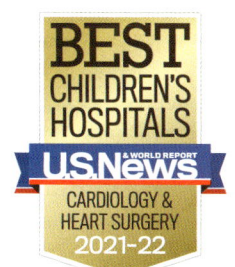

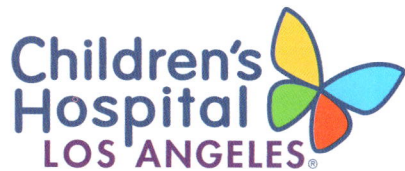

Learn more at CHLA.org/heart

PATIENT POWER

vors are subsequently falling ill with a condition called postural orthostatic tachycardia syndrome, or POTS, that typically follows some type of viral illness and is characterized by a rapid heart rate and lightheadedness (especially when standing up), fatigue and brain fog. "It has a constellation of symptoms that lie on a spectrum from really mild to really debilitating. Some people do get over it, but it's a chronic syndrome that people may have for many years," she says.

The most vexing symptoms may be neurologic. Patients commonly recount dizziness, headache and the loss of taste and smell when first sick, and some experience strokes. But as weeks and months pass, symptoms like confusion, difficulty concentrating, memory loss, seizures and encephalitis – brain inflammation – may crop up, even among asymptomatic patients or those with mild cases. According to a recent study from Northwestern Medicine in Chicago, 85% of patients seeking help for long COVID had four or more neurologic symptoms that affected their quality of life and, in some cases, their cognitive abilities.

When Melissa Bradley, 41, tested positive in July 2020, she had few signs of illness. But Bradley, who lives in a suburb of Atlanta, has since developed crushing fatigue and a constellation

> ❛**I am not who I was prior to having COVID.**❜

of neurologic ills, including headaches, nerve pain, visual changes, agitation and brain fog. "I'll forget words mid-sentence," she says. "I forget the names of people that I work with on a regular basis." Although she continues to work full time in marketing, "my life has completely changed," Bradley says. "I am not who I was prior to having COVID."

Bradley's story is a familiar one to neurologist Dr. Igor Koralnik, director of the Northwestern Medicine Comprehensive COVID-19 Center, which has evaluated and treated long COVID patients from over 30 states. "We think that the long-haul syndrome, or long COVID, is most likely not a direct infection of the brain by the virus," he says, "but a post-infectious autoimmune problem, where the virus has confused the immune system to think that the brain is foreign or abnormal and needs to be attacked."

Pediatric puzzle. Some pediatric survivors suffer from multisystem inflammatory syndrome in children, or MIS-C, a rare condition that occurs several weeks after the acute infection, says Dr. Jacqueline Szmuszkovicz, a pediatric cardiologist with the Heart Institute at Children's Hospital Los Angeles. MIS-C causes different body parts – the heart, lungs, kidneys, brain, gastrointestinal tract – to become inflamed, resulting in gut pain, fever, headache, vomiting, diarrhea, rashes and fatigue. "The symptoms are due to the effects of overwhelming inflammation throughout the body, so we see many organ systems involved," she says. Complications may include decreased heart function, leading to low blood pressure, as well as aneurysms and heart rhythm abnormalities. While most children recover from MIS-C, she says, the long-term outcomes are unknown.

Long haulers have been slow to get relief. Like patients with misunderstood ailments like chronic fatigue syndrome, they struggle to have their symptoms recognized. "Usually, doctors cut me off after three or four symptoms and start trying to fix one thing" rather than look at the symptoms as a whole, says Bradley. At one doctor visit, her rapid heart rate and lightheadedness were blamed on dehydration and anxiety. In June, the Centers for Disease Control and Prevention offered providers guidance on managing long haulers to help alleviate the problem.

The undiagnosed. Circumstances tend to be worse for people who never received an official COVID diagnosis. They "usually get bounced around from one place to the next because people tell them that they don't have COVID," says Koralnik. "And therefore, it's all in their head. That adds insult to injury and stigma for those patients."

But things are beginning to look up, particularly at the post-COVID clinics at Northwestern and Mount Sinai and a growing number of sites, including Penn Medicine's Post-COVID Recovery Clinic in Philadelphia, the UCSF OPTIMAL Clinic in San Francisco and WakeMed Rehab's COVID-19 Recovery Program in Raleigh, North Carolina. (Centers can be searched by state at survivorcorps.com/pccc.) These clinics take a multidisciplinary approach, with pulmonologists, cardiologists, neurologists, physical and respiratory therapists, geriatricians, social workers, pharmacists and mental health professionals often weighing in. In February, the National Institutes of Health launched an initiative to study long COVID, and Congress provided $1.15 billion for the effort. Patients have also found solace and solutions on Facebook and in other survivor support groups.

And there's evidence that vaccines for COVID-19 may relieve some symptoms. In a Survivor Corps survey of members last spring, some 40% of long haulers responding said their symptoms had improved after being vaccinated. The reality is that "recovery involves lots of ups and downs and relapses," Koralnik says. But even long haulers "do tend to get better." •

Do You Or a Loved One Need Cardiac Care?

- **Heart Attack** (Stent, Surgery,) **and Chest Pain**
- **Heart Rhythm Disorder** (AFib Ablation, Implantable Cardioverter-Defibrillator, Pacemaker)
- **Heart Valve Disease** (TAVR, Surgery)

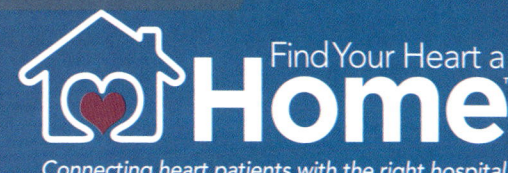

Find Your Heart a **Home**™
Connecting heart patients with the right hospital

For these and other treatments, use the online tool to...

 **SEARCH** over **700 hospitals**

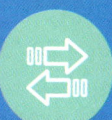 **COMPARE** their **performance**

 **SELECT** the **right hospital**

DON'T DELAY YOUR CARE! Remember that hospitals have safety measures to protect patients from virus infection.

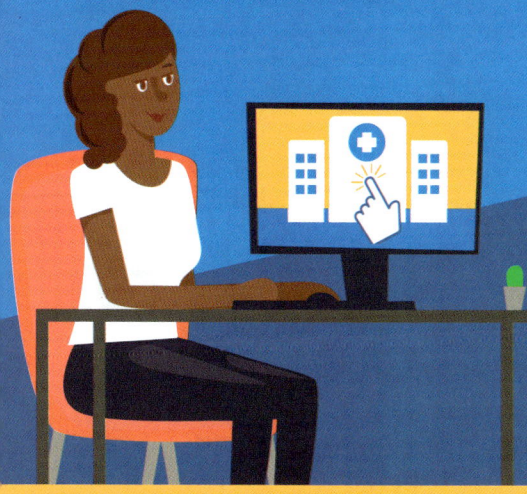

Powered by ACC's NCDR® and CardioSmart®

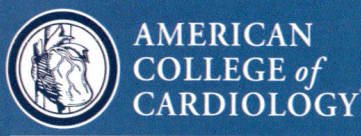

AMERICAN COLLEGE of CARDIOLOGY®
Advancing Heart Care Worldwide

Get Started at *FindYourHeartaHome.org*

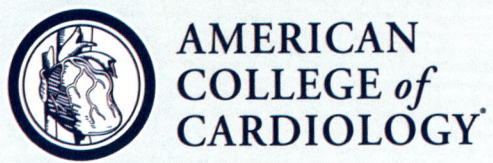

Advancing Heart Care Worldwide

THE HEART OF QUALITY PATIENT CARE

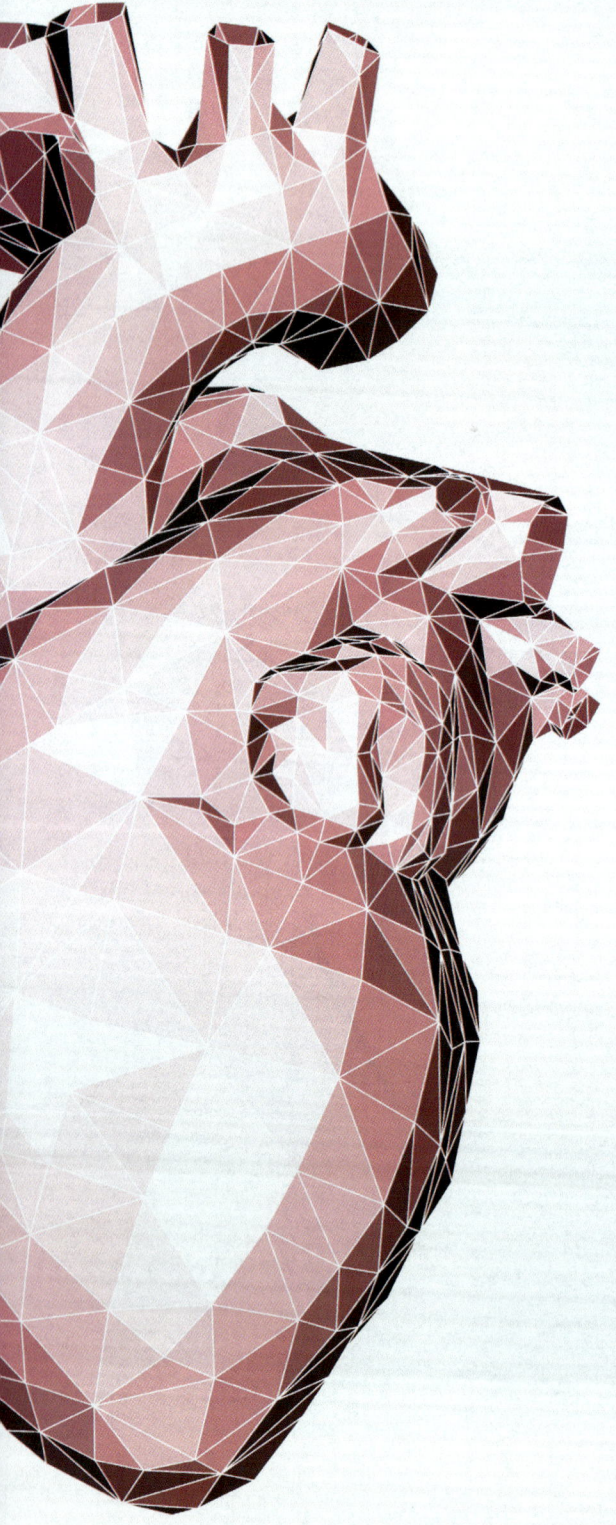

As the global professional organization for the entire cardiovascular care team, the American College of Cardiology (ACC) is committed to supporting patients, caregivers, and health care professionals by ensuring the highest quality care is delivered to every patient, every time.

ACC Accreditation Services™
ACC Accreditation Services links performance improvement to patient outcomes and promotes consistent processes across the care continuum. Working with hospitals and health systems, ACC Accreditation Services partners to build communities of excellence by advancing the highest standards of quality patient care.

NCDR® (National Cardiovascular Data Registry)
The NCDR is ACC's suite of data registries helping hospitals and health systems measure and improve the quality of cardiovascular care they provide. The NCDR utilizes real-world evidence to improve patient outcomes and achieve quality heart care.

MedAxiom, an ACC Company
MedAxiom is the premier source for cardiovascular organizational performance solutions. MedAxiom unites the cardiovascular community via cutting-edge education, networking opportunities and best practices to transform cardiovascular care, together.

FOR CARDIOVASCULAR PROFESSIONALS,
please visit *CVQuality.ACC.org* to learn more about ACC's Quality Improvement for Institutions program. To learn more about cardiovascular organizational peformance solutions, visit *MedAxiom.com*.

FOR PATIENTS AND CAREGIVERS,
please visit *CardioSmart.org* to learn more about ACC's clinician-directed heart health education and resources.

The following pages list more than 2,000 hospitals, centers and health systems that rely on ACC's NCDR and Accreditation Services. Patients and caregivers can trust hospitals and centers that participate in the NCDR, receive the ACC's Accreditation seal of approval, and are recognized with the Chest Pain – MI Registry™ Performance Achievement Award and the HeartCARE Center™ Award for delivering the best cardiovascular patient care.

ACC Accreditation Services

AF Atrial Fibrillation Accreditation
Incorporates evidence-based guidelines and clinical best practices to treat patients with atrial fibrillation.

CL Cardiac Cath Lab Accreditation
Merges the latest evidence-based science and process improvement methodologies, while addressing pre-procedure, peri-procedure and post-procedure care for patients undergoing treatment in the Cath Lab.

CP Chest Pain Center Accreditation
Integrates triage treatment protocols, risk stratification, and best practices for the emergency care of acute coronary syndrome patients.

EP Electrophysiology Accreditation
Links the latest science, process improvement methodologies and patient outcomes across the care continuum for patients undergoing treatment in the EP Lab.

HF Heart Failure Accreditation
Leverages guideline-directed medical therapies and best practices to ensure greater operational efficiency and a more consistent approach to treatment.

TV Transcatheter Valve Certification
Utilizes evidence-based science, real-world patient outcomes and expert recommendations to standardize and improve care for patients requiring transcatheter valve therapies.

NCDR

A AFib Ablation Registry™
(Catheter-based atrial fibrillation ablation procedures) Assesses the prevalence, demographics, acute management and outcomes of patients undergoing atrial fibrillation (AFib) catheter ablation procedures.

C CathPCI Registry®
(Diagnostic cardiac catheterization and percutaneous coronary intervention) Measures adherence to the ACC/AHA clinical practice guideline recommendations, procedure performance standards and appropriate use criteria for coronary revascularization.

CP Chest Pain - MI Registry™
(Acute myocardial infarction treatment) Leverages national evidence-based standards for understanding and improving the quality, safety and outcomes of care provided for heart attack patients.

E EP Device Implant Registry™
(Implantable cardioverter defibrillator and pacemaker procedures) Provides a national standard for understanding patient characteristics, treatments, outcomes, device safety and the overall quality of care for ICD/CRT-D and select novel pacemaker procedures.

IM IMPACT Registry®
(Pediatric and adult congenital treatment procedures) Assesses the prevalence, demographics, management and outcomes of pediatric and adult congenital heart disease patients who undergo diagnostic catheterizations and catheter-based interventions.

L LAAO Registry™
(Left atrial appendage occlusion procedures) Captures data on left atrial appendage occlusion (LAAO) procedures to assess real-world procedural outcomes, short and long-term safety, and comparative effectiveness.

T STS/ACC TVT Registry™
(Transcatheter valve therapy procedures) Monitors real-world outcomes on transcatheter valve therapies leading to improved patient outcomes, enhanced assessment of treatment options and results, and more informed decision making.

Honors

Chest Pain - MI Registry™ Performance Achievement Award
Recognizes hospitals participating in Chest Pain – MI Registry that have demonstrated sustained, top level performance in quality of care and adherence to guideline recommendations.

▲ Platinum
▲ Gold
▲ Silver
♦ **HeartCARE Center™**
Recognizes hospitals that have demonstrated a commitment to world-class cardiovascular care through comprehensive process improvement, disease and procedure-specific accreditation, professional excellence and community engagement.

Hospitals are listed by state and then by level of engagement with the ACC's quality and process improvement programs.

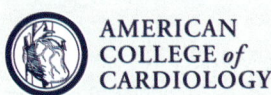

THE HEART OF QUALITY PATIENT CARE

ALABAMA

Hospital	Designations
Grandview Medical Center	C CP E L T CL CP
University of Alabama Hospital	A C CP E L T ▲
Huntsville Hospital	C CP E L T
Shelby Baptist Medical Center	C L T CL TV
Flowers Hospital	C CP CP HF
Riverview Regional Medical Center	C E CL CP
Thomas Hospital	A C CP E
Andalusia Health	E CP HF
Brookwood Medical Center	C L T
Crestwood Medical Center	C CP CP
Health Care Authority for Baptist Health	C E L
Mobile Infirmary Medical Center	C L T
North Alabama Medical Center	C E CP
Princeton Baptist Medical Center	C L T
Providence Hospital	C L T
Southeast Health	L T CP
Springhill Medical Center	C L T
St. Vincent's East	C L T
St. Vincent's Hospital	C L T
DCH Regional Medical Center	C E
DeKalb Regional Medical Center	C CP
East Alabama Medical Center	C T
Gadsden Regional Medical Center	C CP
Jackson Hospital and Clinic	C L
Northeast Alabama Regional Medical Center	C E
South Baldwin Regional Medical Center	C CP
Vaughan Regional Medical Center	C CP
Baptist Medical Center South	CL
Cullman Regional Medical Center	C
Marshall Medical Center	C
Russell Medical Center	E
Shoals Hospital	CP
The Children's Hospital of Alabama	IM
University of South Alabama Cardiology Department	C
Walker Baptist Medical Center	C

ALASKA

Hospital	Designations
Alaska Regional Hospital	C L T AF CP HF
Providence Alaska Medical Center	A C CP T ▲
Fairbanks Memorial Hospital	C E
Mat-Su Regional Medical Center	C CP
Alaska Cardiovascular Surgery Center, LLC	E
Alaska Native Medical Center	C
Central Peninsula Hospital	C

ARIZONA

Hospital	Designations
Abrazo Arizona Heart Hospital	C CP L T AF CL CP HF ▲
Chandler Regional Medical Center	A C CP E L T CP
St. Joseph's Hospital and Medical Center	A C CP L T CP
Abrazo Arrowhead Campus	C CP L T CP
Mercy Gilbert Medical Center	A C CP E CP
Tucson Medical Center	C CP L T CP
Carondelet St. Mary's Hospital	C L T CP
Havasu Regional Medical Center	C E CL CP
Northwest Medical Center	C L T CP
Abrazo Central Campus	C CP CP
Abrazo West Campus	C CP CP
HonorHealth	C L T
Mayo Clinic Arizona	C L T
Mountain Vista Medical Center	C CP CP
Valley View Medical Center	C E CP
Western Arizona Regional Medical Center	C CP CP
Yavapai Regional Medical Center	C L T
Yuma Regional Medical Center	C E T
Abrazo Scottsdale Campus	C CP
Banner - University Medical Center Tucson	L T
Banner Boswell Medical Center	L T
Banner Desert Medical Center	L T
Banner Heart Hospital	L T
Banner Thunderbird Medical Center	L T
Banner University Medical Center - Phoenix	L T
Canyon Vista Medical Center	C E
Carondelet St. Joseph's Hospital	C CP
Flagstaff Medical Center	C L
HonorHealth - Deer Valley Medical Center	C T
Kingman Regional Medical Center	C E
Oro Valley Hospital	C CP
Summit Healthcare Regional Medical Center	C E
HonorHealth John C. Lincoln Medical Center	L
Phoenix Children's Hospital	IM
Tempe St. Luke's Hospital	C
Verde Valley Medical Center	C

ARKANSAS

Hospital	Designations
CHI St. Vincent Infirmary	A C CP L T CP ▲
Mercy Hospital Northwest Arkansas	C CP L T CP ▲
Arkansas Heart Hospital	C CP E L T
Baptist Health - Fort Smith	C CP CP ▲
Baptist Health Medical Center - Little Rock	C CP L T
Northwest Medical Center - Bentonville	C CP L CP
Saline Memorial Hospital	C CP E CP
St. Bernards Medical Center	CP L T ▲
St. Mary's Regional Medical Center	C CP E CP
Washington Regional Medical Center	C CP L T
Baxter Regional Medical Center	C CP E
CHI St. Vincent Hospital Hot Springs	C CP ▲
Mercy Hospital Fort Smith	C CP CP
National Park Medical Center	C CP E
NEA Baptist Memorial Hospital	C CP
Northwest Medical Center - Springdale	C CP CP
Unity Health White County Medical Center	C CP E
Baptist Health Medical Center - North Little Rock	C CP
Baptist Memorial Hospital - Jonesboro	CL CP
CHI St Vincent North	C CP
Conway Regional Medical Center	C CP
Jefferson Regional Medical Center	CP E
Medical Center of South Arkansas	C CP
Arkansas Children's Hospital	IM
Baptist Health Medical Center - Conway	CP
Siloam Springs Regional Hospital	CP
University of Arkansas Medical Sciences	CP
White River Medical Center	CP

CALIFORNIA

Hospital	Designations
Bakersfield Heart Hospital	C CP L T CP HF ▲
California Pacific Medical Center	A C CP E L T ▲
El Camino Health	A C CP L T TV ▲
French Hospital Medical Center	A C CP L T TV ▲
UCLA Health for Ronald Reagan UCLA Medical Center	C CP E IM L T EP
Adventist Health Bakersfield	C CP E CP HF ▲
Adventist Health White Memorial	C E L T AF CP
Antelope Valley Hospital	C CP L T CP ▲
Dignity Health St. Joseph's Medical Center	C CP E L T ▲
Doctors Medical Center of Modesto	C CP L T CP ▲
Loma Linda University Medical Center	C E IM L T CP
NorthBay Medical Center	C CP E T CP ▲
Palomar Center	C CP E T TV
Pomona Valley Hospital Medical Center	C CP L T CP ▲
Temecula Valley Hospital	C CP E T CP ▲
University Of California Davis Medical Center	C CP E IM L T
Adventist Health and Rideout Hospital	C CP E T ▲
Adventist Health Glendale	C E L T CP
Alta Bates Summit Medical Center	A C E L T
Cedars - Sinai Health Systems	C E IM L T
Eisenhower Medical Center	C E L T CP
Hoag Memorial Hospital Presbyterian	A C E L T
Loma Linda University Medical Center - Murrieta	C E L T CP
Marian Regional Medical Center	A C E L EP
Memorial Medical Center Modesto	C CP E T ▲
MemorialCare Long Beach Medical Center	C E IM L T
Mercy General Hospital - Sacramento	A C E L T
Mills - Peninsula Health Services	A C E L T
Riverside Community Hospital	C CP L T CP
Salinas Valley Memorial Healthcare System	CP E L T
St. Bernardine Medical Center	A C L T CP
Sutter Medical Center - Sacramento	C E IM L T
Sutter Santa Rosa Regional Hospital	A C E L T
UC Irvine Health	C CP E L T

Registries
- **A** AFib Ablation Registry™
- **C** CathPCI Registry®
- **CP** Chest Pain - MI Registry®
- **E** EP Device Implant Registry®
- **IM** IMPACT Registry®
- **L** LAAO Registry™
- **T** STS/ACC TVT Registry®

Accreditations
- **AF** Atrial Fibrillation
- **CL** Cardiac Cath Lab
- **CP** Chest Pain Center
- **EP** Electrophysiology
- **HF** Heart Failure
- **TV** Transcatheter Valve

Awards
- ▲ Chest Pain - MI Registry™ Award Platinum
- ▲ Chest Pain - MI Registry™ Award Gold
- ▲ Chest Pain - MI Registry™ Award Silver
- ◆ HeartCARE Center

Participants in ACC's NCDR Registries, Accreditation Services and Awardees

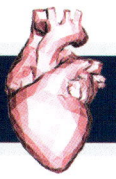

Facility	Codes
University of California San Francisco Medical Center	C E IM L T
Adventist Health St. Helena	C E L T
Community Memorial Hospital	C E L T
Desert Regional Medical Center	C CP L CP
Desert Valley Hospital	C CP E CP
Fresno Heart and Surgical Hospital	C E L T
Keck Medical Center of USC	C E L T
Los Robles Hospital & Medical Center	A C L T
MemorialCare Saddleback Medical Center	C E L T
Saint Agnes Medical Center	C E L T
St. Johns Regional Medical Center	A C L T
Torrance Memorial Medical Center	A C L T
Tri-City Medical Center	C CP L ▲
UC San Diego Health System Sulpizio CV Center	C E L T
Arrowhead Regional Medical Center	C CP E
Bakersfield Memorial Hospital	C L T
Community Hospital of the Monterey Peninsula	C L T
Emanate Health Medical Center	C E T
Emanuel Medical Center	C CP CP
Enloe Medical Center	C E T
Fresno Community Hospital and Medical Center	C E T
Garfield Medical Center	C CP T
Good Samaritan Hospital	C L T
Huntington Hospital	C L T
John Muir Medical Center - Concord Campus	C L T
Kaiser Foundation Hospital Fontana	C E T
Kaiser Permanente Medical Center	C L T
Kaiser Permanente Medical Center	C L T
Kaweah Delta Hospital District	C E T
Marin Health Medical Center	C L T
Memorialcare Orange Coast Medical Center	C E T
Northridge Hospital Medical Center	C L T
PIH Health Good Samaritan Hospital	C L T
Providence Saint John's Health Center	C L T
Providence St. Joseph Hospital	C L T
Santa Barbara Cottage Hospital	C L T
Santa Rosa Memorial Hospital	C L T
Scripps Memorial Hospital - La Jolla	C L T
Scripps Mercy Hospital - San Diego	C L T
Sharp Chula Vista Medical Center	C L T
Sharp Grossmont Hospital	C L T
Sharp Memorial Hospital	C L T
Shasta Regional Medical Center	C T CP
Stanford Healthcare	C E T
Sutter Delta Medical Center	C E CL
Washington Hospital	C E T
Adventist Health and Rideout	CL CP
Adventist Health - Simi Valley	C E
Children's Hospital of Los Angeles	E IM
Community Medical Center - Clovis	C E
Corona Regional Medical Center	C E
Dameron Hospital Association	C E
Dignity Health Dominican Hospital	C T
El Centro Regional Medical Center	E CP
Henry Mayo Newhall Hospital	C T
JFK Memorial Hospital	C CP
Kaiser Foundation Hospital	C E
Kaiser Permanente Irvine Medical Center	C E
Kaiser Permanente Oakland Medical Center	C IM
Lakewood Regional Medical Center	C T
Lucile S Packard Children's Hospital at Stanford University	E IM
Palmdale Regional Medical Center	C E
PIH Health Hospital - Whittier	C T
Providence Little Company of Mary Medical Center	C T
Providence Mission Hospital	C T
Providence St. Jude Medical Center	C T
Providence St. Mary Medical Center	C CP
Riverside University Health System Medical Center	C E
San Antonio Regional Hospital	T CP
Sequoia Hospital	C T
Southern California Hospital At Culver City	C E
Stanford Health Care ValleyCare	C E
Sutter Roseville Medical Center	C E
University of California Santa Monica	C E
Valley Presbyterian Hospital	C E
West Anaheim Medical Center	C CL
West Hills Hospital & Medical Center	C L
Adventist Health Simi Valley	CP
Adventist Medical Center - Hanford	E
Alameda Health System	C
Barstow Community Hospital	CP
California Hospital Medical Center	C
Children's Hospital of Orange County	IM
Chino Valley Medical Center	C
Dignity Health	C
Dignity Health Mercy Medical Center Redding	C
Fountain Valley Regional Hospital	C
Glendale Memorial Hospital and Health Center	C
Hollywood Presbyterian Hospital	C
John Muir Medical Center - Walnut Creek Campus	C
Kaiser Foundation - Roseville Medical Center	C
Kaiser Foundation Hospital South Sacramento	C
Kaiser Permanente Fremont Medical Center	C
Kaiser Permanente Medical Center	E
Kaiser Permanente Modesto Medical Center	C
Kaiser Permanente Orange County - Anaheim Medical Center	E
Kaiser Permanente Sacramento Medical Center	C
Kaiser Permanente San Rafael Medical Center	C
Kaiser Permanente Walnut Creek	C
Kaiser Permanente - Vallejo Medical Center	C
Kaiser Redwood City Medical Center	C
Los Alamitos Medical Center	C
Marshall Medical Center	E
Mercy Medical Center Merced	C
Methodist Hospital of South CA	C
Orange County Global Medical Center	C
Oroville Hospital	C
PIH Health Hospital - Downey	C
Pioneer Memorial Hospital	CP
Placentia Linda Hospital (TENET)	C
Providence Holy Cross Medical Center	C
Providence Saint Joseph Medical Center	C
Providence Tarzana Medical Center	C
Queen of the Valley Medical Center	C
Rady Children's Hospital of San Diego	IM
Rancho Spring Medical Center	E
Regional Medical Center - San Jose	C
Ridgecrest Regional Hospital	E
San Joaquin General Hospital	E
San Ramon Regional Medical Center	C
Santa Teresa Community Hospital	C
Sherman Oaks Hospital	C
Sierra View District Hospital	C
St. Joseph Hospital	C
St. Mary Medical Center	C
St. Mary's Medical Center	C
St. Rose Hospital	C
Sutter Amador Surgery Center	E
Sutter Medical Center Sacramento	TV
Sutter Solano Medical Center	E
UCSF Benioff Children's Hospitals, Oakland	IM
Valley Children's Hospital	IM

COLORADO

Facility	Codes
The Medical Center of Aurora	C CP L T AF CP HF TV ▲ ◆
UCHealth Memorial Hospital	C CP E L T AF CP TV ▲ ◆
Rose Medical Center	A C CP L AF CL CP ▲ ◆
Medical Center of the Rockies	A C CP E L T ▲
Porter Adventist Hospital	A C CP L AF CP HF
Saint Joseph Hospital	C CP L T CP TV
St. Anthony Hospital	A C CP L T CP ▲
St. Mary's Hospital & Medical Center	A C CP L T CP ▲
University of Colorado Hospital Authority	A C CP E L T ▲
Parkview Medical Center	C CP L T CP ▲
Lutheran Medical Center	A C CP CP ▲
North Colorado Medical Center	CP L T TV ▲
Penrose Hospital	C CP L T ▲
Valley View Hospital	A C CP E L
Boulder Community Health	C E L T
Good Samaritan Medical Center	C CP CP ▲
Littleton Adventist Hospital	C CP CP ▲
Parker Adventist Hospital	C CP CP ▲
Platte Valley Medical Center	C CP CP ▲
St. Anthony North Hospital	C CP CP ▲
Swedish Medical Center	C CP T ▲
Longmont United Hospital	C CP ▲
Mercy Regional Medical Center	C CP ▲
Presbyterian/St.Luke's Medical Center	C CP IM
Sky Ridge Medical Center	C CP ▲

Continues on next page

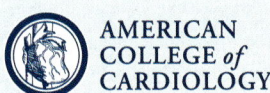

THE HEART OF QUALITY PATIENT CARE

Hospital	Registries/Awards
St. Francis Medical Center	C CP ▲
Avista Adventist Hospital	C CP
Castle Rock Adventist	C CP
Children's Hospital Colorado	E IM
Highlands Ranch Hospital	C CP
McKee Medical Center	CP ▲
Poudre Valley Hospital	CP ▲
Colorado Plains Medical Center	CP
Denver Health Medical Center	L
North Suburban Medical Center	C
UCHealth Longs Peak Hospital	CP
UCHealth Memorial Hospital North	CP

CONNECTICUT

Hospital	Registries/Awards
St. Vincent's Medical Center	C CP E L T ▲
Yale New Haven Hospital	A C IM L T TV
Hartford Hospital	A C E L T
St. Francis Hospital & Medical Center	A C E L T
Bridgeport Hospital	A C L T
Stamford Hospital Health Sciences Library	C E L T
Danbury Hospital	C E T
Trinity Health Of New England	A C E
Waterbury Hospital	C E T
Connecticut Children's Medical Center	E IM
Norwalk Hospital	C E
The Hospital of Central Connecticut	C E
Greenwich Hospital	C
Lawrence & Memorial Hospital	C
Midstate Medical Center	E
University of CT Health Center John Dempsey Hospital	C
William W. Backus Hospital	E

DELAWARE

Hospital	Registries/Awards
Christiana Care Health Services	C CP L T CL CP ▲ ◆
Bayhealth Hospital Kent Campus	C E L T
Beebe Healthcare	C E L T
St. Francis Hospital	A C CP E
Bayhealth Hospital Sussex Campus	C E
Bayhealth Medical Center	TV
Nanticoke Memorial Hospital	C
Nemours Children's Clinic Alfred I duPont Hospital	IM

DISTRICT OF COLUMBIA

Hospital	Registries/Awards
The George Washington University Hospital	A C CP E L T ▲
MedStar Washington Hospital Center	A C E L T
Children's National Medical Center	IM

Registries
- A AFib Ablation Registry™
- C CathPCI Registry™
- CP Chest Pain - MI Registry™
- EP EP Device Implant Registry™
- IM IMPACT Registry®
- L LAAO Registry™
- T STS/ACC TVT Registry™

Accreditations
- AF Atrial Fibrillation
- CL Cardiac Cath Lab
- CP Chest Pain Center
- EP Electrophysiology
- HF Heart Failure
- TV Transcatheter Valve

Awards
- ▲ Chest Pain - MI Registry™ Award Platinum
- ▲ Chest Pain - MI Registry™ Award Gold
- ▲ Chest Pain - MI Registry™ Award Silver
- ◆ HeartCARE Center

FLORIDA

Hospital	Registries/Awards
AdventHealth Ocala	C E L T CL CP HF TV ◆
AdventHealth Tampa	C CP E L T CP HF TV ◆
Bayfront Health St. Petersburg	C CP E L T CL HF ▲
Manatee Memorial Hospital	C CP E L T CP TV ▲
Sarasota Memorial Hospital	A C CP E L T CP TV
AdventHealth Orlando	A C E IM L T TV
UF Health Jacksonville	C CP E L T CP ▲
AdventHealth Waterman	A C CP E T CP
Mount Sinai Medical Center	C CP L T CP ▲
Osceola Regional Medical Center	A C CP L T CP
Physicians Regional Medical Center - Pine Ridge	A C CP L T CP
St. Joseph's & St. Joseph's Children's Hospitals	A C E IM L T
AdventHealth Celebration	A C CP E ▲
AdventHealth Daytona Beach	C E L T TV
Ascension St. Vincent's Riverside	A C E L T
Baptist Health System	A C E L T
Baptist Hospital of Miami	A C L T TV
Broward Health Medical Center	C E L T TV
Holy Cross Hospital	A C E L T
JFK Medical Center	A C L T CP
Lakeland Regional Health	C E L T
Lee Health - HealthPark Med Center	A C E L T
Memorial Hospital Jacksonville	A C L T CP
Morton Plant Hospital	A C E L T
Naples Community Hospital	C CP L T TV
North Florida Regional Medical Center	C L T CP TV
Tampa General Hospital	C L T AF CP
UF Health Shands Hospital	C E IM T CP
University of Miami Hospital and Clinics	A C E L T
West Florida Hospital	C CP AF CP
Winter Haven Hospital	A C E L T
AdventHealth North Pinellas	C CP E CP
AdventHealth Zephyrhills	C CP E CP
Ascension Sacred Heart Pensacola	C E L T
Aventura Hospital and Medical Center	A C L T
Bayfront Health Port Charlotte	C L T CP
Bayfront Health Seven Rivers	C CP CP HF
Boca Raton Regional Hospital	C E L T
Central Florida Regional Hospital	C CP L T
Cleveland Clinic Florida	C E L T
Cleveland Clinic Indian River Hospital	C CP E T
Fort Walton Beach Medical Center	C L T CP
Jackson Memorial Hospital	C E IM T
Jupiter Medical Center	C E L T
Largo Medical Center	A C L T
Leesburg Regional Medical Center	C CP T CP
Northside Hospital	A C L T
Orlando Health	C IM L T
South Miami Hospital	A C L T
Tallahassee Memorial HealthCare	C L T CP
Wellington Regional Medical Center	C CP CP ▲
AdventHealth	C CP E
AdventHealth Dade City	C E CP
AdventHealth Heart of Florida	C E CP
Baptist Hospital	C L T
Bayfront Health Brooksville	C CP CP
Bethesda Health	C L T
Blake Medical Center	C L T
Brandon Regional Medical Center	C L T
Citrus Memorial Hospital	C L T
Cleveland Clinic Martin Health	C E T
Delray Medical Center	C L T
Fawcett Memorial Hospital	C L T
Flagler Hospital	C L T
Florida Medical Center a Campus of North Shore	C L CP
Holmes Regional Medical Center	C L T
Lakewood Ranch Medical Center	C CP CP
Lawnwood Medical Center and Heart Institute	C L T
Mayo Clinic	C L T
Memorial Regional Hospital /South Broward Hospital	C L T
North Okaloosa Medical Center	C CP CP
Ocala Regional Medical Center	C L T
Orange Park Medical Center	C L T
Palm Beach Gardens Medical Center	C L T
Palmetto General Hospital	C L T
Regional Medical Center Bayonet Point	C L T
Rockledge Regional Medical Center	C L T
The Villages Regional Hospital	C CP CP
Venice Regional Bayfront Health	C L T
Westside Regional Medical Center	C L T
Advent Health New Smyrna Beach	C E
AdventHealth Sebring	C E
AdventHealth Tampa	C E
AdventHealth Altamonte Springs	C E
AdventHealth Deland	C E
AdventHealth East Orlando	C E
AdventHealth Fish Memorial	C E
Ascension Sacred Heart Bay	C T
Ascension St. Vincent's Southside	C E
Bartow Regional Medical Center	C E
Bayfront Health Spring Hill	CP CP
Broward Health Imperial Point Medical Center	C E
Capital Regional Medical Center	C CP
Gulf Coast Regional Medical Center	C CP
HCA Oak Hill Hospital	C T
Jackson North Medical Center	C E
Jackson South Community Hospital	C E
Kendall Regional Medical Center	C L
Lake City Medical Center	C E
Lee Health - Gulf Coast Medical Center	C E
Lower Keys Medical Center	C CP
Mease Countryside Hospital	C E
Mercy Hospital	C T
Morton Plant North Bay Hospital	C E
North Broward Medical Center	C E
Northwest Medical Center	C L
Orlando Health Dr. P. Phillips Hospital	C CP

Participants in ACC's NCDR Registries, Accreditation Services and Awardees

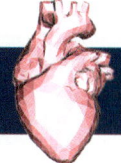

Hospital	Badges
Orlando Health St. Cloud Hospital	C CP
Oviedo Medical Center	C CP
Parrish Medical Center	C E
Physicians Regional HS - Collier	C CP
Sacred Heart on the Emerald Coast	C E
Sebastian River Medical Center	C CP
South Florida Baptist Hospital	C E
St. Anthony's Health Care	C E
St. Joseph's Hospital - North	C E
St. Joseph's Hospital - South	C E
St. Lucie Medical Center	C CP
Wolfson Children's Hospital	E IM
Adventhealth Apopka	E
AdventHealth Lake Wales	CP
AdventHealth Palm Coast	C
Ascension St. Vincent's Clay County	CP
Bayfront Health Punta Gorda	CP
Cape Canaveral Hospital	C
CCC Outpatient Cath Lab	C
Cleveland Clinic Tradition Hospital	C
Doctors Hospital of Sarasota	C
Englewood Community Hospital	C
Good Samaritan Medical Center	C
Halifax Health Medical Center	C
Health Central	C
Heart and Rhythm Institute of Trinity	E
Highlands Regional Medical	C
Joe DiMaggio Children's Hospital	IM
Johns Hopkins All Children's Hospital, Inc.	IM
Medical Center of Trinity	C
Melbourne Regional Medical Center	C
Memorial Hospital of Tampa	C
Memorial Hospital West /South Broward Hospital District	C
Miami Children's Health System	IM
Nemours Children's Hospital	IM
North Shore Medical Center	C
Ocala Regional Medical Center	CP
Palm Bay Hospital	C
Palms of Pasadena Hospital	C
Palms West Hospital	C
Physicians Regional Medical Center - Collier Boulevard	CP
Poinciana Medical Center	C
Putnam Community Medical Center	C
Santa Rosa Medical Center	CP
South Bay Hospital	C
South Lake Hospital	C
South Miami Hospital	TV
South Seminole Hospital	C
West Marion Community Hospital	CP

GEORGIA

Hospital	Badges
AU Medical Center, Inc.	A C E L T CL CP EP
Medical Center Navicent Health	C E L T AF CP HF
St. Joseph's Hospital	C CP E L T CP ▲
University Health Care System	C CP E L T CP ▲
Hamilton Medical Center	C CP E CP ▲
Memorial University Medical Center	C CP L T CP
Redmond Regional Medical Center	C CP L T CP
St. Francis Hospital	C E T CL CP
St. Mary's Hospital	C CP E CP ▲
Phoebe Putney Memorial Hospital	C E L T
Piedmont Athens Regional Medical Center	C L T CP
Piedmont Atlanta Hospital	C L T CP
Piedmont Fayette Hospital	C CP CP ▲
Piedmont Henry Hospital	C CP CP ▲
Piedmont Newnan Hospital	C CP CP ▲
South Georgia Medical Center	C CP E ▲
Wellstar Kennestone Regional Medical Center	C E L T
Emory Saint Josephs Hospital of Atlanta	C L T
Emory University Hospital	C L T
Emory University Hospital Midtown	C L T
Floyd Medical Center	C E CP
Northeast Georgia Health System	C L T
Northside Hospital Gwinnett	C L T
Southern Regional Medical Center	C CP CP
Atlanta Medical Center	C E
Cartersville Medical Center	C CP
Children's Healthcare of Atlanta	E IM
Coliseum Medical Centers	C L
East Georgia Regional Medical Center	C E
Eastside Medical Center	C CP
Grady Health System	C E
Houston Medical Center	C E
Memorial Satilla Health	C CP
Piedmont Rockdale Hospital	C CP
Southeast Georgia Health System	C E
Spalding Regional Hospital	C E
Tanner Medical Center/Carrollton	C CP
Tanner Medical Center/Villa Rica	C CP
Tift Regional Medical Center	C E
Union General Hospital	CP HF
Wellstar Cobb Hospital	C E

Continues on next page

NORTHEAST

Massachusetts
Lawrence General Hospital
Lawrence, MA

New Jersey
Ocean Medical Center
Brick, NJ

JFK Medical Center
Edison, NJ

Southern Ocean Medical Center
Manahawkin, NJ

Jersey Shore University Medical Center
Neptune, NJ

Riverview Medical Center
Red Bank, NJ

New York
St. Joseph's Hospital Health Center
Syracuse, NY

MIDWEST

Indiana
Lutheran Hospital
Fort Wayne, IN

Parkview Heart Institute
Fort Wayne, IN

Ohio
Summa Health System - Akron Campus
Akron, OH

Mercy Medical Center
Canton, OH

Coshocton Regional Medical Center
Coshocton, OH

Firelands Regional Medical Center
Sandusky, OH

Wisconsin
ProHealth Waukesha Memorial Hospital
Waukesha, WI

SOUTH

Alabama
Andalusia Health
Andalusia, AL

Flowers Hospital
Dothan, AL

Florida
Bayfront Health Seven Rivers
Crystal River, FL

AdventHealth Ocala
Ocala, FL

Bayfront Health St. Petersburg
St. Petersburg, FL

AdventHealth Tampa
Tampa, FL

Georgia
Union General Hospital
Blairsville, GA

Medical Center Navicent Health
Macon, GA

Louisiana
Christus St Frances Cabrini Hospital
Alexandria, LA

Our Lady of the Lake Regional Medical Center
Baton Rouge, LA

East Jefferson General Hospital
Metairie, LA

Mississippi
Merit Health Wesley
Hattiesburg, MS

Baptist Memorial Hospital-DeSoto
Southaven, MS

North Carolina
Catawba Valley Medical Center
Hickory, NC

CarolinaEast Medical Center
New Bern, NC

South Carolina
Spartanburg Medical Center
Spartanburg, SC

Texas
CHI St. Luke's Health Memorial Lufkin
Lufkin, TX

Shannon Medical Center South
San Angelo, TX

Metropolitan Methodist Hospital
San Antonio, TX

CHRISTUS Mother Frances Hospital-Tyler
Tyler, TX

United Regional Health Care System
Wichita Falls, TX

Virginia
Augusta Health
Fishersville, VA

Winchester Medical Center
Winchester, VA

WEST

Alaska
Alaska Regional Hospital
Anchorage, AK

Arizona
Abrazo Arizona Heart Hospital
Phoenix, AZ

California
Adventist Health Bakersfield
Bakersfield, CA

Colorado
The Medical Center of Aurora
Aurora, CO

Porter Adventist Hospital
Denver, CO

Nevada
Renown Regional Medical Center
Reno, NV

New Mexico
Lea Regional Medical Center
Hobbs, NM

Memorial Medical Center
Las Cruces, NM

Utah
Ogden Regional Medical Center
Ogden, UT

Wyoming
Sheridan Memorial Hospital
Sheridan, WY

Improving Heart Failure Care Together

Ensure you are receiving the best in heart failure care by finding dedicated patient care champions at facilities that display the ACC Heart Failure Accreditation seal.

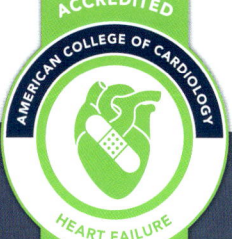

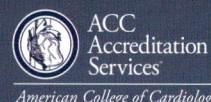

Visit **CardioSmart.org** for:
- Tools to help you and your heart failure care team manage your condition
- Tips for healthy living
- Information to help you research and compare all the heart care services offered at your local hospitals www.cardiosmart.org/find-your-heart-a-home

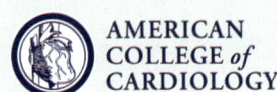

THE HEART OF QUALITY PATIENT CARE

Hospital	Registries/Accreditations/Awards
WellStar North Fulton Hospital	C E
Wellstar Paulding Hospital	C E
WellStar West Georgia Medical Center	C E
Adventist Health System Georgia	C
Atlanta Medical Center South	C
Coffee Regional Medical Center	C
Doctors Hospital - Augusta	C
East Georgia Regional Medical Center	CP
Emory Decatur Hospital	C
Emory Johns Creek Hospital	C
Fairview Park Hospital	C
John D Archbold Memorial Hospital	C
Meadows Regional Medical Center	C
Northeast Georgia Medical Center Braselton	C
Northside Hospital - Forsyth	C
Northside Hospital - Atlanta	C
Northside Hospital - Cherokee	C
Piedmont Columbus Regional Midtown	C
Piedmont Mountainside Hospital	CP
Piedmont Walton Hospital	CP
Polk Medical Center	CP
Upson Regional Medical Center	C
Wellstar Douglas Hospital	C

HAWAII

Straub Medical Center	C E IM L T
The Queen's Medical Center	C E L T
Pali Momi Medical Center	A C E
Hilo Medical Center	C E
Kaiser Permanente - Moanalua Medical Center	C E
Maui Memorial Medical Center	C

IDAHO

Saint Alphonsus Regional Medical Center	A C CP E L T CP
Eastern Idaho Regional Medical Center	C CP L T CP
Kootenai Health	A C E L T
Portneuf Medical Center	C CP L T CP
St. Luke's	A C E L T
Saint Alphonsus Medical Center - Nampa	C CP CP
St. Joseph Regional Medical Center	C CP E
West Valley Medical Center	C CP CP
Idaho Falls Community Hospital	C E
St. Luke's Magic Valley Regional Medical Center	C

ILLINOIS

OSF HealthCare Saint Francis Medical Center	A C CP E IM L T ▲
Riverside Health Care	C CP E L T CP HF ▲
Loyola University Medical Center	A C CP E L T ▲
Copley Memorial Hospital	A C CP E CP
Edward Hospital	C CP E L T ▲
Memorial Hospital Carbondale	C CP E L T ▲
St. Elizabeth's Hospital	C CP L T CP ▲
AMITA Health Adventist Medical Center Hinsdale	C CP E L ▲
AMITA Health Resurrection Medical Center	C E L T CP
AMITA Health Saint Joseph Medical Center	C E L T CP
Memorial Medical Center	C CP L T ▲
OSF Saint Anthony Medical Center	C CP E L T
University of Chicago Medical Center	C CP E L T
AMITA Health Adventist Medical Center GlenOaks	C CP E ▲
AMITA Health Adventist Medical Center La Grange	C CP E ▲
AMITA Health Alexian Brothers Medical Center	C E L T
Blessing Hospital	C L T CP
Carle BroMenn Medical Center	C CP CP
CGH Medical Center	C CP E CP
Highland Park Hospital	A C L T
NorthShore University Health System	A C L T
Northwest Community Hospital	C E L T
Northwestern Medicine McHenry Hospital	C CP T ▲
OSF Saint Joseph Medical Center	C CP E ▲
Protestant Memorial Medical Center	C CP CP ▲
Rush University Medical Center	A C L T
Trinity Medical Center - Rock Island	C CP L T
UnityPoint Health Methodist	C CP E T
University of Illinois Medical Center at Chicago	C E L T
Advocate Christ Medical Center	C L T
Advocate Good Samaritan Hospital	C L T
Advocate Illinois Masonic Medical Center	C L T
Advocate Lutheran General Hospital	C L T
Advocate Sherman Hospital	C L T
AMITA Health Adventist Medical Center Bolingbrook	C CP ▲
AMITA Health Mercy Medical Center	C E L
AMITA Health Saints Mary and Elizabeth Medical Center	C E CP
AMITA Health St. Mary's Hospital Kankakee	C E CP
Carle Foundation Hospital	C L T
Elmhurst Memorial Healthcare	C CP E
Franciscan Health Olympia Fields	C CP
MacNeal Hospital	C CP E
Memorial Hospital Shiloh	C CP
Mercy Hospital & Medical Center	C CP E
Northwestern Lake Forest Hospital	C CP
Northwestern Medicine Huntley Hospital	C CP
Northwestern Memorial Hospital	C L T
Palos Health	C L T
Prairie Heart Institute at St. John's Hospital	C L T
Rush Oak Park Hospital	C CP
UnityPoint Health Methodist	Proctor	C CP E
West Suburban Medical Center	C CP CP
Advocate Condell Medical Center	C L
Advocate Good Shepherd Hospital	C T
AMITA Health Saint Francis Hospital of Evanston	C E
AMITA Health Saint Joseph Hospital Chicago	C E
AMITA Health Saint Joseph Hospital Elgin	C E
AMITA Health St. Alexius Medical Center	C E
Anderson Hospital	C CP
Central DuPage Hospital	C T
Genesis Medical Center, Silvis	C E
Good Samaritan Hospital	C CP
Gottlieb Memorial Hospital	C E
Heartland Regional Medical Center	C CP
Javon Bea Hospital Riverside	C CP
Mount Sinai Hospital	C E
OSF Heart of Mary Medical Center	E CP
Sarah Bush Lincoln Health Center	C E
Silver Cross Hospital	C E
Swedish Covenant Hospital	C E
Advocate Childrens Hospital Oak Lawn	IM
Advocate South Suburban Hospital	C
AdvocateTrinity Hospital	C
Alton Memorial Hospital	C
Delnor Hospital	C
FHN Memorial Hospital	C
Gateway Regional Medical Center	C
Glenbrook Hospital	C
Ingalls Memorial Hospital	CP
Jersey Community Hospital District	E
Katherine Shaw Bethea Hospital	C
Lurie Children's Hospital of Chicago	IM
Northwestern Medicine Kishwaukee Hospital	C
Norwegian American Hospital	C
Red Bud Regional Hospital	CP
Southern Illinois Hospital - Herrin Hospital	CP
SSM Health Good Samaritan Hospital - MT Vernon	CP
St. Mary's Hospital	C
Vista Medical Center	C

INDIANA

Lutheran Hospital	A C CP L T AF CL CP HF TV ♦
Indiana University Health Methodist Hospital	C CP E IM L T CL EP ▲ ♦
Parkview Heart Institute	A C E L T AF EP ▲
Ascension St. Vincent Evansville	C CP E L T ▲
Deaconess Gateway Heart Hospital	C CP E L T ▲
Franciscan Health Indianapolis	C CP L T TV ▲
Indiana University Health Arnett Hospital	C CP E T CP
Indiana University Health Ball Memorial Hospital	C CP E L T ▲
Indiana University Health Bloomington	C CP E L T ▲
Columbus Regional Hospital	C CP E CP ▲
Northwest Health La Porte	A C CP CP EP
Northwest Health Porter	C L T AF CP
Union Hospital	C E L T CP

Registries
- **A** AFib Ablation Registry™
- **C** CathPCI Registry®
- **CP** Chest Pain - MI Registry™
- **E** EP Device Implant Registry™
- **IM** IMPACT Registry®
- **L** LAAO Registry™
- **T** STS/ACC TVT Registry™

Accreditations
- **AF** Atrial Fibrillation
- **CL** Cardiac Cath Lab
- **CP** Chest Pain Center
- **EP** Electrophysiology
- **HF** Heart Failure
- **TV** Transcatheter Valve

Awards
- ▲ Chest Pain - MI Registry™ Award Platinum
- ▲ Chest Pain - MI Registry™ Award Gold
- ▲ Chest Pain - MI Registry™ Award Silver
- ♦ HeartCARE Center

Participants in ACC's NCDR Registries, Accreditation Services and Awardees

Hospital	Codes
Ascension St. Vincent Heart Center	C E L T
Ascension St. Vincent Hospital	C E IM L
Clark Memorial Hospital	C CP E
Community Hospital	C E L T
Deaconess Hospital	C CP E
Goshen Hospital	C CP E ▲
Indiana University Health North Hospital	C CP E ▲
Indiana University Health Saxony Hospital	C CP E ▲
Indiana University Health West Hospital	C CP E ▲
Methodist Hospitals Southlake Campus	C E CL CP
Reid Health	C E L T
Saint Joseph Health System	A C L T
Community Heart and Vascular Hospital	C L T
Dupont Hospital	C CP CP
Elkhart General Hospital	C T CL
Franciscan Health Crown Point	C L CP
Franciscan Health Lafayette East	C CP ▲
Kosciusko Community Hospital	C CP CP
Marion General Hospital	C CP E
Memorial Hospital of South Bend	C L T
Methodist Hospitals Northlake Campus	C CL CP
St. Catherine Hospital	C E CP
St. Mary Medical Center	C L CP
Baptist Health Floyd	C L
Franciscan Health - Dyer	C CP
Franciscan Health - Hammond	C CP
Franciscan Health - Michigan City	C CP
Health and Hospital Corporation of Marion County	C E
Hendricks Regional Health	C CP
Pinnacle Healthcare, LLC	C E
Riley Hospital for Children Indiana University Health	E IM
Riverview Health	C CP
Community Hospital Anderson	C
Community Hospital East	C
Community Hospital South	C
Community Howard Regional Health	C
Franciscan Health Munster	C
Good Samaritan Heart Center	C
Hancock Memorial Hospital	C
Memorial Hospital and Health Care Center	C
Scott Memorial Hospital	CP
St. Elizabeth Dearborn	E
St. Joseph Hospital	CP
St. Vincent Kokomo	CP
Terre Haute Regional Hospital	C
Union Hospital Clinton	CP
Witham Health System	C

IOWA

Hospital	Codes
Mercy Medical Center - Des Moines	A C CP L T CP ▲
UnityPoint Health - St. Luke's Hospital	C CP L T CP TV
Allen Memorial Hospital	C CP T CP ▲
MercyOne North Iowa Medical Center	A C CP E T
MercyOne Siouxland Medical Center	C CP E T ▲
UnityPoint Health - St Luke's Sioux City	A C CP E ▲
Genesis Medical Center, Davenport	C E L T
Iowa Methodist Medical Center	C CP L T
Mercy Iowa City	C CP E ▲
University of Iowa Hospitals and Clinics	C IM L T
MercyOne Waterloo Medical Center	C CP E CP
Trinity Medical Center - Bettendorf	C CP
Trinity Regional Medical Center	C CP
Iowa Lutheran Hospital	C CP
Mercy Medical Center	C T
MercyOne Dubuque Medical Center	C T
The Finley Hospital	C
CHI Health Mercy	C
MercyOne Clinton Medical Center	C
Ottumwa Regional Health Center	C

KANSAS

Hospital	Codes
Advent Health Shawnee Mission	A C CP E L T ▲
The University of Kansas Health System	A C CP E L T ▲
Hays Medical Center	C CP E L CP ▲
Stormont - Vail HealthCare	C CP L T TV ▲
Olathe Medical Center	C CP L T
Overland Park Regional Medical Center	A C CP E L
Providence Medical Center	C CP E CP ▲
Salina Regional Health Center	C E L T CP
University of Kansas Health System St. Francis Campus	C CP E CP ▲
Wesley Medical Center	C CP L T
Via Christi Hospitals in Wichita	C L T
Western Plains Medical Complex	C E CP
Menorah Medical Center	C CP
Mercy Regional Health Center	C E
Newman Regional Health	C E
St. Catherine Hospital	C CP
St. Luke's South Hospital	C E
Kansas Medical Center	E
Lawrence Memorial Hospital	C
Via Christi Hospital - Pittsburgh KS	E
Wesley Woodlawn Hospital and ER	C
William Newton Memorial Hospital	C

KENTUCKY

Hospital	Codes
Baptist Health Lexington	C CP E L T AF CL CP TV ♦
Baptist Health Paducah	C CP E L T CL CP TV ♦
Norton Audubon Hospital	C L T CL CP TV ♦
Pikeville Medical Center	C CP L T CL CP
U of L - Jewish Hospital	C CP E L T CP
Baptist Health Louisville	C CP T CP HF
Saint Elizabeth Healthcare Edgewood	C CP E L T
Saint Joseph Hospital	A C CP E T
University of Kentucky	C CP E IM L T
King's Daughters Medical Center	C E L T CP
Norton Hospital	C L T CL CP
Saint Joseph East	C CP E CL CP
The Medical Center	C E L T CP
Baptist Health Corbin	C CP CP ▲
Ephraim McDowell Regional Medical Center	C CP E CP
Mercy Health Lourdes Hospital	C E L T
Clark Regional Medical Center	C E CP
Harrison Memorial Hospital	C E CP
Hazard ARH Regional Medical Center	C CP E
Highlands ARH Regional Medical Center	C E CP
Lake Cumberland Regional Hospital	C E CP
Norton Brownsboro Hospital	C CL CP
St. Claire Regional Medical Center	C CP E
TJ Regional Health	C E CP
Baptist Health Madisonville	C E
Frankfort Regional Medical Center	C CP
Georgetown Community Hospital	CP HF
Hardin Memorial Hospital	C CP
Jackson Purchase Medical Center	E CP
Meadowview Regional Medical Center	C CP
Owensboro Health Regional Hospital	C L
Saint Joseph London	C E
TriStar Greenview Regional Hospital	C CP
Baptist Health Richmond	C
Bluegrass Community Hospital	CP
Bourbon Community Hospital	CP
CHI Saint Joseph Health System, St. Joseph Berea	CP
Fleming County Hospital	CP
Logan Memorial Hospital	CP
Murray Calloway County Hospital	C
Norton Children's Hospital	IM
Norton Women's & Children's Hospital	CP
Paul B. Hall Regional Medical Center	CP
Spring View Hospital	CP
St. Mary & Elizabeth Hospital	C
Three Rivers Medical Center	CP
University of Louisville Hospital	C

LOUISIANA

Hospital	Codes
CHRISTUS Ochsner St. Patrick Hospital	C CP L T CP TV ▲ ♦
CHRISTUS St. Frances Cabrini Hospital	C CP T CL CP HF
Ochsner Medical Center	A C E IM L T EP
Our Lady of the Lake Regional Medical Center	C CP L T AF HF
St. Francis Medical Center	C CP E L T CP ▲
CHRISTUS Highland Medical Center	C CP L T CP TV
Ochsner - LSU Health Shreveport	A C CP E L T
St. Tammany Health System	C CP E T CP ▲
Tulane University Hospital and Clinic	C CP L T CP ▲
Willis - Knighton Medical Center	A C E L T CP
East Jefferson General Hospital	C E T HF TV
Lafayette General Medical Center	C CP L T ▲

Continues on next page

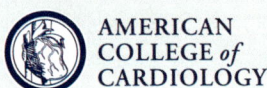

THE HEART OF QUALITY PATIENT CARE

Hospital	Designations
Our Lady of Lourdes Heart Hospital	C CP L T TV
Rapides Regional Medical Center	C CP L T
Terrebonne General Medical Center	C CP E T
Baton Rouge General Medical Center	C L T
Glenwood Regional Medical Center	C T CP
Lake Charles Memorial Hospital	T TV
Lakeview Regional Medical Center, A Campus of Tulane	C CP
Our Lady of Lourdes Regional Medical Center	C CP
University Medical Center New Orleans	C L T
Acadian Medical Center	E
Children's Hospital of New Orleans	IM
Cypress Pointe Surgical Hospital	E
Lane Regional Medical Center	CP
Mercy Regional Medical Center	E
Minden Medical Center	C
North Oaks Medical Center	E
Northern Louisiana Medical Center	CP
Ochsner Baptist Medical Center	C
Ochsner Medical Center - Baton Rouge	C
Ochsner Medical Center - West Bank	C
Ochsner Medical Center - Kenner	C
Ochsner/LSU Health Shreveport Monroe Medical	C
Slidell Memorial Hospital and Medical Center	C
St. Bernard Parish Hospital	C
St. Charles Parish Hospital	C
Touro Infirmary Medical Center	E
West Calcasieu Cameron Hospital	E
West Jefferson Medical Center	C
Willis Knighton Bossier	C
Willis Knighton Pierremont	C

MAINE

Hospital	Designations
Maine Medical Center	C CP E IM L T
Central Maine Medical Center	C E T
Eastern Maine Medical Center	C L T
York Hospital	C E

MARYLAND

Hospital	Designations
Adventist Healthcare White Oak Medical Center	C CP E T CP
Anne Arundel Medical Center	C CP E CP △
Johns Hopkins Hospital	C E IM L T
MedStar Union Memorial Hospital	C E L T
TidalHealth Peninsula Regional, Inc.	C E L T
University of Maryland Medical Center Cardiology	C IM L T
UPMC Western Maryland	C CP E △
Adventist HealthCare Shady Grove Medical Center	C CL CP
MedStar Southern Maryland Hospital Center	C CP E
Sinai Hospital of Baltimore	C L T
Suburban Hospital	C E T
University of Maryland Saint Joseph Medical Center	C L T
Frederick Health Hospital	C E
Holy Cross Hospital of Silver Spring, Inc.	C E
Howard County General Hospital	C E
MedStar Franklin Square Medical Center	C E
Carroll Hospital Center	C
Holy Cross Germantown Hospital	E
Johns Hopkins Bayview Medical Center	C
Meritus Medical Center	C
Prince George's Hospital Center	C
Saint Agnes Hospital	C
UM Baltimore Washington Medical Center	C
UM Upper Chesapeake Medical Center, Inc.	C
University of Maryland Shore Regional Health	C
Walter Reed National Military Medical Center	C

MASSACHUSETTS

Hospital	Designations
Lahey Hospital and Medical Center	A C E L T CL EP ◆
Lawrence General Hospital	C E CL CP HF ◆
Baystate Medical Center	A C E L T
Boston Medical Center	C E L T
Brigham & Womens Hospital	C E L T
Cape Cod Hospital	C E L T
Charlton Memorial Hospital	C E L T
Massachusetts General Hospital	C IM L T
Saint Vincent Hospital	C E L T
Tufts Medical Center	C E L T
UMASS Memorial Medical Center	C E L T
Beth Israel Deaconess Medical Center	C L T
Lowell General Hospital	C E CL
Mount Auburn Hospital	C E T
St. Elizabeths Medical Center	C L T
Anna Jaques Hospital	C E
Berkshire Medical Center, Inc.	C E
Mercy Hospital	C E
Milford Regional Medical Center	C E
Beth Israel Deaconess Hospital - Plymouth, Inc.	C
Beverly Hospital	C
Boston Children's Hospital	IM
Caritas Holy Family Hospital	C
Cooley Dickinson Hospital	C
Good Samaritan Medical Center	C
Melrose - Wakefield Hospital	C
MetroWest Medical Center	C
North Shore Medical Center - Salem Hospital	C
Saint Anne's Hospital	C
Signature Healthcare Brockton Hospital	C
South Shore Health System	C

MICHIGAN

Hospital	Designations
UP Health System - Marquette	C CP E L T CL CP △
Spectrum Health	A C CP IM L T △
MidMichigan Medical Center - Midland	A C CP L T △
Bronson Methodist Hospital	C CP E L T
Edward W. Sparrow Hospital Association	C CP L T △
Mercy Health	A C E L T
St. Joseph Mercy Hospital Ann Arbor	A C E L T
St. Joseph Mercy Oakland	A C E L T
Henry Ford Macomb Hospital	A C L T
McLaren Bay Region	C E L T
McLaren Flint	C E L T
McLaren Greater Lansing	C E L T
McLaren Macomb	C E L T
McLaren Northern Michigan	C E L T
Michigan Medicine	C IM L T
Munson Medical Center	C E L T
Allegiance Health	C L T
Ascension Health	C L T
Ascension Providence Hospital Southfield	C L T
Ascension St. John Hospital	C L T
Beaumont Hospital, Dearborn	C L T
Beaumont Hospital, Royal Oak	C L T
Borgess Medical Center	C L T
Covenant Healthcare	C L T
Harper University Hospital	C L T
Henry Ford Heart and Vascular Institute	C L T
Lakeland HealthCare	A C T
McLaren Port Huron Hospital	C E T
Metro Health Hospital	C CP △
Beaumont Hospital, Troy	C T
Garden City Hospital	C E
Holland Hospital	C CP
Hurley Medical Center	A C
McLaren Oakland	C E
Mercy Health Saint Mary's	C E
Saint Mary Mercy Hospital	C E
Ascension Genesys Hospital	C
Ascension Macomb - Oakland Hospital	C
Ascension Providence Rochester Hospital	C
Beaumont Hospital, Farmington Hills	C
Beaumont Hospital, Grosse Pointe	C
Beaumont Hospital, Trenton	C
Beaumont Hospital, Wayne	C
Henry Ford Health System West Bloomfield	C
Henry Ford Wyandotte Hospital	C
Huron Valley Sinai Hospital	C
Lake Huron Medical Center	C
McLaren Central Michigan	E
McLaren Thumb Region	E
Monroe Regional Hospital	C
ProMedica Monroe Regional Hospital	CL
Providence Park Hospital	C
Sinai - Grace Hospital	C

Registries
- **A** AFib Ablation Registry
- **C** CathPCI Registry
- **CP** Chest Pain - MI Registry
- **E** EP Device Implant Registry
- **IM** IMPACT Registry
- **L** LAAO Registry
- **T** STS/ACC TVT Registry

Accreditations
- **AF** Atrial Fibrillation
- **CL** Cardiac Cath Lab
- **CP** Chest Pain Center
- **EP** Electrophysiology
- **HF** Heart Failure
- **TV** Transcatheter Valve

Awards
- △ Chest Pain - MI Registry Award Platinum
- △ Chest Pain - MI Registry Award Gold
- △ Chest Pain - MI Registry Award Silver
- ◆ HeartCARE Center

Participants in ACC's NCDR Registries, Accreditation Services and Awardees

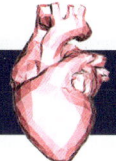

Spectrum Health Butterworth Hospital .... TV
UP Health System - Bell Hospital .... CP
UP Health System - Portage .... CP
Wayne State University - Childrens Hospital of MI ... IM

MINNESOTA

CentraCare Heart & Vascular Center .... A C CP E L T ▲
St. Mary's Medical Center .... C CP L T CP ▲
University of Minnesota Health, Heart Care Minneapolis ... A C IM L T
Mayo Clinic Hospital - Saint Marys Campus .... C IM L T
Mercy Hospital part of Allina Health .... C E L T
Minneapolis Heart Institute at Abbott Northwestern ... C E L T
Minneapolis Heart Institute at United Hospital .... C E L T
North Memorial Health .... C E L T
St Josephs Hospital .... A C L T
St. Luke's Hospital .... C E L T
University of Minnesota Health, Heart Care Edina ..... A C L T
Park Nicollet Methodist Hospital .... C L T
Regions Hospital .... C L T
Sanford Bemidji Medical Center .... C CP
Hennepin County Medical Center .... C E
Children's Minnesota .... IM
Essentia Health - St. Joseph's Medical C
Mayo Clinic Health System Mankato C
Ridgeview Medical Center C
St John's Hospital C
University of Minnesota Health, Heart Care Burnsville ... C

MISSISSIPPI

Merit Health Wesley .... C CP E AF CP HF ▲
Baptist Memorial Hospital - DeSoto .... C CP CL CP HF ▲
Baptist Memorial Hospital - Golden Triangle .... C CP L CL CP ▲
Forrest General Hospital .... C CP E L T ▲
Mississippi Baptist Medical Center .... C CP T CP ▲
North Mississippi Medical Center .... C CP L T ▲
St. Dominic - Jackson Memorial Hospital .... A C CP L T
University of Mississippi Medical Center .... CP L T TV ▲
Anderson Regional Medical Center .... C CP CP ▲
Baptist Memorial Hospital North Mississippi .... C CP T
Magnolia Regional Health Center .... C CP CP ▲
Ocean Springs Hospital .... C CP L T
Merit Health Central .... C CP CP
Merit Health River Oaks .... C CP CP
Merit Health River Region .... C CP CP
Methodist Olive Branch Hospital .... C CP CP
Southwest MS Regional Medical Center .... C CP E
Baptist Memorial Hospital - North Mississippi .... CL CP
Memorial Hospital at Gulfport .... C CP
Merit Health Biloxi .... C CP
Pascagoula Hospital .... C CP
Rush Foundation Hospital .... C CP
Singing River Gulfport .... C CP
Bolivar Medical Center .... CP
Delta Health - Northwest Regional .... CP
Delta Regional Medical Center .... CP
Merit Health Madison .... CP
Merit Health Natchez .... CP
Merit Health Rankin .... CP

MISSOURI

Barnes Jewish Hospital /Washington University ...... A C CP E L T ▲
Mosaic Life Care at St. Joseph .... C CP E L T CP ▲
Research Medical Center .... A C CP E L T ▲
Cox Medical Center South .... C CP E L T ▲
North Kansas City Hospital .... C CP E L T
Saint Francis Medical Center .... C CP L T CP
Centerpoint Medical Center .... C CP E L
Freeman Health System .... C CP L T ▲
Liberty Hospital .... C CP E CP
Mercy Hospital Joplin .... C CP L T
Mercy Hospital South .... C CP L T
MERCY Hospital Springfield .... C CP L T ▲
Mercy Hospital St. Louis .... C CP L T ▲
Saint Luke's Hospital of Kansas City .... A C E L T
Southeast Missouri Hospital .... C CP E T ▲
SSM Health Saint Louis University Hospital .... C CP L T
University of Missouri Hospital and Clinics .... A C E L T
Boone Hospital Center .... C L T TV
Christian Hospital BJC Healthcare .... C CP T
Cox Medical Center Branson .... C CP E
Lee's Summit Medical Center .... C CP E ▲
Poplar Bluff Regional Medical Center - Oak Grove ... C CP CL CP
Saint Joseph Medical Center .... C CP E CP
SSM Health DePaul Hospital - St. Louis .... C CP L T
St Luke's Hospital .... C E L T
St. Mary's Medical Center .... C CP CP
Truman Medical Centers .... C CP E
Capital Region Medical Center .... C CP
Hannibal Regional Hospital .... C CP E
Missouri Baptist Medical Center .... C L T
Noble Health Audrain Community Hospital .... C CP E
SSM Health - St Marys Hospital Jefferson City ...... C CP
SSM St. Joseph Hospital - St. Charles .... C CP E
Children's Mercy Kansas City .... E IM
Citizens Memorial Hospital .... CP
Mercy Hospital Jefferson .... C CP
Mercy Hospital Washington East Community .... C CP
Northeast Regional Medical Center .... C CP
Saint Luke's East Hospital .... C E
Saint Luke's Northland Hospital .... C E
SSM Health St. Clare Hospital - Fenton .... C CP
SSM Health St. Mary's Hospital - St. Louis .... C CP
SSM St. Joseph Hospital West .... C CP
St. Luke's Des Peres Hospital .... C E
Barnes Jewish St. Peters Hospital C
Belton Regional Medical Center .... CP
Bothwell Regional Health Center .... E
Heart Care Center, LLC .... E
Lake Regional Health System C
Moberly Regional Medical Center C
Ozarks Healthcare C
Phelps County Regional Medical Center C
Progress West Healthcare C
SSM Cardinal Glennon Children's Medical .... IM
St. Louis Children's Hospital .... IM

MONTANA

Billings Clinic .... C CP L T CP TV ▲
St. Vincent Healthcare .... A C CP L T CP
Logan Health .... C CP L T
Community Medical Center .... C CP E CP
Providence St. Patrick Hospital .... A C L T
St. James Health Care .... C CP ▲
Bozeman Health .... C CP
Benefis Healthcare C

NEBRASKA

Bryan Medical Center .... C E L T CL EP ◆
Nebraska Medicine .... C CP L T CP ▲
CHI Health CUMC - Bergan Mercy .... A C L T
CHI Health Nebraska Heart .... A C L T
Faith Regional Health Services .... C CP CP ▲
Kearney Regional Medical Center .... C CP T
Nebraska Methodist Hospital .... C L T
Great Plains Health .... C E
Mary Lanning Healthcare .... C CP
Nebraska Medicine Bellevue .... C CP
CHI Health Good Samaritan C
CHI Health Immanuel C
CHI Health Lakeside C
CHI Health St. Francis C
Children's Hospital and Medical Center .... IM

NEVADA

Saint Mary's Regional Medical Center .... C CP E L T CL CP TV ▲ ◆
Renown Regional Medical Center .... C CP L T CP HF
Centennial Hills Hospital Medical Center .... CP E CP ▲
Dignity Health - St. Rose Dominican, Siena Campus ... C CP T CP
MountainView Hospital .... C CP L T
Northeastern Nevada Regional Hospital .... C CP CL CP
Northern Nevada Medical Center .... C CP CP
Spring Valley Hospital Medical Center .... CP E T CP
University Medical Center of Southern Nevada ..... C CP CP ▲
Desert Springs Hospital Medical Center .... CP E CP
Dignity Health - St. Rose Dominican, San Martin Campus ... C CP CP

Continues on next page

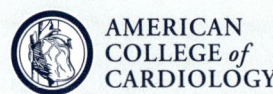

THE HEART OF QUALITY PATIENT CARE

Hospital	Accreditations
North Vista Hospital	C CP CP
Summerlin Hospital Medical Center	CP E CP
Sunrise Hospital and Medical Center	C L T
Valley Hospital Medical Center	CP E CP
Carson Tahoe Regional Medical Center	C E
Henderson Hospital	CP E
Renown South Meadows Medical Center	CP
Southern Hills Hospital	C

NEW HAMPSHIRE

Hospital	Accreditations
Catholic Medical Center	C E L T
Concord Hospital	C L T
Dartmouth Hitchcock Medical Center	C L T
Exeter Hospital	C CL
Parkland Medical Center	C CP
Southern New Hampshire Medical Center	C E
St. Joseph Hospital	C E
Elliot Hospital	C
Wentworth - Douglass Hospital	C

NEW JERSEY

Hospital	Accreditations
Jersey Shore University Medical Center	C CP E L T CL CP HF ▲
JFK Medical Center	C CP CL CP HF ◆
Ocean Medical Center	C CP CL CP HF ▲
Riverview Medical Center	C CP CL CP HF ▲
Cooper University Hospital	C E L T TV
Hackensack University Medical Center	C CP L T CP
Morristown Medical Center	C E L T TV
Newark Beth Israel Medical Center	C E IM L T
St. Francis Medical Center	A C E L T
The Valley Hospital	C CP E L T
Atlanticare Regional Medical Center	C E L T
Bayshore Medical Center	C CP CP ▲
Englewood Health	C CP L T
Robert Wood Johnson University Hospital	C E L T
Southern Ocean Medical Center	C CP CP HF
Deborah Heart & Lung Center	C L T
Saint Barnabas Medical Center	C E L T
Virtua Our Lady of Lourdes	C E L T
Capital Health Medical Center - Hopewell	CP CP
Inspira Medical Center Vineland	CP CP
St. Mary's General Hospital	L CP
St. Michael's Medical Center	E T
University Hospital	E L
CentraState Medical Center	CP
Chilton Medical Center	C
Clara Maass Medical Center	CP
Hackensack UMC Moutainside	C
Hackettstown Medical Center	CP
Hunterdon Healthcare System	C
Inspira Medical Center - Mullica Hill	CP
Inspira Medical Center Elmer Hospital	CP
Inspira Medical Center Woodbury	CP
Monmouth Medical Center	C
Newton Medical Center	C
Overlook Medical Center	C
Raritan Bay Medical Center	CP
Robert Wood Johnson University Hospital Somerset	C
Saint Clare's Hospital	C
St. Joseph's Health	T
Virtua Our Lady of Lourdes Hospital	EP

NEW MEXICO

Hospital	Accreditations
Presbyterian Healthcare Services	A C CP E IM L T ▲
Lovelace Medical Center	C CP L T ▲
Memorial Medical Center	C E CP HF
San Juan Regional Medical Center	C CP E CP
University of New Mexico Hospital	C E L T
Gerald Champion Regional Medical	C CP E
MountainView Regional Medical Center	C CP CP
Carlsbad Medical Center	C CP
Eastern New Mexico Medical Center	C CP
CHRISTUS St. Vincent Regional Medical Center	C
Lea Regional Medical Center	HF
Los Alamos Medical Center	CP

NEW YORK

Hospital	Accreditations
Strong Memorial Hospital	A C CP E IM L T TV ▲
St. Elizabeth Medical Center	C CP E L T CL EP ◆
The Mount Sinai Hospital	C CP E IM L T TV ▲
Bellevue Hospital Center	A C CP E L CL
New York Presbyterian/Queens	C CP E L T
Stony Brook University Hospital	A C CP L T CP
Montefiore Medical Center	C E IM L T
Mount Sinai St Luke's	C CP L T ▲
New York - Presbyterian Weill Cornell Medical Center	C CP IM L T
St. Joseph's Hospital Health Center	C L T CP HF
Vassar Brothers Medical Center	C E L T TV
Westchester County Health Care Corp	C E IM L T
Albany Medical Center Hospital	C E L T
Bassett Medical Center	C E L T
Cayuga Medical Center	C CP CP ▲
Jamaica Hospital Medical Center	C CP E ▲
Mercy Hospital of Buffalo	C E L T
New York - Presbyterian Brooklyn Methodist Hospital	C CP L T
New York - Presbyterian/Columbia University Irving	C CP L T
NYU Langone Health - Tisch Hospital	C IM L T
St. Francis Hospital	C L T TV
Upstate Medical University	C E L T
Arnot Ogden Medical Center	C CP E
Bronx Care Health System	CP E ▲
Ellis Hospital	C L T
Gates Vascular Institute	C L T
Good Samaritan Hospital	C L T
Good Samaritan Hospital Medical Center	C E T
Maimonides Medical Center Division of Cardiology	C L T
New York - Presbyterian Lawrence Hospital	C CP CP
Northwell Health Lenox Hill Hospital	C L T
Northwell Health North Shore University Hospital	C L T
Northwell Health Southside Hospital	C L T
Northwell Health Staten Island Hospital	C L T
NYU Langone Hospital–Long Island	C L T
St. Peter's Hospital	C L T
Wyckoff Heights Medical Center	C CP E
Cohen Children's Medical Center	E IM
Garnet Health	C E
Glens Falls Hospital	C E
Long Island Community Hospital	C E
Montefiore St Lukes's Cornwall	C E
Mount Sinai Beth Israel	C E
Mount Sinai South Nassau Hospital	C E
Northwell Health Long Island Jewish Hospital	C L
Olean General Hospital	C E
Richmond University Medical Center	C CP
Rochester Regional Health System	L T
Stony Brook Southampton Hospital	C E
The Brooklyn Hospital Center	C CP
United Health Services Hospitals /Wilson Regional	L T
UPMC Chautauqua	CP E
UVM Health Network CVPH	C E
Brookdale Hospital & Medical Center	E
Crouse Hospital	L
Montefiore Nyack Hospital	C
New York Presbyterian - Morgan Stanley Children's	IM
Niagara Falls Memorial Medical Center	C
Northern Westchester Hospital	C
Northwell Health Huntington Hospital	C
NYU Langone Hospital - Brooklyn	C
Peconic Bay Medical Center	C
Samaritan Hospital	C
Saratoga Hospital	C
SBH Health System	C
St. Catherine of Siena	C
White Plains Hospital	C

NORTH CAROLINA

Hospital	Accreditations
Carolina East Medical Center	C CP E L T CL CP HF ▲ ◆
University of North Carolina Hospital	A C CP E IM L T CP TV ▲
New Hanover Regional Medical Center	A C CP E L T CL CP
Duke University Hospital	C CP E IM L T ▲
Frye Regional Medical Center	C CP E CL CP ▲ ◆

Registries
- **A** AFib Ablation Registry™
- **C** CathPCI Registry®
- **CP** Chest Pain - MI Registry®
- **E** EP Device Implant Registry®
- **IM** IMPACT Registry®
- **L** LAAO Registry™
- **T** STS/ACC TVT Registry®

Accreditations
- **AF** Atrial Fibrillation
- **CL** Cardiac Cath Lab
- **CP** Chest Pain Center
- **EP** Electrophysiology
- **HF** Heart Failure
- **TV** Transcatheter Valve

Awards
- ▲ (light blue) Chest Pain - MI Registry™ Award Platinum
- ▲ (gold) Chest Pain - MI Registry™ Award Gold
- ▲ (silver) Chest Pain - MI Registry™ Award Silver
- ◆ HeartCARE Center

Participants in ACC's NCDR Registries, Accreditation Services and Awardees

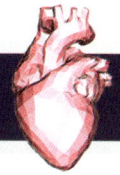

Hospital	Registries
Novant Health Presbyterian Medical Center	A C CP L T CP ▲
Atrium Health's Carolinas Medical Center	C CP IM L T ▲
Cape Fear Valley Medical Center	C CP E T CP ▲
Moses H. Cone Memorial Hospital	C CP E L T ▲
Novant Health Forsyth Medical Center	A C CP L T ▲
UNC REX Healthcare	C CP L T CP ▲
Vidant Medical Center	C CP E IM L T
Wake Forest Baptist Medical Center	C CP IM L T ▲
WakeMed Raleigh Campus	C CP L T CP ▲
CaroMont Regional Medical Center	C CP E L T
UNC Health Southeastern	A C CP E ▲
Alamance Regional Medical Center	C CP E ▲
Atrium Health Cabarrus	C CP T ▲
Catawba Valley Medical Center	C CP CP HF
Duke Raleigh Hospital	C CP E
Duke Regional Hospital	C CP E
Haywood Regional Medical Center	C E CL CP
Mission Hospital - Memorial Campus	C L T CP
Nash UNC Health Care	C CP CP ▲
Sentara Albemarle Medical Center	C CP E ▲
Wake Forest Baptist High Point Medical Center	C CP CP ▲
WakeMed Cary Hospital	C CP CP ▲
Atrium Health Pineville	C CP ▲
Central Carolina Hospital	C CP HF
Margaret R. Pardee Memorial Hospital	C CP CP
Novant Health - Rowan Medical Center	C CP ▲
Novant Health Huntersville Medical Center	C CP ▲
Novant Health Matthews Medical Center	C CP ▲
Watauga Medical Center	C CP E
Wayne UNC Healthcare	C CP ▲
Wilson Medical Center	C E CP
Davis Regional Medical Center	C CP
FirstHealth Moore Regional Hospital	C T
Harris Regional Hospital	C CP
Iredell Memorial Hospital	C CP
Johnston Health	C CP
Lake Norman Regional Medical Center	C CP
Maria Parham Health	C CP
Atrium Health Union	C
Betsy Johnson Hospital	CP
Caldwell Memorial Hospital	C
Carteret Health Care	C
Central Harnett Hospital	CP
DLP Cardiac Partners LLC/BRC	C
Halifax Regional Medical Center	C
Johnston Health Clayton	CP
Person Memorial Hospital	CP
Rutherford Regional Health System	CP
Scotland Healthcare System	C
Swain County Hospital	CP
Wayne Memorial Hospital	CP

NORTH DAKOTA

Hospital	Registries
Essentia Health Fargo	C CP L T CP ▲
Sanford Medical Center Bismarck	C CP L T CP ▲
Sanford Medical Center Fargo	C CP L T CP ▲
Altru Health System	C CP L T ▲
Trinity Hospitals	C CP E
CHI St. Alexius Health	A C

OHIO

Hospital	Registries
ProMedica Toledo Hospital	C CP E L T CL CP ▲
Summa Health System - Akron Campus	C CP L T CP HF TV ▲
Southwest General Health Center	A C CP E L T ▲
Aultman Hospital	C CP L T CP
Firelands Regional Medical Center	C CP E CP HF ▲
Mercy Health - Fairfield Hospital	C CP E T CL CP
Mercy Health - West Hospital	C CP E L CL CP
St. Rita's Medical Center	C CP E L T TV
The Jewish Hospital - Mercy Health	C CP E L CL CP
The University of Toledo Medical Center	C CP E L T ▲
Bethesda Hospital	A C E L T
Cleveland Clinic	C E IM L T
Fairview Hospital	C CP E CP ▲
Genesis Hospital	C L T CL CP
Hillcrest Hospital	C CP E CP ▲
Kettering Medical Center	A C E L T
Mercy Medical Center	C E T CL HF
Mount Carmel East Hospital	C E L T EP
Saint Elizabeth Youngstown Hospital	C CP E L T
The MetroHealth System	C CP L T ▲
Atrium Medical Center	C E L CP
Cleveland Clinic Akron General	C E L T
Fairfield Medical Center	A C E T
Fort Hamilton Hospital	C CP E ▲
Grandview Medical Center	A C E L
Knox Community Hospital	C CP CP ▲
Lima Memorial Health System	C E T CP

Continues on next page

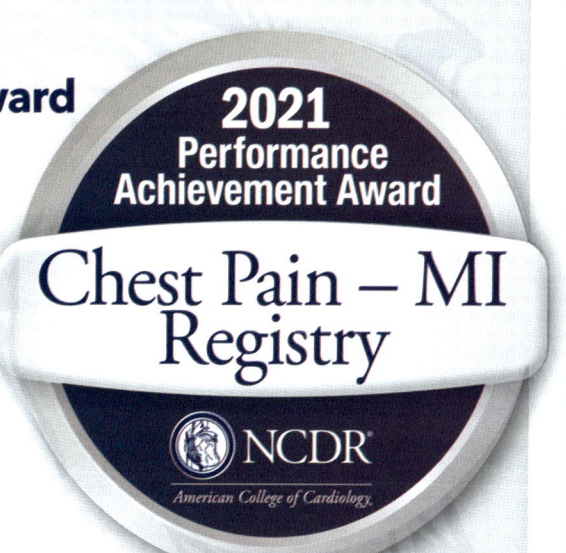

Congratulations to the recipients of the
Chest Pain – MI Registry Performance Achievement Award
Rewarding Excellence. Driving Success.

The Chest Pain – MI Registry™ Performance Achievement Award recognizes a hospital's success in sustaining a superior standard of care for patients experiencing a heart attack.

The Registry helps hospitals improve patient outcomes using ACC/AHA clinical guidelines to measure care and provide real-time data to drive decision making.

As the nation's largest and most authoritative quality improvement registry, the Chest Pain – MI Registry is committed to improving health outcomes for patients.

View hospitals participating in the registry at CardioSmart.org/ChestPainMI

©2021, American College of Cardiology B21052

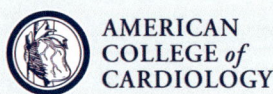

THE HEART OF QUALITY PATIENT CARE

Hospital	Registries/Accreditations/Awards
Mercy Health - Anderson Hospital	C CP E CL
Miami Valley Hospital	C E L T
Springfield Regional Medical Center	C CP E T
Summa Health System - Barberton Campus	C CP CP ▲
University Hospitals Cleveland Medical Center	C CP L T
University Hospitals St. John Medical Center	C CP CP ▲
The Christ Hospital Health Network	C L T TV
Adena Regional Medical Center	C CP L
Blanchard Valley Hospital	C E CP
Grant Medical Center	C L T
Lake West Medical Center	C E CP
McLaren St. Luke's	C E CP
Mount Carmel Grove City	C E EP
Mount Carmel St Ann's Hospital	C E EP
OhioHealth Mansfield Hospital	C L T
Riverside Methodist Hospital	C L T
The Ohio State University Medical Center	C L T
Trinity Medical Center West	A C E
Trumbull Regional Medical Center	C E CP
University Hospitals Ahuja Medical Center	C CP CP
University Hospitals Elyria Medical Center	C CP CP
University Hospitals Geauga Medical Center	C CP CP
University Hospitals Parma Medical Center	C CP CP
University Hospitals Portage Medical Center	C CP CP
University of Cincinnati Medical Center	C L T
Community Hospital and Wellness Center	C E
Coshocton Regional Medical Center	CP HF
Good Samaritan Hospital	C E
Holzer Cardiovascular Institute	C E
Marietta Memorial Hospital	C E
Mercy Health Lorain Hospital	C E
Mercy St Vincent Medical Center	C T
Nationwide Children's Hospital	E IM
Soin Medical Center	C E
Wooster Community Hospital	C CP
Ashtabula County Medical Center	E
Avita Ontario Hospital	C
Children's Hospital Medical Center of Akron	IM
Cincinnati Children's Hospital Medical Center	IM
Clinton Memorial Hospital	C
Doctors Hospital	C
East Liverpool City Hospital	CP
Fisher - Titus Medical Center	C
Galion Community Hospital	C
Licking Memorial Hospital	C
Mary Rutan Hospital	C
Memorial Health	C
Mercy Health - Clermont Hospital	CP
Mercy St. Anne Hospital	C
Mercy Tiffin Hospital	C
Miami Valley Hospital South	C
OhioHealth Marion General Hospital	C
Promedica Flower Hospital	C
Rainbow Babies & Children's Hospital	IM
Southern Ohio Medical Center	C
Summa Western Reserve Hospital	CP
Taylor Station Surgical Center	E
UC Health - West Chester Hospital	C
University Hospital East	C
University Hospitals Bedford Medical Center	CP
University Hospitals Conneaut Medical Center	CP
University Hospitals Geneva Medical Center	CP
University Hospitals Richmond Medical Center	CP
University Hospitals Samaritan Medical Center	CP
Upper Valley Medical Center	C
Wilson Memorial Hospital	C

OKLAHOMA

Hospital	Registries/Accreditations/Awards
Hillcrest Hospital South	C CP E CL CP ▲ ♦
St John Medical Center	C CP E L T TV
Norman Regional HealthPlex	C CP E T CP ▲
Oklahoma Heart Institute at Hillcrest Medical Center	C CP E L T ▲
INTEGRIS Baptist Medical Center	C CP E L T
Oklahoma Heart Hospital	C E L T
Oklahoma Heart Hospital South	C E L T
AllianceHealth Midwest	C CP CP
INTEGRIS Baptist Medical Center Portland Avenue	C CP CP
INTEGRIS Southwest Medical Center	C CP E
OU Medicine, Inc.	C IM T
Saint Francis Hospital	C L T
St. Anthony Hospital	C L T
AllianceHealth Durant	C CP
Jane Phillips Memorial Medical Center	C E
Northeastern Health System	C E
AllianceHealth Clinton	CP
AllianceHealth Madill	CP
AllianceHealth Ponca City	CP
AllianceHealth Seminole	CP
Integris Grove Hospital	C
McAlester Regional Health Center	C
Mercy Hospital Ardmore, Inc.	C
Oklahoma State University Medical Center	E
Oklahoma Surgical Hospital LLC	E
Saint Francis South, LLC	C
St Mary's Regional Medical Center	CP
St. Anthony Shawnee Hospital Inc.	C
Stillwater Medical Center	C

OREGON

Hospital	Registries/Accreditations/Awards
Oregon Health & Science University	A C CP IM L T
Asante	C CP L T ▲
Bay Area Hospital	C CP CP ▲
Kaiser Sunnyside Medical Center	C E L T
Legacy Emanuel Medical Center	C E L T
PeaceHealth Sacred Heart Medical Center at RiverBend	C L T CP
St. Charles Health System	C CP L T
Mckenzie Willamette Medical Center	C CP T
Providence Saint Vincent Medical Center	C L T
Salem Hospital	C L T
Adventist Health Portland	A CP
CHI Mercy	C E
Good Samaritan Regional Medical Center	C T
Legacy Good Samaritan Medical Center	C E
Legacy Meridian Park Medical Center	C E
Providence Medford Medical Center	C CP
Legacy Mount Hood Medical Center	C
Providence Portland Medical Center	C
Tuality Healthcare	C
Willamette Valley Medical Center	CP

PENNSYLVANIA

Hospital	Registries/Accreditations/Awards
Chester County Hospital	C CP E T CL CP EP ▲ ♦
Conemaugh Memorial Medical Center	C CP E L T CL CP HF ♦
Albert Einstein Medical Center	C CP E L T CL EP ♦
Doylestown Hospital	A C CP E L T CP ▲
Regional Hospital of Scranton	C CP L T CL CP TV ♦
UPMC Altoona	C CP E L T CL CP EP
Butler Memorial Hospital	C CP E L T CP ▲
St. Mary Medical Center	A C CP E L T CP
Hospital of the University of Pennsylvania	C CP E L T ▲
Penn Presbyterian Medical Center	C CP E L T ▲
Saint Vincent Hospital	C CP E L T CP
UPMC Harrisburg	C CP E L T ▲
Washington Health System	C CP E L T ▲
Allegheny General Hospital	C CP E L T
Excela Health Westmoreland Hospital	A C E L T
Mercy Fitzgerald Hospital	C CP E CP ▲
Penn State Health St. Joseph	C CP L T ▲
Penn State Hershey Medical Center	C E IM L T
Pennsylvania Hospital	C CP E L ▲
Reading Hospital	A C E L T
Sharon Regional Medical Center	C CP T CP ▲
St. Luke's University Hospital - Bethlehem Campus	C E L T CP
Temple University Hospital	C CP E L T
The Guthrie Clinic	A C E L T
UPMC Hamot	C CP E L T
UPMC Memorial	C CP E CP ▲
UPMC Passavant Hospital	C CP E L T
Wilkes - Barre General Hospital	C CP L CL CP
Crozer Chester Medical Center	C CP L T
Einstein Medical Center Montgomery	C E T CP
Geisinger Medical Center	C IM L T
Jeanes Hospital	C CP E
Jefferson Hospital	C CP E A

Registries
- **A** AFib Ablation Registry™
- **C** CathPCI Registry®
- **CP** Chest Pain - MI Registry™
- **E** EP Device Implant Registry™
- **IM** IMPACT Registry®
- **L** LAAO Registry™
- **T** STS/ACC TVT Registry™

Accreditations
- **AF** Atrial Fibrillation
- **CL** Cardiac Cath Lab
- **CP** Chest Pain Center
- **EP** Electrophysiology
- **HF** Heart Failure
- **TV** Transcatheter Valve

Awards
- ▲ Chest Pain - MI Registry™ Award Platinum
- ▲ Chest Pain - MI Registry™ Award Gold
- ▲ Chest Pain - MI Registry™ Award Silver
- ♦ HeartCARE Center

Participants in ACC's NCDR Registries, Accreditation Services and Awardees

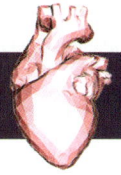

Hospital	Codes
Lehigh Valley Health Network	C E L T
Penn Medicine/Lancaster General Health	C E L T
UPMC Hanover	C CP E ▲
UPMC Presbyterian Hospital	C CP E L
UPMC Shadyside Hospital	C E L T
UPMC Susquehanna	C CP E T
UPMC West Shore	C CP E
WellSpan York Hospital	C L T CP
West Penn Hospital	C CP E ▲
Abington Memorial Hospital	C L T
Conemaugh Nason Medical Center	C E CP
Forbes Hospital	C CP E
Geisinger Wyoming Valley Medical Center	C L T
Lankenau Medical Center	C L T
Lehigh Valley Health Network Muhlenberg	C E L
Meadville Medical Center	C CP ▲
Nazareth Hospital	C CP CP
Penn State Health Holy Spirit Medical Center	C L T
St. Clair Hospital	C E T
Thomas Jefferson University Hospital	C L T
UPMC East	C CP E
UPMC MERCY	C CP E
ACMH Hospital	C CP
Bryn Mawr Hospital	C L
Chambersburg Hospital	C CP
Children's Hospital of Philadelphia	E IM
Geisinger Community Medical Center	C T
Indiana Regional Medical Center Cardiology Department	C E
J.C. Blair Memorial Hospital	C E
Jefferson Torresdale	C L
Lehigh Valley Hospital - Pocono	C E
Mount Nittany Medical Center	C E
Phoenixville Hospital	C L
Somerset Hospital	C CP
St. Luke's Hospital - Allentown Campus	C CP
St. Luke's Hospital - Monroe Campus	C CP
The Uniontown Hospital	C E
UPMC Lititz	C E
UPMC McKeesport	C E
Berwick Hospital Center	CP
Chan Soon - Shiong Medical Center at Windber	C
Conemaugh Meyersdale Medical Center	CP
Conemaugh Miners Medical Center	CP
Easton Hospital	CP
Ephrata Community Hospital	C
Evangelical Community Hospital	C
Grand View Hospital	C
Heritage Valley Beaver	T
Holy Redeemer Hospital	C
Jefferson Bucks	C
Lehigh Valley Hospital - Hazleton	CP
Lehigh Valley Hospital - Schuylkill East Norwegian Street	CP
Lower Bucks Hospital	C
Monongahela Valley Hospital	C
Moses Taylor Hospital	CP
Paoli Hospital	C
Penn Highlands Dubois	C
Pottstown Hospital Tower Health	CP
Prime Healthcare	C
Riddle Hospital	C
St. Christopher's Hospital For Children	IM
St. Luke's Hospital - Lehighton Campus	CP
St. Luke's Hospital - Miners Campus	CP
St. Luke's University Health Network - Anderson	C
The Good Samaritan Hospital	C
Tyler Memorial Hospital	CP
UPMC Children's Hospital of Pittsburgh	IM
UPMC Jameson	C
Wayne Memorial Hospital	C
Wellspan Gettysburg Hospital	C
Wexford Hospital	C

PUERTO RICO

Hospital	Codes
Cardiovascular Center of Puerto Rico	E L T CP
Hospital Pavia Santurce	E L T
Hospital Menonita Cayey	L T
Saint Luke's Memorial Hospital	E T
Bayamon Medical Center	T
Doctors Center Hospital	CP
Hospital Auxilio Mutuo	CP
Hospital Damas	T
VA Caribbean Healthcare System	CP

RHODE ISLAND

Hospital	Codes
Rhode Island Hospital	C L T
Kent Hospital	C E
Landmark Medical Center	C E
Miriam Hospital	C

SOUTH CAROLINA

Hospital	Codes
Lexington Medical Center	C CP E L T CL CP TV ▲ ◆
Spartanburg Regional Healthcare System	A C CP E L T CP HF ▲ ◆
AnMed Health Medical Center	A C CP L T CP ▲
McLeod Regional Medical Center	C CP E L T CP ▲
Self Regional Healthcare	C CP E L T CP ▲
Prisma Health Richland Hospital	C CP L T CP ▲
Providence Health	C CP E L T CP
Bon Secours St. Francis Health System	C CP L T
Greenville Memorial Hospital	C L T CP
Medical University of South Carolina	C IM L T
Trident Medical Center	A C L T
Beaufort Memorial Hospital	C CP ▲
Conway Medical Center	C CP E
Grand Strand Health	C L T
Hilton Head Hospital	C CP ▲
Roper Hospital	C L T
Carolina Pines Regional Medical Center	E CP
Kershaw Medical Center	E CP
Tidelands Georgetown Memorial Hospital	C CP
Aiken Regional Medical Center	C
Cherokee Medical Center	CP
Conway Medical Center	CP
East Cooper Medical Center	C
MUSC Health Florence Medical Center	C
MUSC Health Lancaster Medical Center	CP
MUSC Health Marion Center	CP
Piedmont Medical Center	C
Providence Health Northeast	CP
Spartanburg Medical Center - Mary Black Campus	CP

SOUTH DAKOTA

Hospital	Codes
Avera Heart Hospital of South Dakota	C CP L T CP ▲
Monument Health	C CP E L T ▲
Sanford Medical Center	C CP L T CP ▲
Avera St. Luke's	C CP
Prairie Lakes Healthcare	C CP
Avera Sacred Heart Hospital	E
Sanford Aberdeen Medical Center	CP

TENNESSEE

Hospital	Codes
CHI Memorial	A C CP L T CP ▲
Jackson - Madison County General Hospital	C CP E T CP TV
Turkey Creek Medical Center	A C CP L T ▲
Baptist Memorial Hospital - Memphis	C CP L T CP
Chattanooga - Hamilton County Hospital Authority	C CP E L T ▲
Methodist Le Bonheur Germantown Hospital	A C E L T CP
Methodist University Hospital	A C CP E CP ▲
University of Tennessee Medical Center	C CP E L T ▲
Vanderbilt University Medical Center	C CP L T CP ▲
Holston Valley Medical Center	C CP L T ▲
Maury Regional Medical Center	C CP E CP ▲
Parkridge Medical Center	A C L T CP
TriStar Centennial Medical Center	A C L T CP
Ascension Saint Thomas Hospital West	C E L T
Cookeville Regional Medical Center	C L T CP
Johnson City Medical Center	C CP L T
North Knoxville Medical Center	C CP CP ▲
Portsmouth Regional Hospital	A C T CP
Saint Francis Hospital	C CP T CP
Vanderbilt Tullahoma - Harton Hospital	C CP CP ▲
Ascension Saint Thomas Hospital Midtown	C E L
Blount Memorial Hospital	CP CP
Bristol Regional Medical Center	C CP
Methodist North Hospital	C E CP
Saint Francis Hospital - Bartlett	C CP CP
Southern Tennessee Regional Health System Winchester	C E CP
Sumner Regional Medical Center	C E CP
Ascension Saint Thomas Rutherford	C E
NorthCrest Medical Center	C CP
Parkwest Medical Center	L T
Tennova Healthcare - Clarksville	C CP

Continues on next page

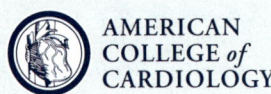

THE HEART OF QUALITY PATIENT CARE

Hospital	Registries/Awards
Tennova Healthcare - Cleveland	C CP
TriStar Hendersonville Medical Center	C CP
TriStar Horizon Medical Center	C CP
TriStar Skyline Medical Center	C CP
TriStar Southern Hills Medical Center	C CP
TriStar StoneCrest Medical Center	C CP
TriStar Summit Medical Center	C CP
Baptist Memorial Hospital - Tipton	CP
Baptist Memorial Hospital Carroll County	CP
Baptist Memorial Hospital - Union City	CP
CHI Memorial Hospital Hixson	CP
Erlanger Medical Center	CP
Erlanger-Chattanooga Hamilton County Hospital - East Campus	C
Hardin Medical Center	CP
Le Bonheur Children's Hospital	IM
Livingston Regional Hospital	CP
Memphis Hospital	C
Parkridge East Hospital	CP
Riverview Regional Medical Center	CP
Southern Tennessee - Sewanee	CP
Southern Tennessee Regional Health System - Lawrenceburg	CP
Southern Tennessee Regional Health System - Pulaski	CP
Starr Regional Medical Center	CP
Tennova - Jefferson Memorial Hospital	CP
Trousdale Medical Center	CP
Vanderbilt Wilson County Hospital	CP
West Tennessee Healthcare Dyersburg Hospital	CP
West Tennessee Healthcare Volunteer Hospital	CP

TEXAS

Hospital	Registries/Awards
CHRISTUS Mother Frances Hospital - Tyler	C CP E L T CL CP HF TV ▲ ◆
Baylor St. Luke's Medical Center	A C CP E L T CL EP ▲ ▲
CHI St. Luke's Health Memorial Lufkin	C CP E L CL CP EP HF ◆
The Hospitals of Providence Sierra Campus	C CP L T CL CP HF ▲ ▲
Doctors Hospital at Renaissance	CP E IM L T CP HF TV
Methodist Hospital	A C CP IM L T CP ▲
Methodist Texsan Hospital	C CP E L CL EP ▲ ▲
HCA Houston Healthcare Kingwood	C CP L T AF CP
Houston Methodist Willowbrook Hospital	C CP E L CL CP
Metropolitan Methodist Hospital	A C CP CL CP HF ▲
University Health System	C CP L T CL CP ▲
Woodland Heights Medical Center	C E L CL CP EP ◆
Ascension Seton Medical Center Austin	C CP E L T ▲
Ben Taub Hospital	C CP E T CP
HCA Houston Healthcare Conroe	C CP L T CP
Houston Methodist Hospital	C CP E L T ▲
Houston Methodist The Woodlands Hospital	C CP E L T ▲
Houston Methodist West Hospital	C CP E L T CP
Medical Center Hospital	C CP E L T CP
Medical City Dallas Hospital	A C IM L T CP
Memorial Hermann Hospital TMC	C CP IM L T ▲
Northeast Baptist Hospital	C CP E L CP ▲
Northeast Methodist Hospital	A C CP L CP ▲
Providence Health Center	C CP E L T ▲
United Regional Health Care System	CP E T CP HF ▲
University of Texas Southwestern Medical Center	C CP E L T ▲
UT Health - Tyler	C CP E L T CP
Baptist Medical Center	C CP E T CP
Baylor Scott & White Health	C CP L T ▲
Baylor Scott & White Heart and Vascular - Dallas	C CP L T ▲
Baylor Scott & White Medical Center - Round Rock	C CP L T ▲
CHI St. Luke's Hospital - The Vintage Hospital	C CP E CL CP
CHRISTUS Good Shepherd Medical Center	C CP L T ▲
CHRISTUS Santa Rosa Hospital - New Braunfels	A C CP L CP
CHRISTUS Santa Rosa Hospital - Westover Hills	C CP L CP ▲
CHRISTUS Spohn Hospital Corpus Christi - Shoreline	C CP L T CP
Corpus Christi Medical Center - Bay Area	C CP L T CP
HCA Houston Healthcare Clear Lake	C CP L T CP
HCA Houston Healthcare Medical Center	C CP L T CP
HCA Houston Healthcare Southeast	C CP L CP ▲
Houston Methodist Sugar Land Hospital	C CP E L T
Memorial Hermann Memorial City Hospital	C CP L T ▲
Memorial Hermann The Woodlands Medical Center	C CP L T ▲
North Central Baptist Hospital	C CP E CP ▲
Seton Medical Center Harker Heights	C CP E CL CP
St. David's South Austin Medical Center	A C E L T
St. Luke's Baptist Hospital	C CP E CP ▲
Texas Health Harris Methodist Fort Worth	C CP L T ▲
Texas Health Presbyterian Hospital of Dallas	C CP L T ▲
Texoma Medical Center	C E L T CP
University Medical Center of El Paso	C CP E L CP
Valley Regional Medical Center	C CP L CL CP
AdventHealth Central Texas	C CP E
Ascension Seton Medical Center Hays	C CP E ▲
Ascension Seton Medical Center Williamson	C CP E ▲
Baylor Scott & White Medical Center - College Station	C CP T ▲
BSA Health System	C E T CP
CHI/ St. Luke's the Woodlands Hospital	C CP E T
Covenant Health	A C E T
Dallas Regional Medical Center	CP E CP ▲
Dell Seton Medical Center at The University of Texas	C CP E ▲
DeTar Hospital Navarro	C CP CP ▲
HCA Houston Healthcare - West	C CP L CP
HCA Houston Healthcare Mainland	C CP CP ▲
Heart Hospital of Austin	A C L T
Hillcrest Baptist Medical Center	C CP L ▲
Houston Methodist Clear Lake Hospital	C CP E ▲
McAllen Heart Hospital	CP E T CP
Memorial Hermann Southwest Hospital	C CP L T
Methodist Dallas Medical Center	C CP L T
Methodist Richardson Medical Center	C CP L T
Methodist Stone Oak Hospital	C CP E CP
Mission Trail Baptist Hospital	C CP E CP
Paris Regional Medical Center	C CP E CP
Resolute Health Hospital	C CP E CP
Rio Grande Regional Hospital	C CP CP ▲
Shannon Medical Center	C CP T ▲
Shannon Medical Center South	C CP CP HF
St. David's Medical Center	A C E L
St. Joseph Medical Center	C CP E CP
Tarrant County Hospital District	C CP E ▲
Texas Health Heart and Vascular Hospital	C CP T ▲
The Heart Hospital Baylor Plano	C CP L T
University Medical Center	C E L T
University of Texas Medical Branch at Galveston	C E L T
Baylor Scott & White - Grapevine	C CP ▲
Baylor Scott & White Medical Center Irving	C CP ▲
Baylor Scott and White All Saints Medical Center	CP T ▲
CHI St. Joseph Health Regional Hospital	A C L
CHI/St. Luke's Patients Medical Center	C CP E
CHI/St. Luke's Sugar land Hospital	C CP E
CHRISTUS St. Michael Health System	C CP CP
City Hospital at White Rock	C CP E
HCA Houston Healthcare North Cypress	C CP CP
HCA Houston Healthcare Northwest	C CP CP
HCA Houston Healthcare Pearland	C CP CP
HCA Houston Healthcare Tomball	C CP CP
Hendrick Medical Center North	C L T
Hendrick Medical Center South	C CL CP
Houston Methodist Baytown Hospital	C CP E
Lake Pointe Medical Center	C CP ▲
Las Palmas Medical Center	C CP L
Longview Regional Medical Center	C L T
Medical City Arlington	C CP CP
Medical City Denton	C CP CP
Medical City Fort Worth	C L T
Memorial Hermann Southeast Hospital	C CP T
Methodist Mansfield Medical Center	C CP ▲

Registries
- A: AFib Ablation Registry
- C: CathPCI Registry
- CP: Chest Pain - MI Registry
- E: EP Device Implant Registry
- IM: IMPACT Registry
- L: LAAO Registry
- T: STS/ACC TVT Registry

Accreditations
- AF: Atrial Fibrillation
- CL: Cardiac Cath Lab
- CP: Chest Pain Center
- EP: Electrophysiology
- HF: Heart Failure
- TV: Transcatheter Valve

Awards
- ▲ Chest Pain - MI Registry Award Platinum
- ▲ Chest Pain - MI Registry Award Gold
- ▲ Chest Pain - MI Registry Award Silver
- ◆ HeartCARE Center

Participants in ACC's NCDR Registries, Accreditation Services and Awardees

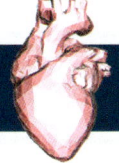

Facility	Codes
Odessa Regional Medical Center	C CP CP
Palestine Regional Medical Center	C E CP
Parkland Health & Hospital System	C E L
Southwest General Hospital	C CP CP
Texas Health Harris Methodist HEB	C CP ▲
Texas Health Harris Methodist Hospital Southwest Fort Worth	C CP ▲
Texas Health Huguley Hospital	C CP E
Texas Health Presbyterian Denton	C CP ▲
Texas Health Presbyterian Hospital Plano	C CP ▲
The Heart Hospital Baylor Denton	C CP ▲
The Medical Center of Southeast Texas	C CP CP
The University of Texas Medical Branch Clear Lake Campus	C E L
Wadley Regional Medical Center	C CP CP
Baptist Hospital of Southeast Texas	L T
Baylor Scott & White Heart and Vascular - FW	C L
Baylor Scott & White Medial Center - Lakeway	C CP
Baylor Scott & White Medical Center - Centennial	C CP
Cedar Park Regional Medical Center	C CP
CHI St. Joseph Health College Station Hospital	A C
CHI/St. Luke's Lakeside Hospital	C E
CHRISTUS Hospital - St Elizabeth	C CP
CHRISTUS San Marcos	C CP
CHRISTUS Santa Rosa Hospital - Medical Center	C CP
Citizens Medical Center	CP CP
Corpus Christi Medical Center - Doctors Regional	CP CP
Del Sol Medical Center	C CP
Doctors Hospital of Laredo	E CP
Harlingen Medical Center	C E
Hospitals of Providence - Memorial Campus	C CP
Hospitals of Providence East Campus	C CP
Huntsville Memorial Hospital	C E
Lake Granbury Medical Center	C CP
Laredo Medical Center	C CP
Lubbock Heart Hospital	C E T
Medical City Alliance	C CP
Medical City Plano	C CP
Medical City Weatherford	C CP
Memorial Hermann Cypress Hospital	CP ▲
Memorial Hermann Greater Heights Hospital	CP ▲
Memorial Hermann Katy Hospital	CP ▲
Memorial Hermann Northeast	CP ▲
Memorial Hermann Pearland	CP ▲
Memorial Hermann Sugar Land	CP ▲
Methodist Charlton Medical Center	C CP
Round Rock Medical Center	A C
Texas Regional Medical Center at Sunnyvale	C CP
The Heart Hospital of Northwest Texas	C L
Valley Baptist Medical Center - Brownsville	C CP
Wise Health System	C CP
Ascension Providence	TV
Baylor Medical Center At McKinney	CP
Baylor Scott & White Health, Marble Falls	C
Baylor Scott & White Medical Center Waxahachie	CP
Children's Hospital of San Antonio	IM
Children's Medical Center of Dallas	IM
CHRISTUS Santa Rosa San Marcos	CP
CHRISTUS Spohn Hospital Alice	C
CHRISTUS St. Michael Hospital - Atlanta	CP
Cigarroa Interventional Institute	E
Cook Children's Medical Center	IM
Dell Children's Medical Center of Central Texas	IM
Ennis Regional Medical Center	CP
Guadalupe Regional Medical Center	C
Houston Methodist Clear Lake	CP
Hunt Regional Medical Center	C
Matagorda Regional Medical Center	E
Medical City Frisco	C
Medical City Heart and Spine Hospitals	CP
Medical City Las Colinas	C
Medical City Lewisville	C
Medical City Mckinney	C
Medical City North Hills	C
Methodist Speciality and Transplant Hospital	C
Midland Memorial Hospital	E
Nacogdoches Medical Center	C
Nacogdoches Memorial Hospital	E
Navarro Regional Hospital	CP
North Austin Medical Center	C
Parkview Regional Hospital	CP
Peterson Regional Medical Center	C
Texas Children's Hospital	IM
Texas Health Harris Methodist Hospital Alliance	C
Texas Health Presbyterian Hospital Allen	C
The Hospitals of Providence Transmountain Campus	C
University of Texas MD Anderson Cancer Center	E
Valley Baptist Medical Center	C
Valley Baptist Medical Center Brownsville	CP
Wise Health Surgical Hospital at Parkway	E
Wise Health System - East Campus	CP

UTAH

Facility	Codes
Ogden Regional Medical Center	C CP AF CP HF ▲
St. Mark's Hospital	C CP L T CP ▲
University of Utah Health	C CP L T
Lakeview Hospital	C CP CP
Timpanogos Regional Hospital	C CP L CP
Intermountain Health St. George Regional Hospital	C L T
Intermountain Healthcare	C L T
Intermountain Medical Center	C L T
McKay - Dee Hospital Center	C L T
Mountain View Hospital	C CP CP
Davis Hospital and Medical Center	C CP
Salt Lake Regional Medical Center	C L
Ashley Regional Medical Center	CP
Brigham City Community Hospital	CP
Castleview Hospital	CP
Intermountain Primary Children's Hospital	IM
Jordan Valley Medical Center	C
Jordan Valley Medical Center - West Valley Campus	C
Lone Peak Hospital	CP
Mountain Point Medical Center	C
Mountain West Medical Center	CP

VERMONT

Facility	Codes
The University of Vermont Medical Center	A C E L T
Central Vermont Medical Center Inc	E

VIRGINIA

Facility	Codes
Inova Fairfax Medical Campus IHVI	A C CP E IM L T ▲
Winchester Medical Center	C CP E L T CP HF ▲
Carilion Roanoke Memorial Hospital	C CP E L T CP ▲
Centra Lynchburg General Hospital	C CP E L T CP ▲
VCU - Medical College of Virginia	C CP E IM L T ▲
Sentara Norfolk General Hospital	C CP E L T
Sentara Rockingham Memorial Hospital	C CP E L T ▲
SOVAH Health - Danville	C CP E CL CP HF
Augusta Health	C CP CP HF ▲
Bon Secours Southside Medical Center	C CP CL CP ▲
Chesapeake Regional Medical Center	C CP E CP ▲
CJW Medical Center	A C CP L T
Sentara Martha Jefferson Hospital	C CP E CP ▲
Sentara Williamsburg Regional Medical Center	C CP E CP ▲
Sovah Health - Martinsville	C E CL CP HF
University of Virginia Medical Center	A C E L T
Virginia Hospital Center	C CP E L T
Inova Alexandria Hospital	C CP E ▲
Inova Loudoun Hospital	C CP E ▲
LewisGale Medical Center	C CP T CP
Reston Hospital Center	C CP CP ▲
Riverside Regional Medical Center	C E L CP
Sentara Careplex Hospital	C CP E ▲
Sentara Halifax Regional Hospital	C CP E
Sentara Leigh Hospital	C CP E
Sentara Northern Virginia Medical Center	C CP E ▲
Sentara Virginia Beach General Hospital	C CP E ▲
Bon Secours - Memorial Regional Medical Center	C L T
Bon Secours Mercy Health - St. Marys Hospital	C L T
Henrico Doctors Hospital	C L T
LewisGale Hospital Montgomery	C CP CP
Mary Washington Healthcare	C L T
Novant Health UVA Prince William Hospital	C CP ▲
Sentara Obici Hospital	C CP E
Sentara Princess Anne Hospital	C CP ▲
Fauquier Health	C E CP
Bon Secours Maryview Medical Center	C CP
Carilion New River Valley Medical Center	C E

Continues on next page

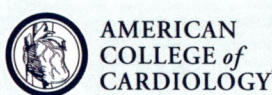

THE HEART OF QUALITY PATIENT CARE

Hospital	Codes
Children's Hospital of The King's Daughters, Inc.	E IM
Clinch Valley Medical Center	C CP
Johnston Memorial Hospital	C CP
Spotsylvania Regional Medical Center	C CP
Stonesprings Hospital Center	C CP
Warren Memorial Hospital	C CP
Bon Secours DePaul Medical Center	C
Bon Secours St Francis Medical Center	C
Centra Southside Community Hospital	C
John Randolph Medical Center	CP
LewisGale Hospital Alleghany	CP
LewisGale Hospital Pulaski	CP
Mary Immaculate Hospital	C
Page Memorial Hospital	CP
Riverside Walter Reed Hospital	CP
Shenandoah Memorial Hospital	CP
Southampton Memorial Hospital	CP
Southern Virginia Regional Medical Center	CP
Stafford Hospital	C
Twin County Regional Healthcare	CP
Virginia Commonwealth University Medical Center	CP
Wythe County Community Hospital	CP

WASHINGTON

Hospital	Codes
Deaconess Hospital MultiCare Health System	C CP L T ▲
MultiCare Tacoma General Hospital	C CP L T ▲
Virginia Mason Medical Center	C CP L T ▲
Confluence Health Central Washington Hospital & Clinics	C CP E T
PeaceHealth St. Joseph Medical Center	C L T TV
Providence Regional Medical Center Everett	A C L T
Providence Sacred Heart Medical Center	C IM L T
St. Joseph Medical Center	A C L T
St. Michael Medical Center	A C L T
Swedish Health Services	A C L T
MultiCare Auburn Medical Center	C CP
MultiCare Good Samaritan Hospital	C CP
Overlake Hospital Medical Center	C E T
PeaceHealth Southwest Medical Center	C L T
Providence St. Peter Hospital	C L T
University of Washington Medical Center - Montlake	C L T
Capital Medical Center	C E
Evergreen Healthcare	C E
Legacy Salmon Creek Medical Center	C E
Astria Sunnyside Hospital	C
CHI Franciscan Health St. Anne Hospital	C
Grays Harbor Community Hospital	C
Kadlec Regional Medical Center	C
Providence St. Mary's Medical Center	C
Seattle Children's Hospital	IM
St. Francis Hospital	C
St. John Medical Center	C
Swedish Edmonds Hospital	C
Trios Health	C
University of Washington Medical Center - Northwest	C
Valley Medical Center	C
Virginia Mason Memorial	C

WEST VIRGINIA

Hospital	Codes
Mon Health Medical Center	C CP E L T AF CP ♦
Wheeling Hospital	A C CP E L T CP ▲
St. Mary's Medical Center	C CP L T CP ▲
WVU Medicine Camden Clark Medical Center	C CP E CL CP ♦
Charleston Area Medical Center	C CP E L T
Raleigh General Hospital	C CP E CP
WVU Medicine	C E L T
Berkeley Medical Center	C E
CAMC Memorial Hospital	CL CP
St. Francis Hospital	C E
Thomas Memorial Hospital	C E
Weirton Medical Center	C E
WVU Medicine United Hospital Center	C E
Beckley Appalachian Regional Healthcare	C
Cabell Huntington Hospital	CP
Greenbrier Valley Medical Center	C
Logan Regional Medical Center	CP
Princeton Community Hospital	C
Reynolds Memorial Hospital	C

WISCONSIN

Hospital	Codes
Aurora St. Luke's Medical Center	A C CP L T CP TV ▲
Marshfield Medical Center	A C CP E L T ▲
UW Health	C CP E IM L T ▲
Waukesha Memorial Hospital	A C L T CL CP HF
Gundersen Lutheran Health System	C CP E L T ▲
Marshfield Medical Center - Weston	A C CP E T ▲
Mercyhealth Hospital and Trauma Center - Janesville	C CP E L T CP
ThedaCare Regional Medical Center - Appleton	C E L T CL CP
Aurora BayCare Medical Center	A C CP CL ▲
Aurora Medical Center in Grafton	A C CP CP ▲
Froedtert Hospital	C E L T CP
SSM Health St. Mary's Hospital - Madison	C CP L T ▲
Ascension Columbia St. Mary's Hospital Milwaukee	C CP L T
Aurora Medical Center in Summit	C CP CP ▲
St. Agnes Hospital	C E L T
UnityPoint Health - Meriter	C CP E ▲
Aspirus Wausau Hospital	C L T
Bellin Memorial Hospital	C L T
Holy Family Memorial	C CP ▲
Watertown Regional Medical Center	C E CP
Ascension Columbia St. Mary's Hospital Ozaukee	C CP
Ascension NE Wisconsin St. Elizabeth Hospital	C T
Aurora Medical Center - Kenosha	C CP
Beloit Memorial Hospital	C E
Froedtert South, Inc.	C E
HSHS Sacred Heart Hospital	C T
HSHS St. Vincent Hospital	C T
Marshfield Medical Center - Eau Claire	C CP
Mayo Clinic Health System - Eau Claire Hospital	C T
The Monroe Clinic	C E
Ascension NE Wisconsin Mercy Hospital	C
Ascension St. Michael's Hospital	C
Aurora Lakeland Medical Center	CP
Aurora Medical Center Oshkosh	C
Aurora Sheboygan Memorial Medical Center	C
Children's Hospital of Wisconsin	IM
Community Memorial Hospital	C
Froedtert West Bend Hospital	CP
HSHS St. Mary's Hospital	C
Mayo Clinic Health System - Franciscan Healthcare	C
Mercyhealth Hospital and Medical Center - Walworth	CP
Oconomowoc Memorial Hospital	C
Wheaton Franciscan - St Joseph Campus	C
Wheaton Franciscan Healthcare - Franklin, Inc	C
Wheaton Franciscan Healthcare - All Saints, Inc.	C
Wheaton Franciscan Healthcare - St. Francis, Inc.	C
Wheaton Franciscan Inc. Elmbrook Memorial Campus	C

WYOMING

Hospital	Codes
Wyoming Medical Center	C CP E T ▲
Campbell County Health	C CP E ▲
Cheyenne Regional Medical Center	C CP ▲
Sheridan Memorial Hospital	C E HF
SageWest Healthcare - Lander	C CP
Cody Regional Health	C
Evanston Regional Hospital	CP
SageWest Health Care at Riverton	CP

To learn more about hospitals and centers near you, visit *FindYourHeartaHome.org*.

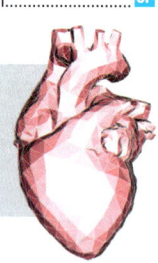

PATIENT POWER

Strengthened Defenses

Long term, here are a few ways to boost your immune system

by **Heidi Godman** *and* **Lisa Esposito**

DURING THE PANDEMIC, getting vaccinated against COVID-19 has been the most pressing way to help your immune system fend off serious illness. But in the long run, how can you continue to bolster the cells, tissues and organs that protect you from disease in their fight against all the other threats they face?

The best immune boosters don't suddenly rev up the body's defenses; they support and optimize them over the long haul. "You want to give the immune system a chance to react in its appropriately designed way. You don't want to get in the way of it," says Dr. John McCarty, director of the Cellular Immunotherapies and Transplant program at VCU Massey Cancer Center in Richmond, Virginia.

You can help your immune system do its job by:

1 Reducing stress

When the brain senses danger, it triggers the body's "fight or flight" response, preparing the muscles, heart and lungs to get you out of harm's way. "Stress works to increase certain hormones, particularly cortisol, which ask the immune system to stand down so they can do the temporary job of addressing the existential threat," explains Dr. Rachel Franklin, vice chair and medical director in the department of Family and Preventive Medicine at the University of Oklahoma College of Medicine. But when stress is chronic, it hurts immunity. "If allowed to circulate, stress hormones make the immune system sluggish when faced with a challenge," Franklin says.

Stress reduction, then, becomes an important immune booster. To ease chronic stress, you might consider meditation, exercise and psychotherapy.

2 Eating a healthy diet

When you eat a Western diet rich in refined grains, sugary beverages and fatty and processed foods, you do two things to your immune system: deprive it of the antioxidants and nutrients it needs to function properly, and change the gut flora – the microbiome – in your GI tract, home to a significant number of immune cells. "A Western diet reduces diversity in the gut microbiome and is associated with bad health outcomes," McCarty says.

Health risks of a Western diet include chronic inflammation, lingering activation of the immune system even when there's no threat, an increased risk of chronic diseases such as heart disease and Type 2 diabetes, and an increased risk of obesity (defined as a body mass index of 30 or more).

Those consequences affect your ability to fend off harmful microbes. "Obesity increases inflammation. Chronic inflammation and chronic disease make the immune response less effective," says Dr. Heidi Zapata, an immunologist, infectious diseases specialist and assistant professor at the Yale School of Medicine.

Many nutrients form the foundation of immune health, including Omega-3 fatty acids, vitamin C and D and zinc. How do they help? Take vitamin C: "We know that

PATIENT POWER

vitamin C not only regulates white blood cells but also helps them do a better job of defending the body from viruses and bacteria. Vitamin C is also an excellent antioxidant. It protects our body from inflammation and the negative effects of an overactive immune system," says Alexander Michels, a research associate at Oregon State University's Linus Pauling Institute.

Unless you have a nutrient deficiency, a healthy and varied diet is all you need to get your fill of nutrients. A Mediterranean-style diet (story, Page 103), for example, includes lots of immune-boosting foods such as fruits, vegetables, legumes, nuts and seeds, whole grains, lean protein, low-fat dairy and olive oil. What if there's a gap in your diet? "Taking a multivitamin is not a bad thing," Zapata says, "but getting vitamins in natural ways, from vegetables or fruits, is more potent."

Will taking supplements boost immune system health if you suddenly get sick? The jury is still out on that one. When it comes to vitamin C, Michels says, taking some before symptoms appear "may reduce the duration of the common cold." But it's best to get at least the recommended amounts every day to see the greatest benefits, he says. "At least 200 mg per day is acceptable. The Linus Pauling Institute recommends 400 mg a day from diet and supplement sources."

3 Exercising

Just like a Western diet, a sedentary lifestyle is associated with an increased risk for chronic disease and obesity, as well as chronic inflammation.

The antidote – exercise – appears to increase the diversity of gut bacteria, flushes out stress hormones and reduces the risk for obesity and chronic disease. Exercising regularly also leads to better heart and lung health, increased metabolism, lower blood pressure and better blood sugar control.

The recommended amount of exercise is at least 150 minutes per week of moderate-intensity activity, such as brisk walking. "But even people who get a minimal amount of exercise seem to have improved microbiome diversity," McCarty points out.

> 'To ease chronic stress, consider meditation, exercise and therapy.'

4 Getting enough sleep

Making a habit of getting too little sleep leads to increased levels of cortisol, chronic inflammation, an increased risk for chronic disease – and decreased immune function. In fact, getting enough sleep, especially at night, is one of the body's best immune boosters. "We know that the number of circulating and patrolling immune cells peaks at night," Zapata says.

How much sleep do you need? "Children need 10 to 12 hours of sleep," Franklin says. "Adults need six or seven hours."

5 Getting recommended vaccinations

When you're exposed to a harmful new microbe, it takes time to build up defenses. "By the time the body makes the tools to fight it, the body has been damaged by infection," Franklin explains.

Vaccinations give your system the upper hand. "They allow the immune system to preview a microbe signature so the body can work better and faster once it actually encounters a pathogen," Zapata says. Some vaccinations are recommended annually, such as flu shots. But check with your doctor and your children's doctor to see if everyone is up to date on their other shots.

6 Limiting alcohol intake and quitting smoking

Smoking and heavy drinking are very harmful to immunity. "In people with cirrhosis and liver disease, I'd in many ways consider them immunocompromised," Zapata says. And "there's nothing worse you could do for your immune system than smoke," Franklin says. When that system "should be on patrol looking for something it needs to fight," she says, you've instead "sent it to your lungs, sinus passages, mouth and throat to fight the poison you just ingested." You can't expect your body's defenders to "fight battles on multiple fronts and do it effectively," she says. ●

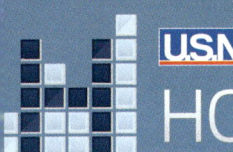

HOSPITAL DATA INSIGHTS | PEDIATRICS

hdi.usnews.com | An Analytics Platform from *U.S. News & World Report*

115+ HOSPITALS

2,500+ METRICS

500,000+ DATA POINTS

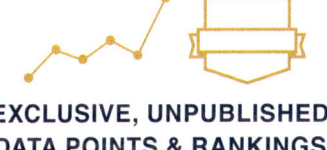
EXCLUSIVE, UNPUBLISHED DATA POINTS & RANKINGS

UNLIMITED PEER GROUPS

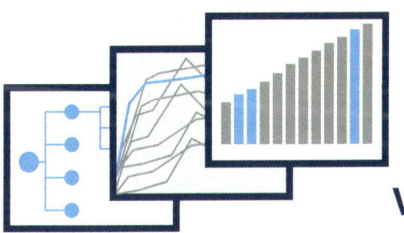
9 CUSTOM VISUALIZATIONS
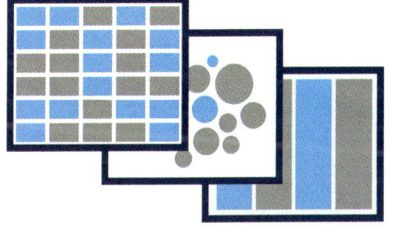

Why Hospital Data Insights Pediatrics?

- Best-in-class analytics
- Superior benchmarking
- Extract charts and graphs easily for detailed analysis
- Study year on year data trends to drive clinical improvements

For more information or to request a demo, contact us at

hdi.usnews.com

✉ hdi@usnews.com
☎ 202.955.2171

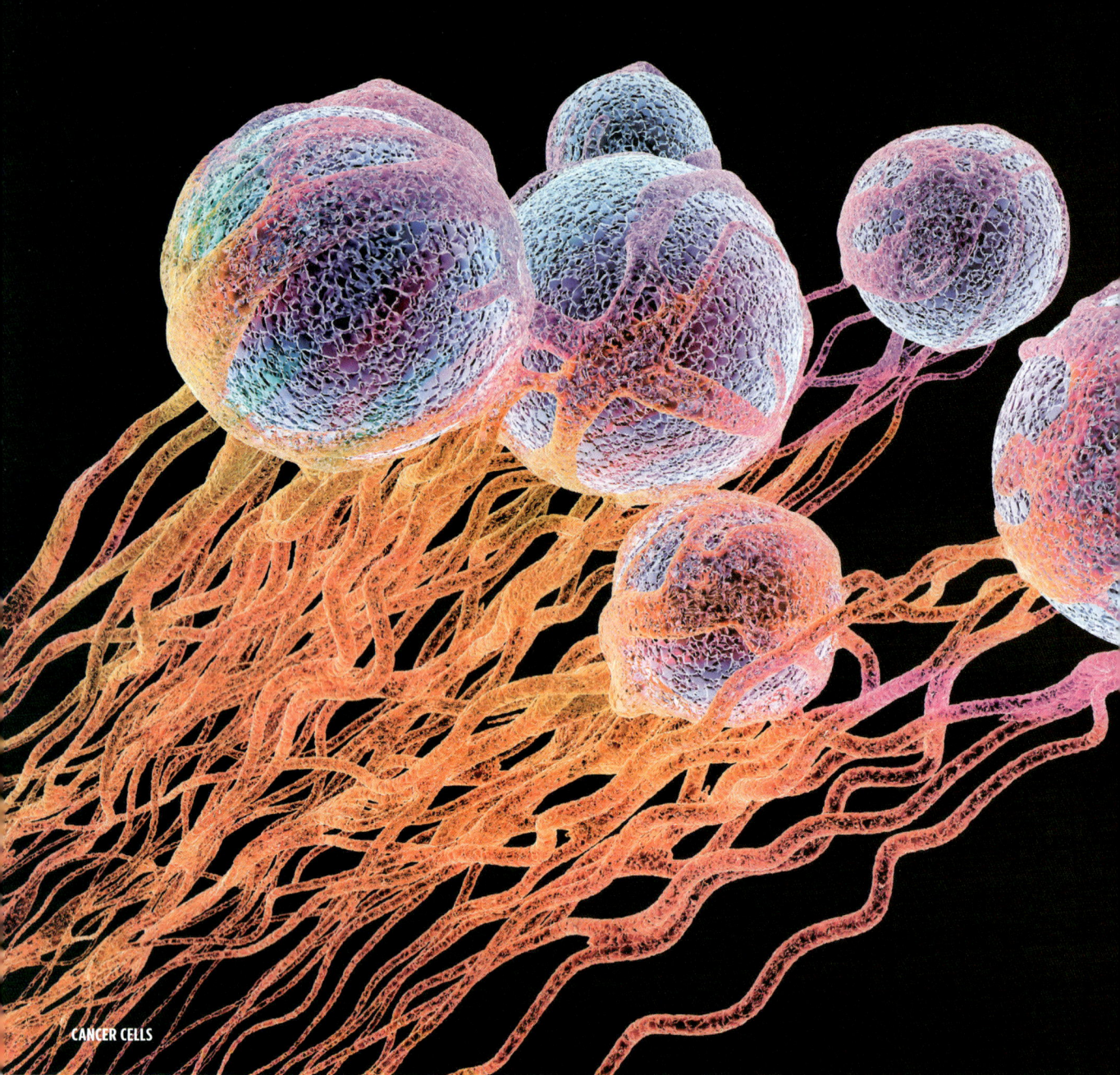

CANCER CELLS

Measuring Cancer's Unequal Impact

Overall, the prospects may be brighter – but not for everyone

PATIENT POWER

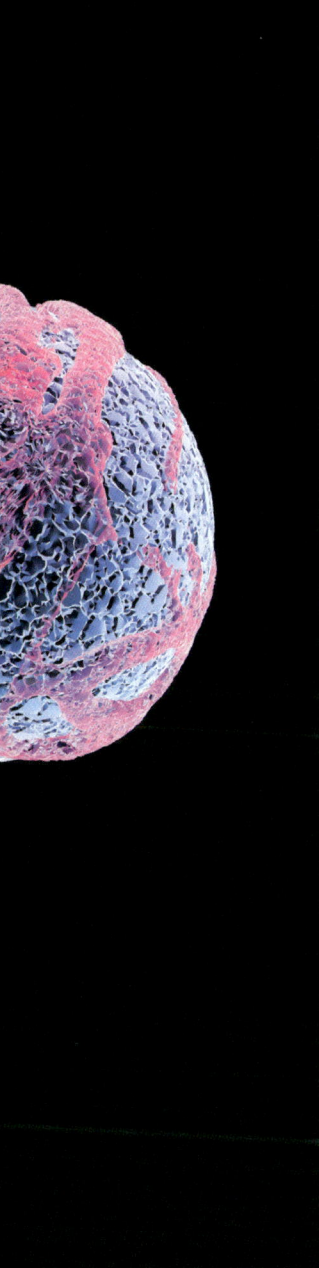

by **Lisa Esposito**

IN MANY WAYS, the U.S. cancer picture is getting better. Cancer is becoming increasingly curable or survivable as a manageable, chronic condition. However, barriers in access to care, noninclusive research, unequal reliance on preventive measures like screening, and findings of differences in treatment and outcomes among people with similar disease are signs of much work yet to be done. In its first report on the state of progress against cancer disparities, the American Association for Cancer Research late last year highlighted a number of inequities persisting even as overall death rates have been declining. Some of the findings:

- The cancer mortality rates remain disproportionate, though gaps are narrowing. For more than four decades, African Americans have had the highest overall cancer death rate of any racial or ethnic group in the U.S. In 2016, the cancer death rate was 14% higher for African Americans compared with whites. The rate was 33% higher for African Americans in 1990.
- Bisexual women are 70% more likely than heterosexual women to be diagnosed with cancer, according to the AACR report. However, more data are needed on disparities affecting the LGBTQ community. One issue is that patient intake forms don't always ask about sexual orientation.
- African American women have a 39% higher risk of dying from breast cancer than their white peers. "African American women are nearly twice as likely as white women to be diagnosed with triple-negative breast cancer, which is one of the more aggressive ones," points out Monica Baskin, a professor in the department of medicine and the associate director for community outreach and engagement at O'Neal Comprehensive Cancer Center at the University of Alabama at Birmingham.
- African Americans with colorectal cancer have a death rate topping 18%, compared with a 13.5% death rate for whites.
- Hispanic children are 20% more likely to develop leukemia than non-Hispanic white children, and that gap increases to 38% in adolescents.
- African American men with prostate cancer die at twice the rate of men of any other race or ethnicity. Overall, patients with the most common type of localized liver cancer who don't have health insurance survive only half as long as patients with private health insurance.

One problem is that minorities are seriously underrepresented in clinical studies. As a result, the understanding of how cancer develops in those populations is significantly lacking. Making clinical research more inclusive is a must for achieving equity in outcomes, says Dr. Carol Brown, chief health equity officer at Memorial Sloan Kettering Cancer Center and a gynecologic oncologist at MSK in New York City.

Unequal access to the latest advances in care is also key. "Another area where underserved patients – particularly racial and ethnic minorities – have not been historically included is in the realm of precision medicine," Brown says. Within the last five years or so, she says, "we've learned that all cancers, even if they're the same type and of the same organ, can be very different in their genetic makeup."

A targeted tumor-sequencing test developed by MSK researchers can identify mutations in more than 450 genes related to cancer, potentially indicating targets for cancer therapies. However, patients of different races and ethnicities haven't typically had an opportunity to participate in these types of studies, Brown says. "So we really haven't learned about the genetic makeup of these patients' cancers." Brown is working to change that dynamic.

PROGRESS CLOSING GAPS RELIES ON DOING A BETTER JOB OF ENGAGING COMMUNITIES IN PREVENTION.

Unequal access to clean air and water, healthy food, educational opportunity and secure employment, among other social factors underpinning health, may also contribute to cancer outcome disparities.

Baskin says her work is motivated by the loss of her father to colorectal cancer while she was a senior in high school. The cancer wasn't detected until it was too advanced to have a good chance of responding to treatment, and he died at 51. "Colorectal cancer is absolutely one that we can prevent," she says. "Making sure that everyone understands the progression of the disease, how we can go in to get screened, and making sure that people have access to that screening is really critical."

Unconscious bias that can affect decision-making by health care providers is another critical issue for Baskin. "It's important to educate providers around potential biases that might limit recommendations for certain

PATIENT POWER

patients to get certain treatments," she says.

A study on health care bias published in 2016 in the Journal of Clinical Oncology examined interactions between Black patients and non-Black oncologists who had previously completed a survey measuring their unconscious racial bias. Researchers noted that oncologists measuring higher in bias had shorter, less supportive exchanges with patients. Patients, who were asked how patient-centered the oncologists were and what they had taken from the interaction in terms of information, feelings of distress or trust and treatment perceptions, reported less confidence in recommended treatments and greater perceived difficulty in going though those treatments after interacting with more biased physicians.

"I'm motivated in my work," Baskin says, "just to call that out and help people to understand how important it is for everyone to have access to high-quality care."

"We all deserve to have equal outcomes regardless of the color of our skin or where we live or what access we may have to health insurance," says Kathy Briant, a public health researcher and program administrator for the Office of Community Outreach and Engagement at Fred Hutchinson Cancer Research Center in Seattle. "It's a human right. That's why disparities matter and why we do this work."

Beyond research and treatment, progress closing gaps relies on doing a better job of engaging communities in prevention. And true inclusion involves bringing people from the community to the table, Briant says. One Fred Hutch field office is located in Sunnyside in eastern Washington, a primarily agricultural area, she explains. For nearly 20 years, the bilingual, bicultural health education team has been running cancer prevention initiatives. "Because the people that have been hired are from the community, they're trusted, they're respected," she says. "So, it makes it really easy for them to engage different stakeholders."

Designing studies and deciding what kind of cancer research takes priority is a two-way street. "Through the community action board there, we've brought ideas about projects researchers want to work on, but the community members have also brought ideas," Briant says. "Such as, 'We believe obesity is important, but we're really worried about pesticides. We want to work at looking at: What does it do to us as farmworkers, being exposed and bringing pesticides home?'"

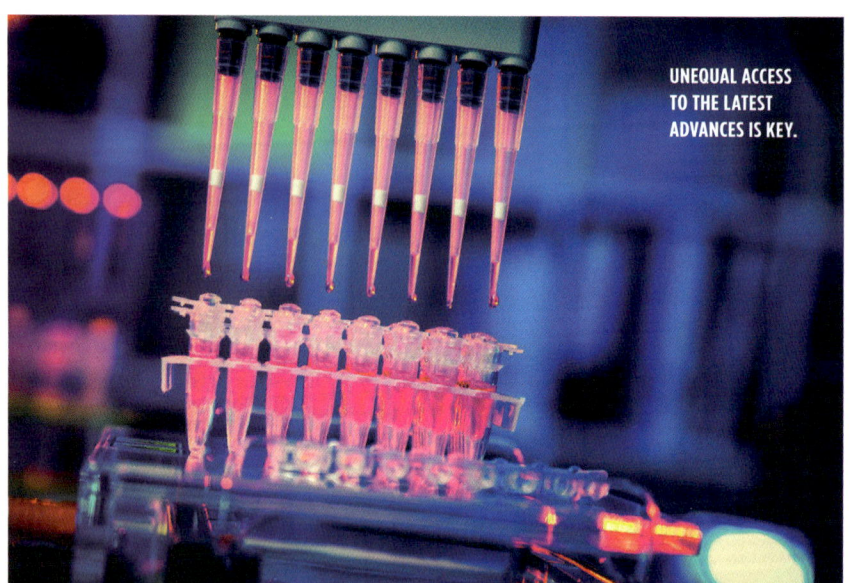

UNEQUAL ACCESS TO THE LATEST ADVANCES IS KEY.

What can you do? As an individual, you can take certain steps to make yourself and your loved ones less vulnerable to inequitable care:

Know your family history. With a father who died of colon cancer at a young age, and who also lost an eye to cancer earlier, Baskin knows that it's "really critical" for her to share that information with her health care provider so together they can "make decisions about when it's appropriate for me to get screened and what risk factors I have. Knowing that family history of cancer and other chronic conditions that run in families is really key."

Get recommended screenings and vaccinations. Age-appropriate cancer screening and vaccines – such as HPV vaccination against the human papillomavirus – may save your life. "It's really critical to catch cancer as early as possible to allow for treatment, as well as to maintain efforts to prevent individuals from actually having cancer," Baskin says.

Improve lifestyle behaviors. Maintaining a healthy diet, getting regular physical activity, managing your weight, quitting smoking, limiting alcohol and protecting yourself from ultraviolet radiation all represent efforts toward cancer prevention.

If diagnosed with cancer, ask about clinical trials. "Participating in a clinical trial is one of the most important ways that an individual patient can address these issues of disparities," Brown says. When you join a trial, she says, you will be followed extremely closely as a patient and receive the latest available advances in treatment and diagnosis. ●

> **"One problem is that minorities are seriously underrepresented in clinical studies."**

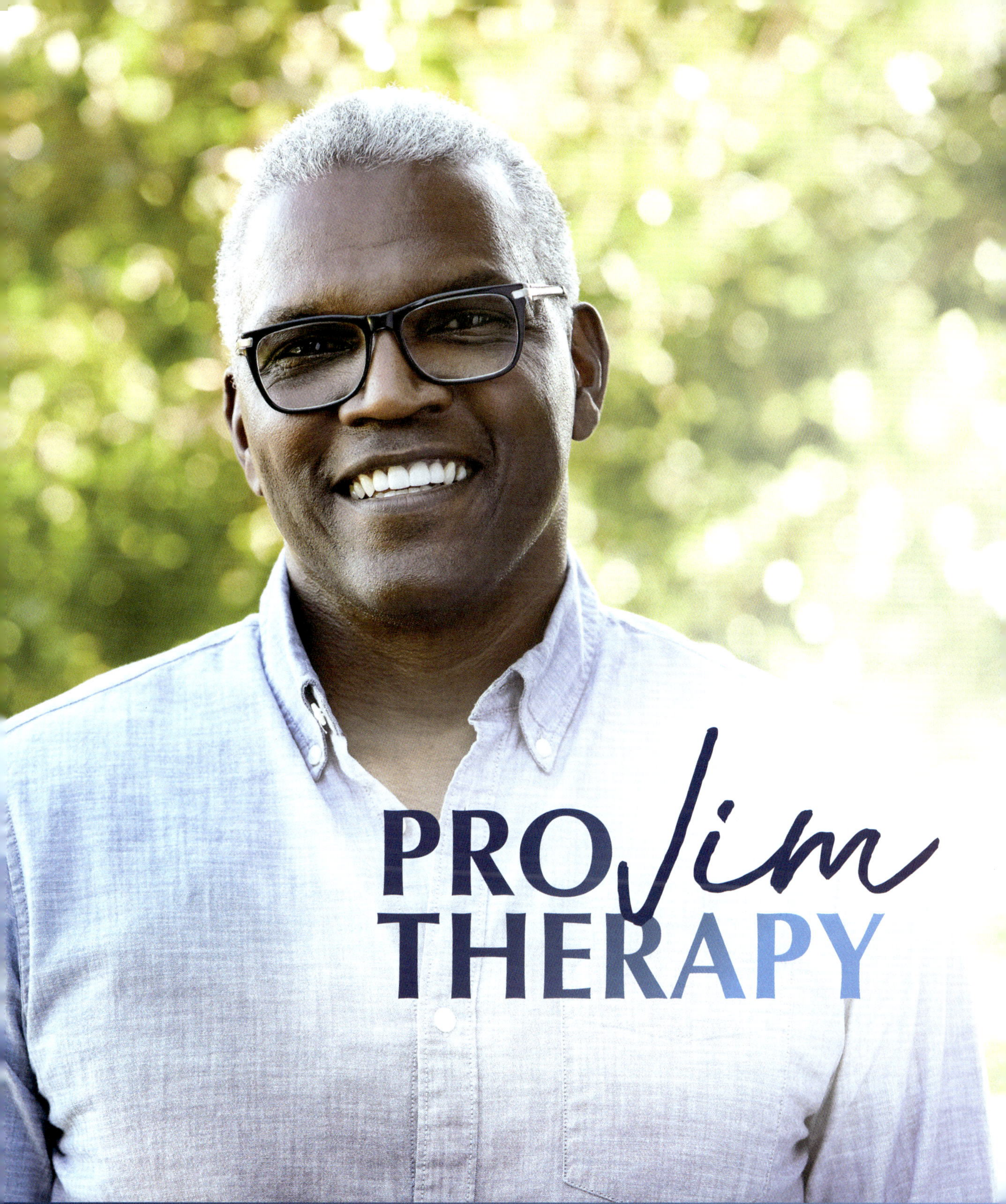

PRO*Jim* THERAPY

PROTON THERAPY is PRO YOU therapy.

We've added the country's top cancer-destroying technology for the simplest of reasons: to ensure your quality of life when you need it the most. To find out if this revolutionary new procedure can treat your cancer, visit **inova.org/protontherapy**.

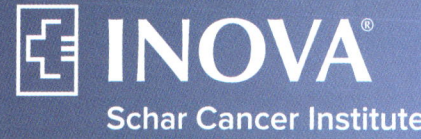

PATIENT POWER

Building Strength With a Purpose

Functional fitness training can help you reach your performance goals

by **Lisa Esposito**

A **WOMAN WANTS TO JOIN** her family on backpacking hikes. A golfer would like to strike the ball farther and avoid back soreness. A grandfather longs to lift his small grandchildren with confidence. An elite athlete is interested in pitching a baseball better. A virtual employee has become deconditioned and is suffering shoulder pain. An older adult needs to reduce the risk of falls and stay independent.

People in these scenarios have something in common: They all stand to benefit from functional fitness training. By learning proper movement patterns and strengthening key muscle groups, they can build power, coordination, balance and agility to reach their goals.

Definitions of functional training vary, to put it mildly. While group classes may promote boot-camp style training to build strength or improve your body shape, fitness experts emphasize the individualized, targeted nature of functional training programs, and goals that center on performing a specific activity.

Functional fitness consistently lands among the top 20 worldwide fitness trends in the yearly survey of health professionals conducted by ACSM's Health & Fitness Journal, published by the American College of Sports Medicine. (It hit the No. 14 spot in 2021.) So what does it entail? It starts with a goal or desired outcome regarding a specific function, such as an activity of daily living or a sport-related skill. A trainer assesses an individual's baseline – measuring muscular strength, range of motion, flexibility, reflexes, coordination and areas of pain or discomfort – to design an effective program, which will incorporate core functional movements such as squatting, bending, lifting, pulling and twisting.

A focus on patterns. Exercises combine several muscle groups and multiple joints rather than feature isolated movements like bicep curls. Movement patterns rather than individual muscles are the focus. Muscles are gradually strengthened and lengthened, and range of motion increased. Equipment tends to be simple:

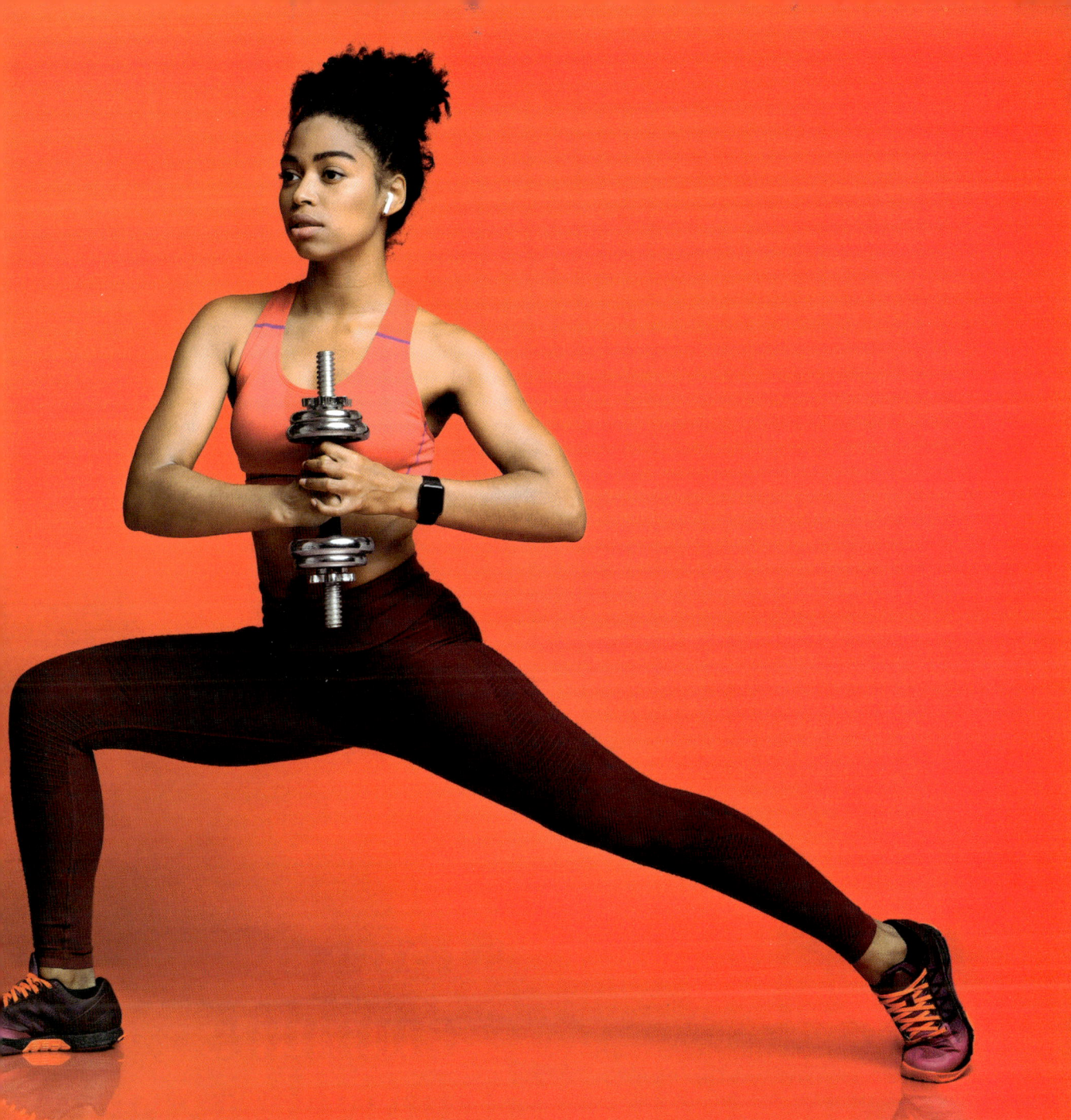

resistance bands, tubing, kettlebells, household items (like a dish), light weights and body weight itself.

"Functional training is all about movement quality," says Brad Roy, executive director of the Summit Medical Fitness Center at Kalispell Regional Healthcare in Montana. "Functional training is really neuromuscular training. It's training the mind, body and muscular system to work together to produce some kind of an outcome." While jogging, lifting weights or riding a bike can boost your overall fitness, they don't themselves constitute functional training (although they could be part of a functional program), notes Roy, who is also editor-in-chief of ACSM's Health & Fitness Journal.

This mode of exercise can be beneficial at any age. In fact, Roy argues, "resistance training and movement quality are really important and need to be emphasized at an equal level with cardiovascular fitness – and in some cases, maybe even emphasized more."

Function is a key focus of physical therapy, notes Clare Safran-Norton, an orthopedic specialist in physical therapy and clinical supervisor of the physical and occupational therapy ambulatory service at Brigham and Women's Hospital. "What are the activities you need to do in your life? It can be as simple as putting a shirt on or off, fastening a bra strap, or reaching for a cup or putting plates away in a cupboard," she says. "It can be getting on or off a chair, in and out of a car, or up and down stairs."

Training begins with a comprehensive assessment of

PATIENT POWER

"the function for the individual person," Safran-Norton says. "Then we test all the strength for all the muscles, the length of the muscles, whether they're tight or not, as well as range of motion."

These data points inform a tailored plan with the goal always in mind. "We balance the muscles that are tight, the muscles that are weak," Safran-Norton says. "Then, as we restore those individual muscles, we start to couple them with other muscles to restore back the function. So in the end, we're using a band with resistance to simulate the tennis swing, or we're using a golf club to simulate the golf swing. Or we're practicing putting the dish back into the cupboard." For functional training by a physical therapist, you need a medical diagnosis and physician referral.

The moves. Squatting, bending, lifting, pushing, pulling, rocking, turning and twisting are the types of core functional movements that are incorporated in a functional fitness training routine. "When we go to do an activity in life, we are always involving the whole body," says Cedric X. Bryant, president and chief science officer of the American Council on Exercise, or ACE (and a contributor to U.S. News). "Whether it's pushing a grocery cart or carrying groceries, what functional training tries to do is get the body to work in a coordinated fashion. So a lot of movements are going to focus on multi-joint exercises where you're involving multiple parts of the body to overcome the resistance. You're typically going to be working your upper and lower body and combining muscle groups."

The differences between what's traditionally considered fitness and functional fitness are "subtle and nuanced," Bryant says. "Fitness tends to focus on eliciting improvements in the different components, whether you improve your cardio performance or your abilities to either lift more weight or do more repetitions." By contrast, he says, functional fitness is focused on enhancing one's ability to perform certain activities "with greater ease, less discomfort and less risk for injury."

Functional fitness instructors can come from a variety of backgrounds. Clinical exercise physiologists, athletic trainers and physical therapists are skilled in aspects of functional training, Roy notes. Organizations such as ACSM and ACE offer certification for these professionals. "You want somebody who either has a degree in the field of exercise science and/or certifications from accredited agencies," says Leslie Stenger, an exercise physiologist and an assistant professor of kinesiology, health and sport science at Indiana University of Pennsylvania.

In her own life, Stenger has a functional training "client" she works with continually: her mother. Locomotion – moving from one point to another – is a problem. "She doesn't propel herself forward – she shuffles side to side," putting all her weight on one hip, Stenger says. So together they focus on the concept of forward propulsion, with proper weight-shifting from heel to toes throughout the foot.

Arthritis makes people change their gait, Stenger says. They tend to look down at their feet and stoop over. Resistance band exercises help them focus on pulling back their shoulders and squeezing their shoulder blades together, along with reminders to hold their head up. Practice leads to improvement. "Those neuromuscular

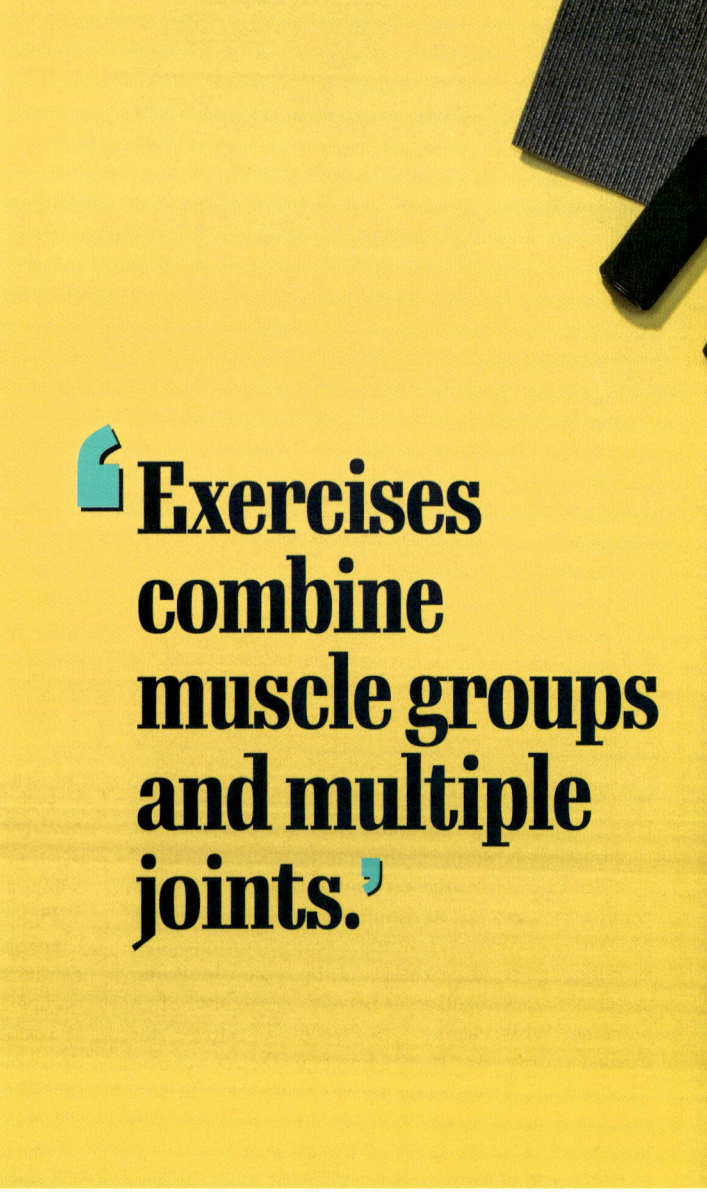

'Exercises combine muscle groups and multiple joints.'

pathways are established," she says. "With more repetition, it's going to happen."

At the opposite end of the spectrum, functional fitness can help people thrive in physically demanding occupations such as firefighting and the military. For example, high-intensity functional training, or HIFT, is used "to physically prepare military personnel for the unknown in terms of the types of movement patterns they will need when called to a job or emergency," Stenger says. This type of class would not be appropriate for everyone, she notes.

In between those extremes, people can take advantage of functional training for recreational sports, from prepping to run their first 5K to improving their game. For instance, you could have your tennis serve dissected and corrected. "They would look at that tennis serve from a biomechanical standpoint," Stenger says. "Eye-hand coordination, timing, reaction time – making sure you can get the ball up and hit it at the same time." Core development and rotation exercises would help your rotational movement, while working on acceleration and power would help you translate all your force up from the ground to the tennis racket, get more speed behind your ball and put it into the service box.

Meanwhile, "there's a whole area of youth development," Roy says, that could potentially help cut down on the plethora of overuse injuries in young athletes. "There are kids out there playing sports and specializing too young," Roy says. "They often drop out, they don't exercise later in life." Adding to the need, he says, is the fact that schools often don't offer much physical education. "So kids are not, at early ages, getting the right movement patterns and learning how to do these different kinds of movements correctly."

Kids need to learn basics, such as how to run correctly. "Teaching running techniques, how to change directions, is really important," Roy says. "How not just to jump, but also how to land." Activities and games that build these skills can lead to success later on in whichever sports young people want to do, he says.

Meaningful results. With functional training, Bryant finds, "the results – because they really connect to the individual's 'why' – are more meaningful. And they really have much greater impact on motivating the individual to continue down that path still more. Because rather than just looking at numbers and saying, 'OK, I can lift more weight – so what?' if you can say, 'Boy, I can experience the joy of more life,' that's a big deal." Some of Bryant's most rewarding work is with more mature clients who've had limitations in mobility, he says. "It kind of causes them to be prisoners in their own body."

The training can also do a lot of good for someone who's been quite sedentary and lost muscular function, he says. "You might have that person just practice getting up and out of a chair – maybe try to do it 10 times during commercials if they're watching television." Next, the person could work on getting out of the chair and reaching overhead.

"It can start that simply," Bryant says. As a person becomes stronger, "you can introduce some resistance in terms of doing it with a light weight, introduce some type of balance challenge." The declines didn't occur overnight, he points out, and fixing them is also going to take time. ●

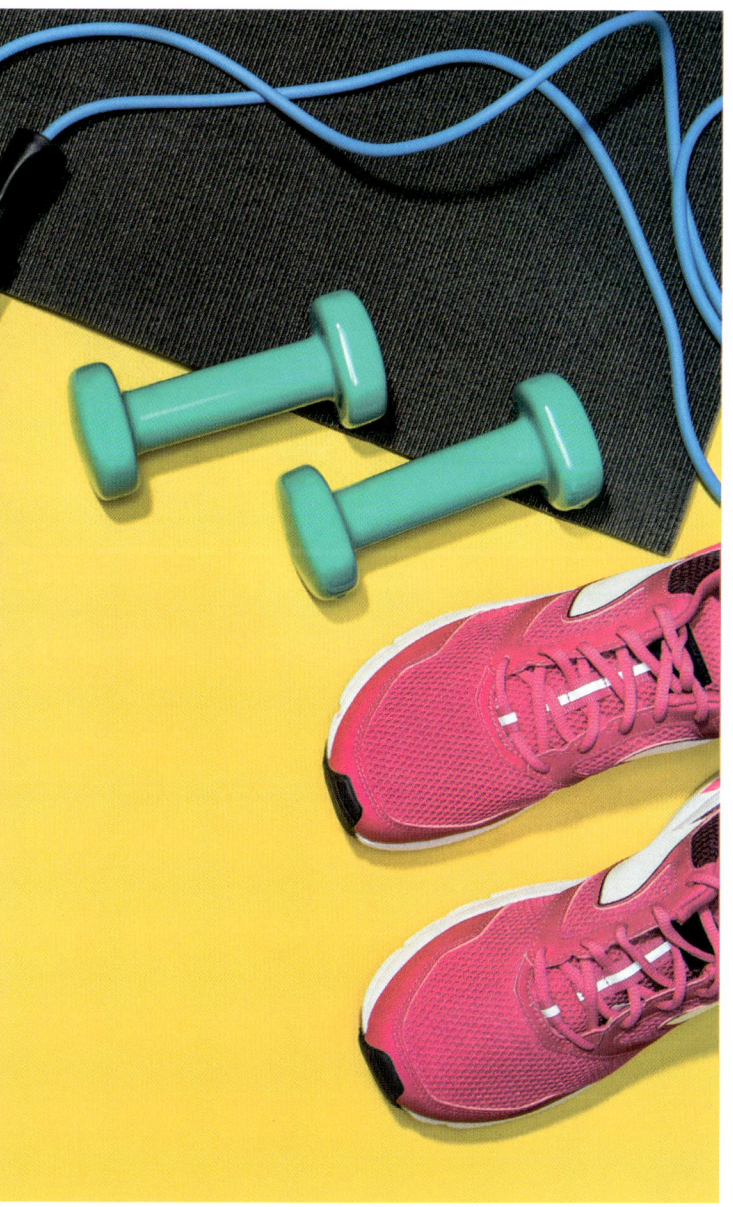

PATIENT POWER

Best Diets of 2021

Your goal: to find the plan that will work for you

by **Angela Haupt**

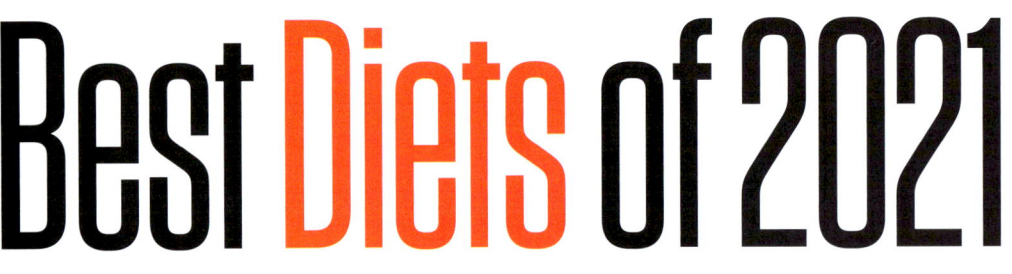

WHAT MAKES A DIET "BEST"? In the latest set of exclusive rankings from U.S. News weighing the merits and shortcomings of 39 eating plans, the Mediterranean diet beat out the competition to win the "Best Diets Overall" crown. Among the 15 commercial diet programs marketed to the public, WW (Weight Watchers) came out on top. We also ranked the diets on likelihood of weight loss, ability to prevent and control diabetes and heart disease, healthiness and how easy they are to follow.

Our analysis puts hard numbers on the commonsense belief that no diet is ideal for everybody.

Take DASH, which tied with Flexitarian as the No. 2 Best Diet Overall. It wasn't created as a way to drop pounds, but as a means of combating high blood pressure; the name stands for Dietary Approaches to Stop Hypertension. If losing weight is your primary goal, a diet in our Best Weight-Loss Diets rankings would be a more likely choice. Each diet was scored by a panel of experts in short-term and long-term weight loss, on how easy it is to follow, how well it conforms to current nutrition standards and on health risks it may pose – plus its soundness as a diabetes and as a heart-healthy diet.

At usnews.com/bestdiets, you'll find a detailed profile of each diet that tells you how it works, what evidence supports (or refutes) its claims, a nutritional snapshot – right down to daily milligrams of potassium – and, of course, a close look at the food you'd eat.

Once you've whittled down your eligible diets to a few, consider your personality and lifestyle. If you're a foodie, you probably won't be happy with a plan built around frozen dinners, or mostly just-add-water meals. If cutting carbs will make you cranky, you'll want to stay away from low-carb diets such as Atkins and South Beach.

Then think about what did and didn't work the last time you were on a diet. Was it too restrictive? Lots of diets we covered don't consider any food off-limits. Didn't provide enough structure? Some plans will tell you exactly what to eat and when. Ask yourself: How long can I stay on this? If you can't stick with it in the long run, you'll be back where you started after a couple months.

We're not going to tell you what diet you should be on, but we can help lead you to a winner – the best diet for you. ●

How We Rank Diets

U.S. News and a panel of experts rated 39 eating plans

AS MANY DIETERS have painfully learned, taking off weight can be a serious challenge. This is why U.S. News produces its Best Diets rankings, based on the views of nationally recognized experts (Page 102) who considered the effectiveness of some of the best-known eating plans. Our panelists reviewed the research, added their own fact-finding, and rated the diets from 1 to 5 (the top score) in a number of areas: short-term weight loss (the likelihood of losing significant weight during the first 12 months); long-term weight loss (the likelihood of maintaining significant weight loss for two years or more); diabetes prevention and management; heart health (effectiveness at preventing cardiovascular disease and reducing risk for heart patients); ease of compliance; nutritional completeness (how well a plan meets federal dietary guidelines); and safety (whether, for example, a diet omits key nutrients).

Which plan can help you achieve your goals? Check out the results in these pages. For more on the plans, visit usnews.com/bestdiets.

How the Plans Compare Overall

Thirty-nine diets were rated from 1 to 5 on multiple measures. Rank is based on a score compiled from panelists' average scores for each measure. The results:

Rank	Diet	Overall score	Short-term weight loss	Long-term weight loss	For diabetes	For heart health	Nutrition	Safety	Easy to follow
1	Mediterranean	4.2	3.0	3.1	3.6	4.3	4.8	4.8	3.8
2	DASH	4.1	3.0	3.4	3.5	4.3	4.8	4.8	3.3
2	Flexitarian	4.1	3.6	3.5	3.6	4.0	4.6	4.8	3.5
4	WW (Weight Watchers)	3.9	3.9	3.4	3.3	3.3	4.6	4.5	3.6
5	Mayo Clinic	3.8	3.4	3.2	3.5	3.5	4.5	4.4	3.1
5	MIND	3.8	2.7	2.7	3.3	3.7	4.5	4.5	3.4
5	TLC	3.8	3.0	2.8	3.0	4.0	4.5	4.6	2.8
5	Volumetrics	3.8	3.7	3.4	3.3	3.3	4.5	4.5	3.1
9	Nordic	3.6	2.8	3.0	3.0	3.2	4.5	4.5	2.5
9	Ornish	3.6	3.5	3.0	3.3	4.3	4.2	4.2	2.0
9	Vegetarian	3.6	3.2	3.0	3.2	3.7	4.3	4.2	2.7
12	Jenny Craig	3.5	3.7	3.0	3.4	3.0	3.9	4.0	3.2
12	Noom	3.5	3.3	2.9	2.8	2.8	4.2	4.2	3.1
14	Anti-Inflammatory	3.4	2.6	2.5	3.0	3.5	3.9	4.0	2.7
14	Asian	3.4	2.9	2.9	2.6	3.1	4.3	4.3	2.6
14	Fertility	3.4	2.4	2.2	3.0	2.9	4.1	4.0	3.3
17	Nutritarian	3.3	3.3	2.7	3.2	3.3	3.8	3.9	2.0
17	Vegan	3.3	3.6	3.3	3.5	4.0	3.1	3.6	1.8
19	Engine 2	3.2	3.5	2.9	3.3	3.6	3.4	3.5	1.8
20	Biggest Loser	3.0	3.8	2.2	2.8	2.7	3.5	3.5	2.3
20	Glycemic-Index	3.0	2.8	2.3	2.9	2.4	3.5	3.8	2.1
20	Nutrisystem	3.0	3.7	2.5	2.9	2.5	3.2	3.5	2.6
20	South Beach	3.0	3.3	2.5	2.8	2.7	3.3	3.3	2.8
20	Zone	3.0	3.2	2.4	2.6	2.7	3.4	3.5	2.2
25	Macrobiotic	2.9	3.0	2.6	3.0	3.2	3.1	3.3	1.7
26	HMR Program	2.8	4.0	2.2	2.6	2.4	3.0	3.0	2.6
26	SlimFast	2.8	3.7	2.4	2.7	2.3	2.9	3.0	2.8
28	Optavia	2.6	3.8	2.2	2.8	2.6	2.5	2.8	2.1
29	Acid Alkaline	2.5	2.3	1.8	2.2	2.3	2.8	3.1	2.0
30	Fast	2.4	3.1	2.1	2.1	2.2	2.5	2.5	2.2
31	Paleo	2.3	3.0	2.1	2.5	1.9	2.1	2.6	1.8
32	Raw Food	2.2	3.7	2.8	2.8	2.6	2.0	2.0	1.1
33	AIP	2.1	2.3	1.7	2.0	1.7	1.8	2.8	1.6
33	Atkins	2.1	3.9	2.1	2.6	1.9	1.7	2.1	1.7
35	Modified Keto	2.0	3.5	2.1	2.4	1.6	1.6	2.1	1.4
35	Whole30	2.0	2.9	1.7	1.9	1.7	1.9	2.4	1.4
37	GAPS	1.9	2.2	1.8	2.0	1.8	1.7	2.4	1.3
37	Ketogenic	1.9	3.8	2.1	2.6	1.8	1.3	1.9	1.4
39	Dukan	1.8	3.0	1.8	1.8	1.4	1.5	2.0	1.3

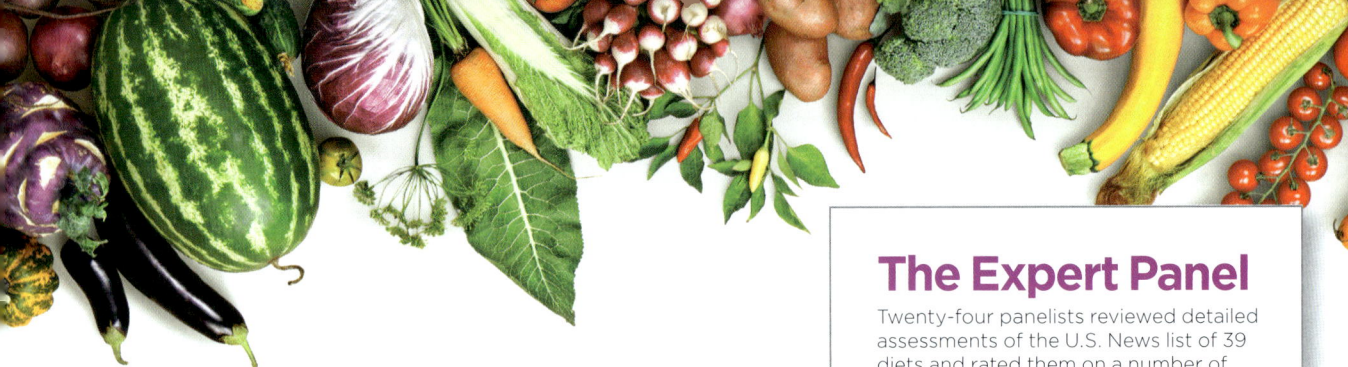

Best Weight-Loss Diets

Diets are ranked by the average of the scores experts assigned them for producing short- and long-term results.

Rank	Diet	Avg. score
1	Flexitarian	3.6
1	(WW) Weight Watchers	3.6
3	Vegan	3.5
3	Volumetrics	3.5
5	Jenny Craig	3.4
6	Mayo Clinic	3.3
6	Ornish	3.3
6	Raw Food	3.3
9	DASH	3.2
9	Engine 2	3.2

Best Diabetes Diets

These plans scored highest for both managing and preventing the condition.

Rank	Diet	Avg. score
1	Flexitarian	3.6
1	Mediterranean	3.6
3	DASH	3.5
3	Mayo Clinic	3.5
3	Vegan	3.5
6	Jenny Craig	3.4
7	Engine 2	3.3
7	MIND	3.3
7	Ornish	3.3
7	Volumetrics	3.3
7	(WW) Weight Watchers	3.3

Easiest-to-Follow Diets

The ranking is based on ease of implementation and ability to deliver weight loss and nutrition.

Rank	Diet	Avg. score
1	Mediterranean	3.8
2	(WW) Weight Watchers	3.6
3	Flexitarian	3.5
4	MIND	3.4
5	DASH	3.3
5	Fertility	3.3
7	Jenny Craig	3.2
8	Mayo Clinic	3.1
8	Noom	3.1
8	Volumetrics	3.1

Best Diets for the Heart

With these plans, you can take aim at cholesterol, blood pressure and triglycerides, as well as weight.

Rank	Diet	Avg. score
1	DASH	4.3
1	Mediterranean	4.3
1	Ornish	4.3
4	Flexitarian	4.0
4	TLC	4.0
4	Vegan	4.0
7	MIND	3.7
7	Vegetarian	3.7
9	Engine 2	3.6
10	Anti-Inflammatory	3.5
10	Mayo Clinic	3.5

Best Plant-Based Diets

These diets emphasize minimally processed foods from plants and are good bets for weight loss.

Rank	Diet	Avg. score
1	Mediterranean	4.2
2	Flexitarian	4.1
3	Nordic	3.6
3	Ornish	3.6
3	Vegetarian	3.6
6	Anti-Inflammatory	3.4
6	Asian	3.4
8	Nutritarian	3.3
8	Vegan	3.3
10	Engine 2	3.2

Best Commercial Diets

Nutritional value, ease of use and safety are counted, as well as weight-loss effectiveness.

Rank	Diet	Avg. score
1	(WW) Weight Watchers	3.9
2	Mayo Clinic	3.8
3	Jenny Craig	3.5
3	Noom	3.5
5	Nutritarian	3.3
6	Engine 2	3.2
7	Nutrisystem	3.0
7	South Beach	3.0
7	Zone	3.0
10	HMR Program	2.8
10	SlimFast	2.8

The Expert Panel

Twenty-four panelists reviewed detailed assessments of the U.S. News list of 39 diets and rated them on a number of key measures, described on Page 101.

Louis Aronne
Professor of metabolic research at Weill Cornell Medical College

Katherine Beals
Associate professor, clinical, department of nutrition and integrative physiology, University of Utah

Amy Campbell
Nutrition and wellness consultant and writer

Lawrence Cheskin
Chair, Department of Nutrition and Food Studies, George Mason University

Michael Dansinger
Founding director of the Diabetes Reversal Program at Tufts Medical Center

Michael Davidson
Professor, director of the Lipid Clinic, University of Chicago Pritzker School of Medicine

Meredith Dillon
Certified diabetes educator and registered dietitian, Children's Hospital of Philadelphia

Teresa Fung
Professor of nutrition, Simmons College

Christopher Gardner
Professor of medicine, Stanford University

Hollie Gelberg
Private practice/consultant dietitian at Healthy Eating and Training Inc.

Andrea Giancoli
Nutrition communications consultant

Michael Greger
Physician, author and internationally recognized speaker on nutrition, food safety and public health issues

David Katz
President, True Health Initiative

Penny Kris-Etherton
Distinguished professor of nutrition, Pennsylvania State University

JoAnn Manson
Professor of women's health, Harvard Medical School

Yasmin Mossavar-Rahmani
Associate professor of clinical epidemiology and population health, Albert Einstein College of Medicine

Elisabetta Politi
Nutrition director, Duke Diet and Fitness Center

Rebecca Reeves
Adjunct assistant professor, University of Texas School of Public Health

Eric Rimm
Professor of epidemiology and nutrition, and director of the Program in Cardiovascular Epidemiology at the Harvard T.H. Chan School of Public Health

Lisa Sasson
Clinical associate professor of nutrition, food studies and public health, New York University

Toby Smithson
Founder of DiabetesEveryDay.com and Diabetes EveryDay YouTube channel

Laurence Sperling
Founder and director of the Heart Disease Prevention Center at Emory University

Anne Thorndike
Assistant professor of medicine at Harvard Medical School and an associate physician at Massachusetts General Hospital

Jill Weisenberger
Author, health and wellness coach, and internationally recognized expert in nutrition and diabetes

PATIENT POWER

Mediterranean Moves

An expert's view of the pleasures of the 2021 top diet overall

by **Kelly Toups**

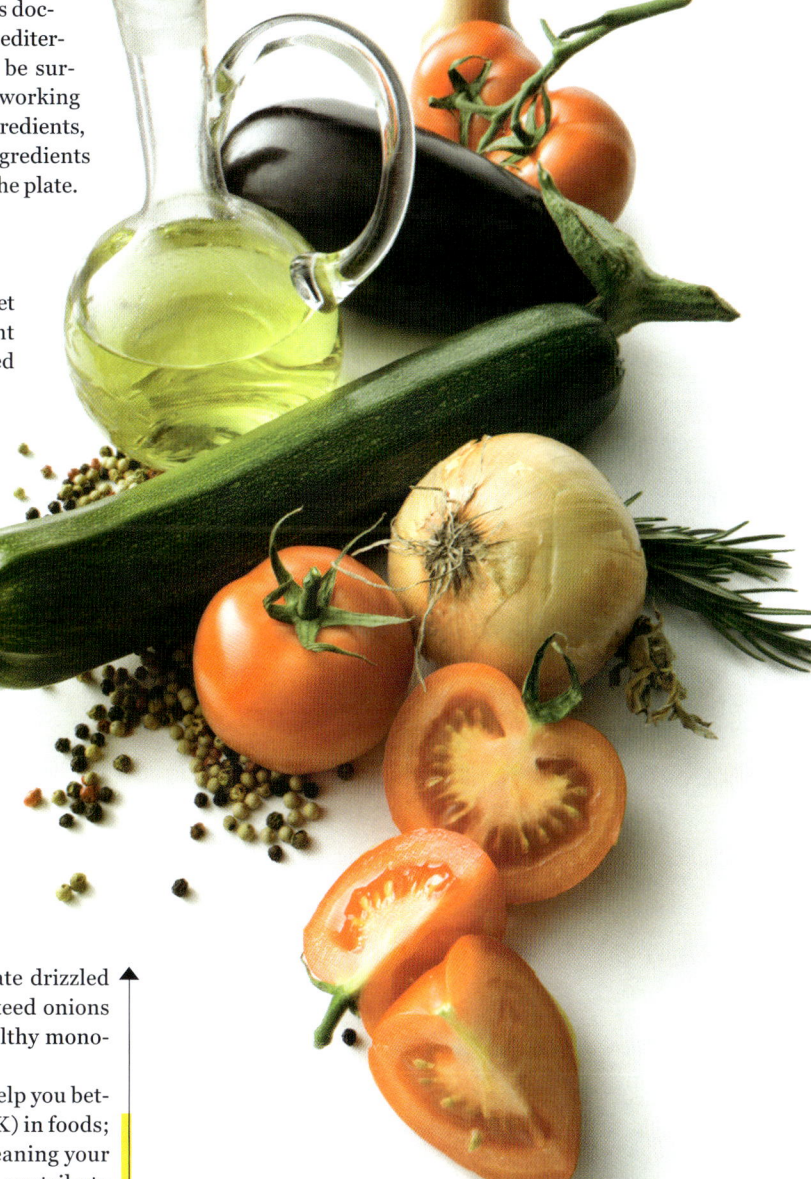

YOU DON'T HAVE to hop on an airplane to enjoy the numerous documented health benefits of a Mediterranean diet. In fact, you may be surprised to learn that you'll be working with many already familiar ingredients, such as pasta. The difference lies in how these ingredients are served – and what they're partnered with on the plate. Here are a few tips to help you get started:

1. Put flavor first.

One of the best things about the Mediterranean diet is that it really isn't a "diet" at all. Flavor is front and center in this style of eating, which is steeped in a rich culinary and cultural heritage. Mediterranean vegetables in particular steal the show in dishes like Pantescan salad with capers (a flavorful tomato and potato salad), orecchiette con cime di rapa (pasta with broccoli rabe and chile peppers) or fattoush (a vegetable and pita bread salad).

To give ordinary foods a Mediterranean flair, brighten them with a squeeze of fresh lemon or orange juice, add a drizzle of extra virgin olive oil and season them with a generous handful of fresh herbs. Not only do these ingredients add acidity, richness and inviting aromas, but also they're a healthy way to season dishes without relying too heavily on salt.

2. Opt for olive oil.

Olive oil is your go-to fat. It's just as appropriate drizzled over vegetable salads as it is as the base of sauteed onions and tomatoes. Olive oil is a source of heart-healthy monounsaturated fats and polyphenols.

Having a little bit of fat with your meals can help you better absorb the fat soluble vitamins (A, D, E and K) in foods; can reduce the glycemic response of a meal, meaning your blood sugar won't spike as much; and can also contribute

PATIENT POWER

GETTY IMAGES

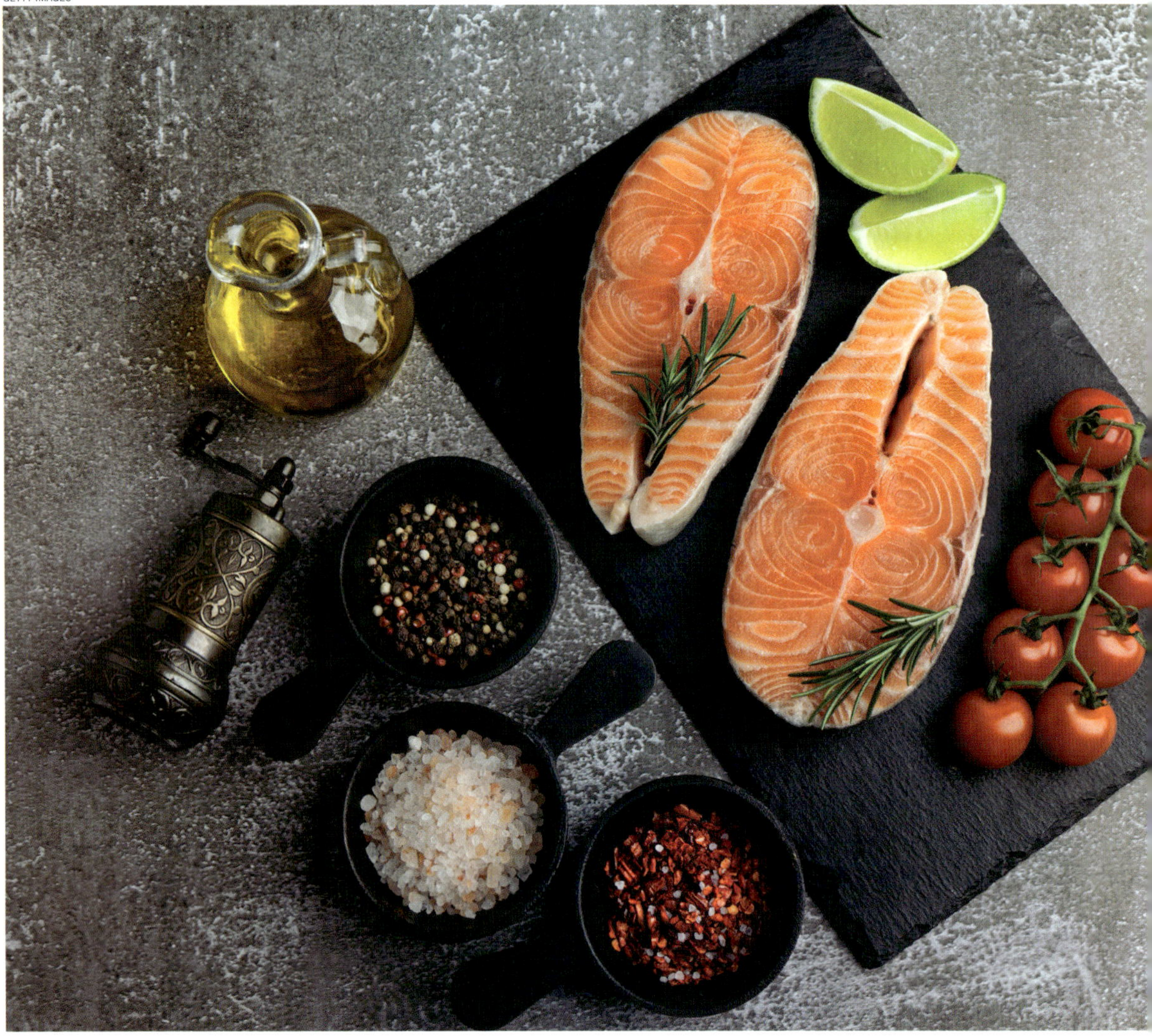

to satiety, so you aren't immediately hungry again. In one study of more than 90,000 people, those eating more than ½ tablespoon of olive oil per day had a 14% to 17% lower risk of heart disease compared with people who didn't eat olive oil. The scientists also found that replacing 5 grams per day of butter, margarine, mayonnaise or dairy fat with the equivalent amount of olive oil was linked with a 5% to 7% lower risk of heart disease.

A product labeled "extra virgin olive oil" was naturally extracted (cold processed) with no heat or chemicals and has more of its original flavors and nutrients intact. Extra virgin is the highest-quality virgin olive oil, meeting both chemical (acidity) and sensory (taste and smell) standards set by the International Olive Council.

For the best health benefits, it's important to store olive oil without exposure to light, heat and oxygen, and to use it before the best-by date on the bottle.

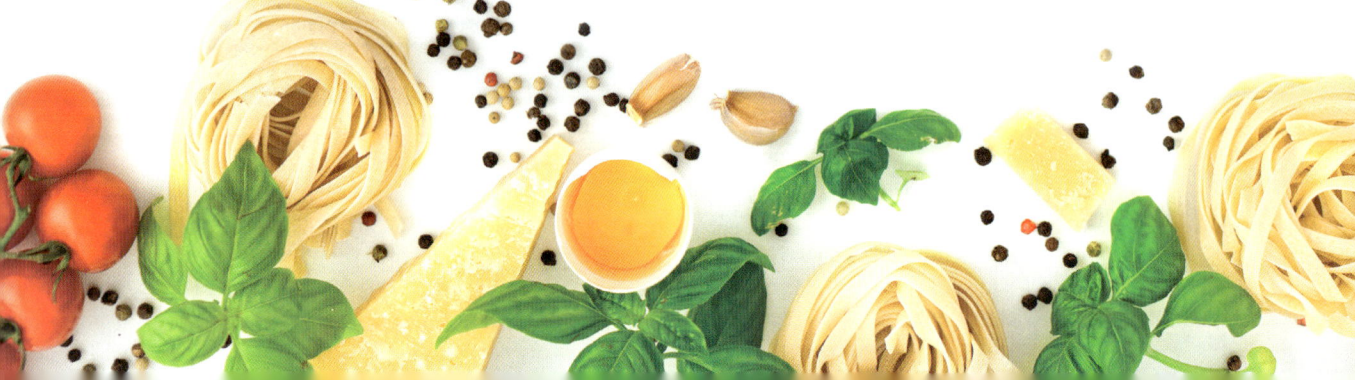

3. Feast on fish.

While most Americans generally eat enough protein, we tend to over-sample from the meat and poultry categories and fall short on seafood and plant-based proteins like legumes. One easy way to embrace the Mediterranean diet is to have seafood-based meals a few times per week.

Not all fish are created equal in the flavor and texture department. Grilled shrimp and grilled octopus have a pleasant, meaty texture, while salmon can be buttery and almost steak-like in its richness. Pan-fried sardine or salmon patties are also a delicious choice. For an affordable and easy weeknight option, turn to canned or pouched tuna or salmon.

4. Bring on the beans.

There are plenty of plant-based Mediterranean dishes that provide protein. Many popular recipes feature this combination of protein and fiber, among them pasta e fagioli (an Italian pasta and bean soup) and espinacas con garbanzos (a Spanish dish made of stewed chickpeas and spinach).

Try using lentils in a casserole or vegetarian Bolognese sauce, mixing chickpeas or cannellini beans into pasta or grain bowls, or choosing hummus or a nut-based trail mix as a snack. Additionally, walnuts and flaxseed offer plant-based sources of omega-3 fatty acids and are important to eat if fish is not frequently on your menu.

5. Find fermented dairy foods.

In the traditional Mediterranean diet, milk spoiled quickly, so it was often enjoyed in small amounts in its fermented form – as yogurt or artisan cheese. Fermented foods are linked with healthy changes to the gut microbiome.

Although dairy is important in a Mediterranean diet, the focus is on quality over quantity. A small amount of a flavorful cheese can be the perfect finishing touch to a mixed green and tomato salad or a warm bowl of whole wheat pasta. Creamy, protein-filled Greek yogurt is delightful in a breakfast bowl with fresh fruit, mixed nuts and a drizzle of honey. To explore the savory side of yogurt, make a tzatziki sauce with Greek yogurt, garlic and fresh herbs and serve it as a dip for fresh or roasted vegetables.

6. Embrace the rest of the lifestyle, too.

The base of the Mediterranean diet pyramid we use at Oldways depicts images of people eating together, cooking together and being active to illustrate that these practices are an important part of an overall Mediterranean lifestyle that can help us manage stress and maintain our health. Traditionally, Mediterranean meals were not rushed eating occasions in a cubicle or drive-through, but rather were a time for socializing with loved ones. And in places like Italy, Spain and Greece, dinner is often followed by an evening walk. While many people have sacrificed mindful meals in managing their busy lifestyles, the tide may be turning. For some families, the COVID-19 pandemic has created space to reclaim mealtime and savor home-cooked recipes with loved ones. No matter where you are, you can take a Mediterranean staycation by embracing the key elements of the diet and lifestyle – and be well on your way to better health and well-being. ●

Kelly Toups is a registered dietitian and director of nutrition at Oldways, a nonprofit organization that inspires people to rediscover the joys of the old ways of eating.

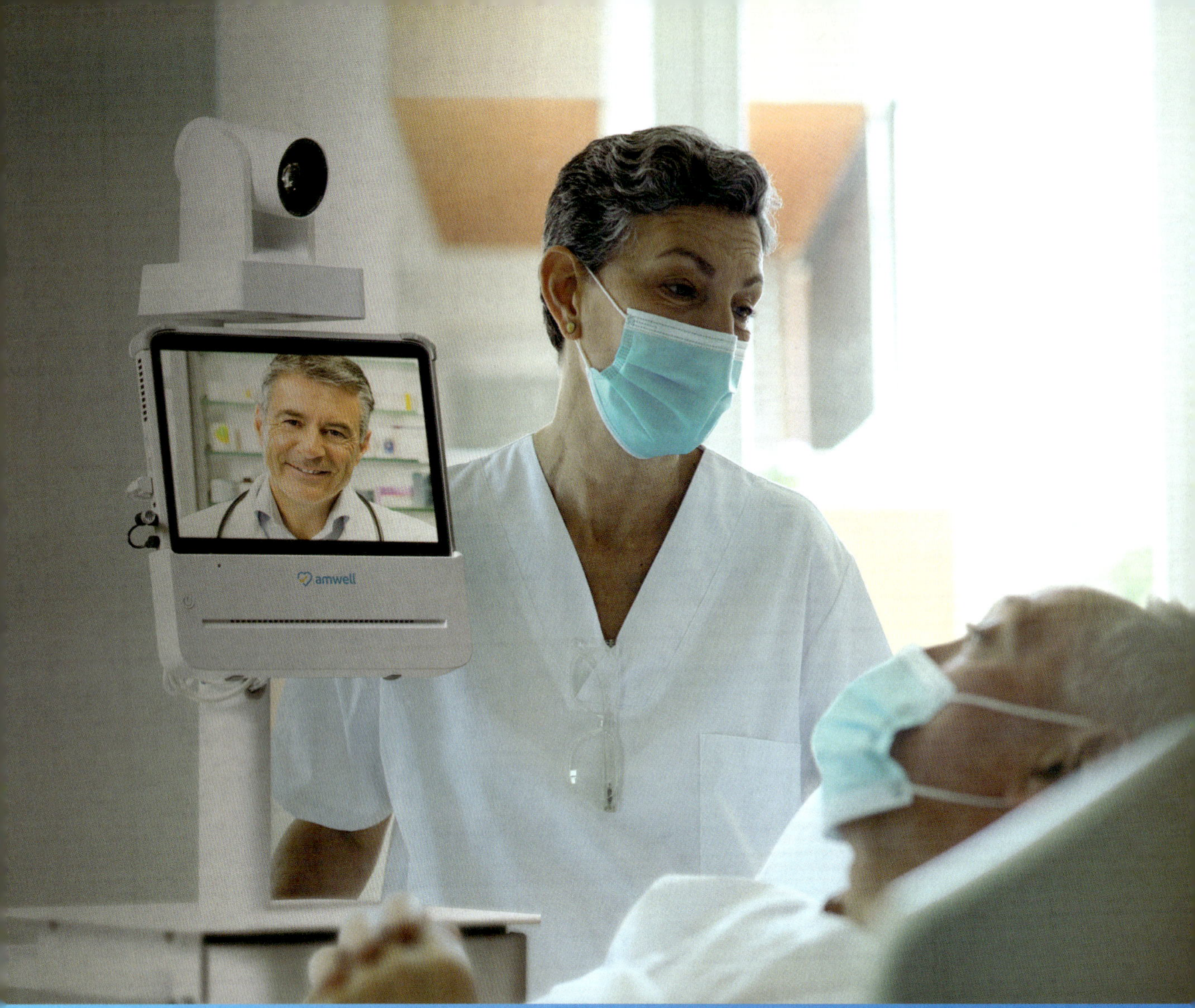

CONGRATULATIONS
TO THE 2021-22 BEST HOSPITALS!

Amwell is a proud partner of the nation's leading health systems and hospitals, working together to transform healthcare through digital care delivery.

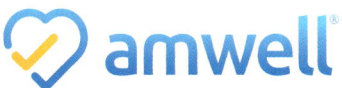

amwell.com

CHAPTER 3

Best Hospitals

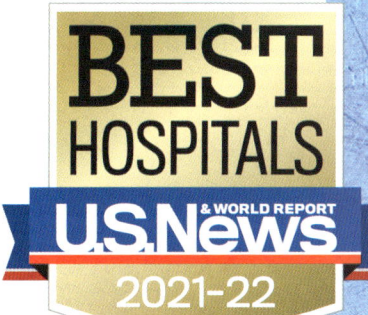

- 108 The Honor Roll
- 110 A Guide to the Rankings
- 114 Cancer
- 118 Cardiology & Heart Surgery
- 124 Diabetes & Endocrinology
- 126 Ear, Nose & Throat
- 130 Gastroenterology & GI Surgery
- 131 Geriatrics
- 132 Gynecology
- 134 Neurology & Neurosurgery
- 136 Orthopedics
- 140 Pulmonology & Lung Surgery
- 142 Rehabilitation
- 144 Urology
- 146 Ophthalmology, Psychiatry, Rheumatology

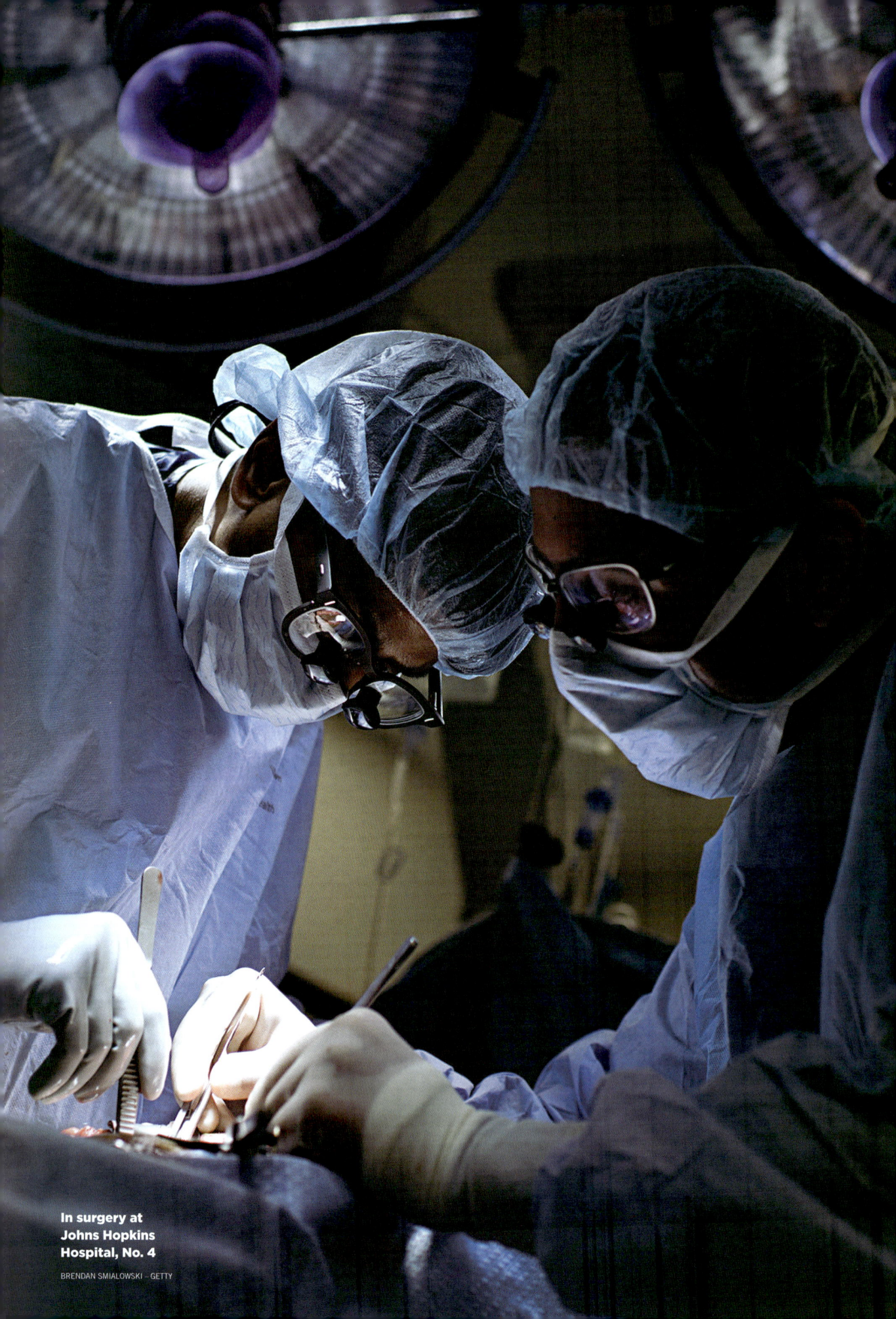

In surgery at Johns Hopkins Hospital, No. 4

BRENDAN SMIALOWSKI — GETTY

U.S. NEWS & WORLD REPORT

Best Hospitals
HONOR ROLL

BEST HOSPITALS U.S. News & WORLD REPORT HONOR ROLL 2021-22

The 20 medical centers below excel in treating patients with complex diagnoses and those with relatively routine needs. Each is nationally ranked in 9 or more of the 15 Best Hospitals specialties and is rated "high performing" in most or all of 17 common procedures and conditions (full ratings at usnews.com/best-hospitals). Honor Roll standing is based on points. A hospital that was ranked No. 1 in all specialties and rated high performing in all procedures and conditions would have received 507 points. The 20 highest scorers qualified for the Honor Roll.

1 Mayo Clinic
Rochester, Minnesota
456 points

2 Cleveland Clinic
419 points

3 UCLA Medical Center
Los Angeles
406 points

4 Johns Hopkins Hospital
Baltimore
405 points

5 Massachusetts General Hospital
Boston, 386 points

6 Cedars-Sinai Medical Center
Los Angeles, 379 points

7 New York-Presbyterian Hospital-Columbia and Cornell
New York, 364 points

8 NYU Langone Hospitals
New York
360 points

9 UCSF Medical Center
San Francisco
331 points

10 Northwestern Memorial Hospital
Chicago
316 points

11 University of Michigan Hospitals-Michigan Medicine
Ann Arbor, 313 points

12 Stanford Health Care-Stanford Hospital
Stanford, California
309 points

13 Hospitals of the University of Pennsylvania-Penn Presbyterian
Philadelphia
304 points

14 Brigham and Women's Hospital
Boston, 299 points

15 Mayo Clinic-Phoenix
291 points

16 Houston Methodist Hospital
277 points

17* Barnes-Jewish Hospital
St. Louis
272 points

17* Mount Sinai Hospital
New York
272 points

19 Rush University Medical Center
Chicago, 252 points

20 Vanderbilt University Medical Center
Nashville, Tennessee
251 points

*Denotes a tie

BEST HOSPITALS

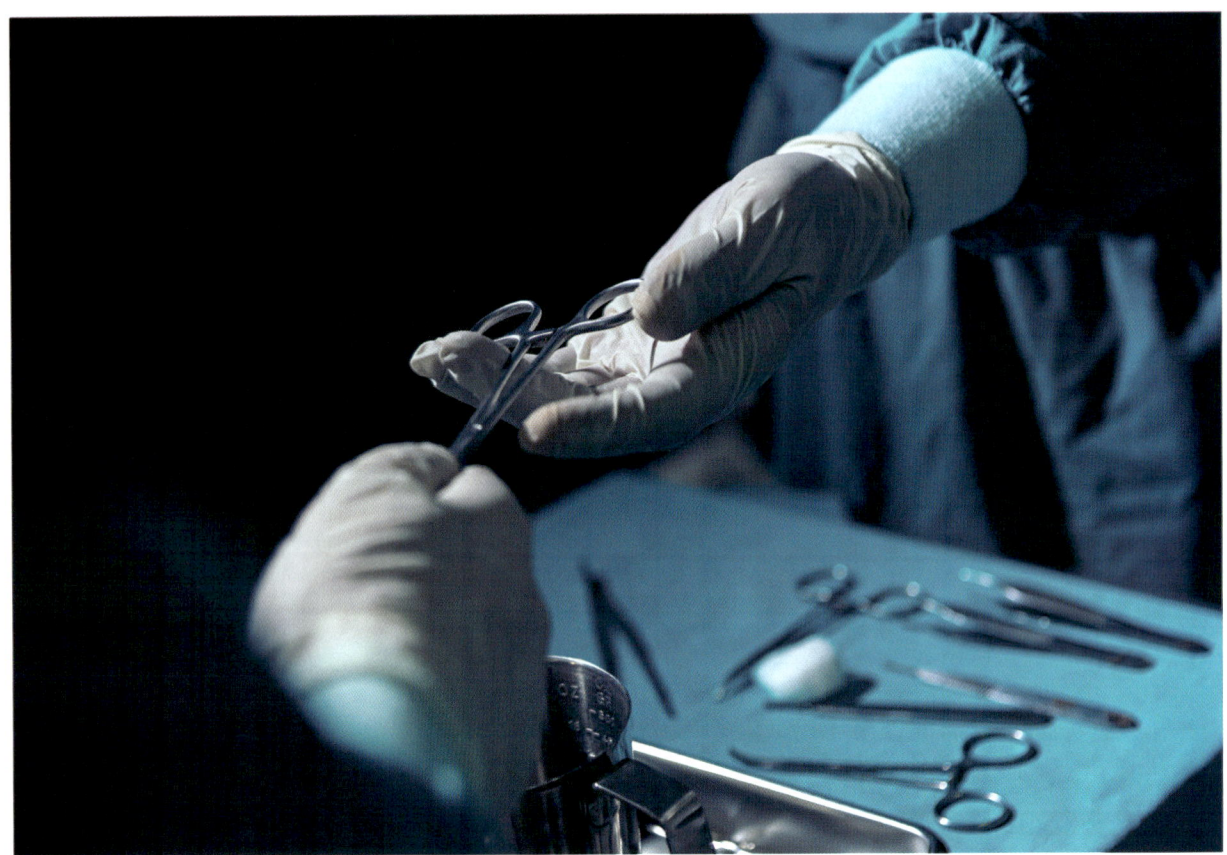

A Guide to the Rankings

How we identified 165 outstanding hospitals in 15 specialties

by **Ben Harder**

OR MORE THAN three decades, the mission of the Best Hospitals rankings has been to help guide patients, in consultation with their doctors, to the right place when they need a high level of specialty care. These are patients whose surgery or condition is complex. Or whose advanced age, physical infirmity or existing medical condition limits their options.

Such people account for a small fraction of hospital patients, but they add up to millions of individuals, and many hospitals may not be able to meet their needs. A hospital ranked by U.S. News in cancer, say, is likely to have the expertise and capability to enroll an elderly patient with a metastatic tumor into a clinical trial for an unproven but innovative treatment. Some community hospitals also can provide access to such experimental therapies. But not all.

The following pages offer hospital rankings in 15 specialties, from cancer to urology. Of more than 4,500 hospitals evaluated by U.S. News this year, only 165 performed well enough to be ranked in any specialty. In 12 of 15 specialties, analysis of objective data from the federal government and other sources generated the main factors determining whether a hospital was ranked. Some kinds of data, such as death rates, are intimately related to quality. Numbers of patients and the balance of nurses to patients are examples of data that are also important, although the quality connection may seem less evident. To capture medical experts' opinions, we also factored in results from annual surveys of specialist physi-

We are honored to be

#6 in the nation.

We're proud to be #6 on U.S. News and World Report's Best Hospitals Honor Roll and to be among the very best in 11 specialties. At the heart of this remarkable achievement is our commitment to providing you and your family the finest expert care available.

NATIONWIDE RANKINGS:

#2 GASTROENTEROLOGY & GI SURGERY

#3 CARDIOLOGY & HEART SURGERY

#3 ORTHOPAEDICS

#3 PULMONOLOGY & LUNG SURGERY

#7 UROLOGY

#9 CANCER

#10 GERIATRICS

#11 NEUROLOGY & NEUROSURGERY

#12 GYNECOLOGY

#18 EAR, NOSE & THROAT

#21 DIABETES & ENDOCRINOLOGY

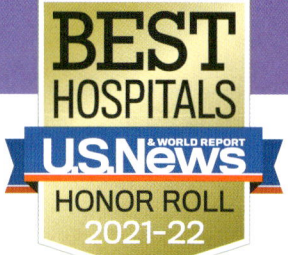
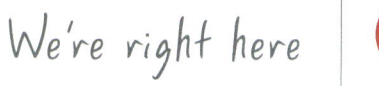
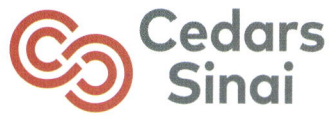

BEST HOSPITALS

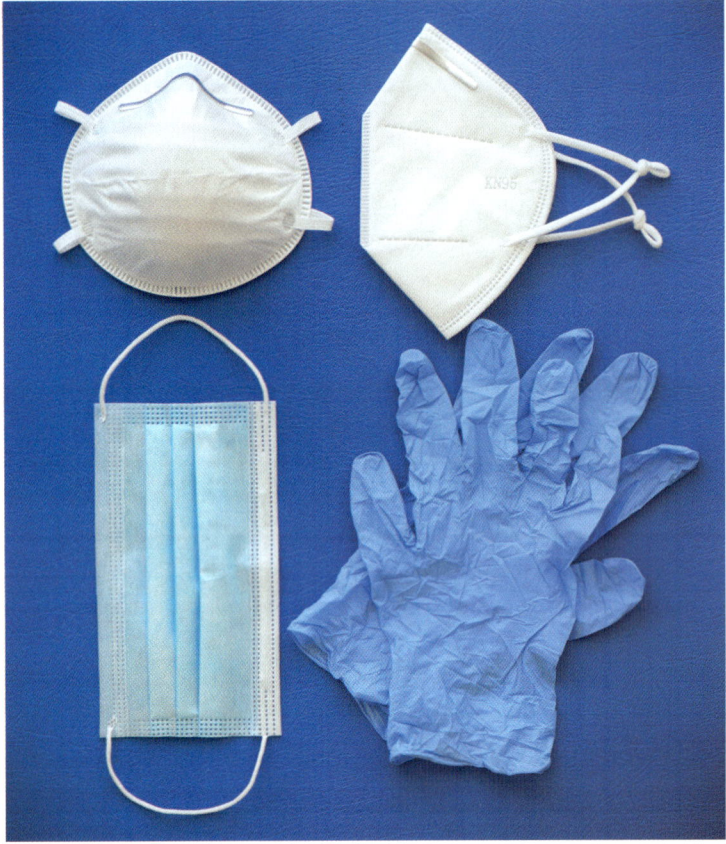

> **"No hospital is best for every patient."**

cians who were asked to name hospitals they consider best in their specialty at handling difficult cases. Hospitals in the other three specialties (ophthalmology, psychiatry and rheumatology) were ranked solely on the basis of the annual physician surveys. That's because reliable objective data aren't available for those areas of care.

Based on input from experts and medical studies, we have revised the ranking methodologies over time to improve the rankings' usefulness to consumers. This year, for example, we incorporated objective data for the first time into the rankings in rehabilitation,

USNEWS.COM/BESTHOSPITALS

Visit usnews.com regularly while researching your health care choices, as U.S. News often adds content aimed at helping patients and families make decisions about their medical care. We also update the Best Hospitals, Best Children's Hospitals and Best Regional Hospitals content and data on the website when new content and data become available.

using a methodology developed specifically for that specialty.

Beyond the specialty rankings, we expanded a set of hospital ratings that give patients information about which hospitals excel in specific procedures, such as hip replacement or colon cancer surgery, or in caring for patients with certain conditions, such as stroke or kidney failure. The kidney failure ratings, new this year, replace a ranking in nephrology that was published in the past. Hospital performance in these areas can be found in the Best Regional Hospitals rankings (Page 198), which combine data from the specialty rankings and the procedures and conditions ratings to help consumers identify hospitals with expertise in numerous areas of care. More detail is available at usnews.com/best-hospitals.

To be considered for ranking in 11 of the data-driven specialties, a hospital had to meet any of four criteria: It had to be a teaching hospital, or be affiliated with a medical school, or have at least 200 beds, or have at least 100 beds and offer at least four out of eight advanced medical technologies.

The hospitals next had to meet a volume requirement in each specialty – a minimum number of Medicare inpatients from 2017 to 2019 who received certain procedures and treatment for specific conditions. A hospital that fell short was still eligible if nominated in the specialty by at least 1% of physicians responding to the expert opinion survey.

At the end of the process, 1,880 hospitals remained candidates for ranking in at least one specialty. Each received a U.S. News score of 0 to 100 based on four elements, described below. The top 50 in each specialty were ranked. Scores and data for the rest are at usnews.com. The four elements and their weights in most specialties:

Patient outcomes (37.5%). Success at keeping patients alive and getting them home was judged by the proportion of Medicare inpatients with certain conditions in 2017, 2018 and 2019 who died within 30 days of admission or were discharged to another health care facility. Both rates were adjusted to account for the severity of patients' illnesses, the complexity of their care, and risk-elevating factors such as advanced age, obesity, high blood pressure and poverty (as reflected by whether they received Medicaid).

A widely used approach to so-called risk adjustment was employed to adjust each patient's risk in calculating odds of a good outcome. To avoid penalizing institutions receiving the sickest patients, we excluded from our analysis patients transferred in from another hospital. A score of 5 indicates the best chance of survival or discharge to home (and 1 the worst) relative to other hospitals.

Patient experience (5%). Most hospitals are required to assess patients' satisfaction with their experience using a survey known as the Hospital Consumer Assessment of Healthcare Providers and Systems, or HCAHPS. The score reflects how many patients had a positive overall experience during hospitalization.

Other care-related indicators (30%). The balance of patients per nurse and the hospital's number of patients – an indicator of its degree of experience in a specialty – are examples of these factors.

Expert opinion (27.5%). Specialists were asked to name up to five hospitals that they consider best in their area of expertise for patients with the most difficult medical problems. In the 2021 survey alone, responses were tallied from more than 30,000 physicians. The figures shown under "% of specialists recommending hospital" in the tables are the average percentages of specialists in 2019, 2020 and 2021 who recommended a hospital. In rehabilitation, expert opinion carried a weight of 50%. In the three specialties based entirely on expert opinion, a hospital had to be cited by at least 5% of responding physicians in the latest three years of U.S. News surveys to be ranked. That created lists of 13 hospitals in ophthalmology, 11 in psychiatry and 11 in rheumatology.

If you've consulted past editions of Best Hospitals, you may notice that a hospital you're considering has risen or fallen in the rankings. A decline shouldn't automatically be interpreted as a decline in performance; rather, it may be because of changes to the methodology or because other hospitals improved.

No hospital, no matter how excellent, is best for every patient. You'll want to add your own fact-gathering to ours and consult with your doctor or other health professional as you weigh your options. ●

A Glossary of Terms

Discharge to home score: reflects proportion of patients who, at discharge, went home rather than to a nursing home or other facility.

FACT accreditation level: hospital meets Foundation for the Accreditation of Cellular Therapy standards as of March 1, 2021, for harvesting and transplanting stem cells from a patient's own bone marrow and tissue (level 1) and from a donor (level 2) to treat cancer.

CARF: accredited by the Commission on Accreditation of Rehabilitation Facilities International as of March 1, 2021.

Completion of care rate: how often a hospital avoids needing to transfer patients to an acute-care hospital during their rehabilitation.

Flu vaccination rate: percentage of hospital's staff who received a seasonal flu vaccine.

NAEC epilepsy center: designated by the National Association of Epilepsy Centers as of March 1, 2021, as a regional or national referral facility (level 4) for staffing, technology and training in epilepsy care.

NCI cancer center: designated by the National Cancer Institute as of March 1, 2021, as a clinical or comprehensive cancer hospital.

NIA Alzheimer's center: designated by the National Institute on Aging as of February 12, 2021, as an Alzheimer's Disease Center, indicating high quality of research and clinical care.

Number of patients: except in rehabilitation, estimated number of Medicare inpatients in 2017, 2018 and 2019 who received certain high-level care as defined by U.S. News. Based on an adjustment to the number of such patients with traditional Medicare insurance. In geriatrics, only patients ages 75 and older are included. In rehabilitation, only patients treated in 2019 are included.

A Nurse Magnet hospital: recognized by the American Nurses Credentialing Center as of January 2, 2021, for nursing excellence.

Nurse staffing score: relative balance of nonsupervisory registered nurses (inpatient and outpatient) to average daily number of all patients. Inpatient staffing receives greater weight. Agency and temporary nurses are not counted.

Patient experience: percentage of patients who responded positively to a survey about the overall quality of their stay.

Patient services score: number of services offered out of the number considered important to quality (such as genetic testing in cancer and an Alzheimer's center in geriatrics).

% of specialists recommending hospital: percentage of physicians responding to U.S. News surveys in 2019, 2020 and 2021 who named the hospital as among the best in their specialty for especially challenging cases and procedures, setting aside location and cost.

Public transparency: indicates whether hospital publicly reports its performance through the American College of Cardiology, the American Heart Association and the Society of Thoracic Surgeons (in cardiology & heart surgery) or the American Heart Association (in neurology & neurosurgery).

Rank: based on U.S. News score except in ophthalmology, psychiatry and rheumatology, where specialist recommendations determined rank.

Readmission prevention rate: how often hospital keeps patients from being readmitted to an acute-care hospital within the 30 days following discharge.

Successful discharge rate: how often patients go directly home from this hospital and remain at home, rather than requiring further institutional care.

Survival score: reflects patient survival rate in the specialty within 30 days of admission.

Technology score: reflects availability of technologies considered important to a high quality of care, such as PET/CT scanner in pulmonology and diagnostic radioisotope services in urology.

Trauma center: indicates Level 1 or 2 trauma center certification. Such a center can care properly for the most severe injuries.

U.S. News score: summary of quality of hospital inpatient care. In most specialties, survival is worth 30%, discharge to home 7.5%, operational quality data such as nurse staffing and patient volume 30%, specialists' recommendations 27.5%, and patient experience 5%.

BEST HOSPITALS

Cancer

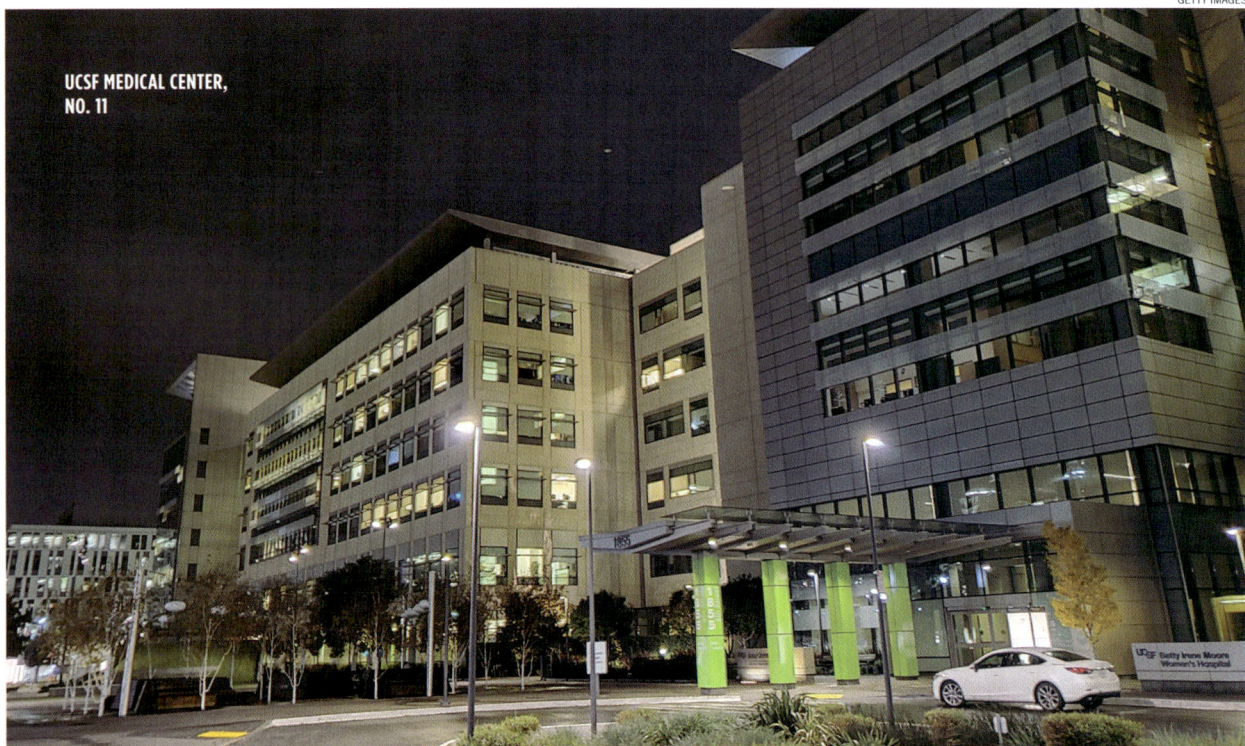

UCSF MEDICAL CENTER, NO. 11

GETTY IMAGES

Rank	Hospital	U.S. News score	Survival score (5=best)	Discharge to home score (5=best)	Patient experience (% positive responses)	Number of patients	Nurse staffing score (higher is better)	NCI cancer center	FACT accreditation level (2=best)	Patient services score (8=best)	% of specialists recommending hospital
1	University of Texas MD Anderson Cancer Center, Houston	100.0	5	5	95%	13,006	1.9	Yes	2	8	37.6%
2	Memorial Sloan Kettering Cancer Center, New York	82.8	5	5	94%	6,514	2.4	Yes	2	8	34.7%
3	Mayo Clinic, Rochester, Minn.	78.2	5	5	95%	4,343	2.7	Yes	2	8	17.7%
4	Dana-Farber/Brigham and Women's Cancer Center, Boston	76.5	5	5	96%	4,289	2.3	Yes	2	8	22.6%
5	Cleveland Clinic	73.1	5	5	92%	3,308	2.3	Yes	2	8	7.0%
6	Johns Hopkins Hospital, Baltimore	68.6	5	5	93%	2,374	2.4	Yes	2	8	14.5%
6	Northwestern Memorial Hospital, Chicago	68.6	5	5	92%	2,532	1.9	Yes	2	7	2.0%
8	UCLA Medical Center, Los Angeles	68.2	5	5	93%	1,918	3.1	Yes	2	8	5.5%
9	Cedars-Sinai Medical Center, Los Angeles	66.5	5	5	91%	2,195	2.6	No	2	8	1.5%
10	Hosps. of the U. of Pennsylvania-Penn Presby., Philadelphia	65.0	5	5	92%	3,522	2.5	Yes	2	8	5.9%
11	UCSF Medical Center, San Francisco	64.8	5	5	93%	2,434	2.5	Yes	2	8	5.2%
12	Stanford Health Care-Stanford Hospital, Stanford, Calif.	64.7	5	5	91%	2,417	2.6	Yes	2	8	4.7%
13	City of Hope Helford Clinical Research Hosp., Duarte, Calif.	63.7	5	5	94%	3,427	2.7	Yes	2	8	5.2%
13	Siteman Cancer Center at Barnes-Jewish Hospital, Saint Louis	63.7	5	5	90%	4,301	2.3	Yes	2	8	3.8%
15	New York-Presbyterian Hospital-Columbia and Cornell, N.Y.	63.3	5	5	89%	5,553	3.0	Yes	2	8	2.8%
16	Mayo Clinic-Phoenix	63.0	5	5	96%	1,499	3.2	Yes	2	8	2.4%
17	UC San Diego Health-Moores Cancer Center	62.2	5	5	91%	1,472	2.0	Yes	2	8	1.8%
18	Massachusetts General Hospital, Boston	61.4	5	5	92%	3,572	2.6	Yes	2	8	9.1%
18	UPMC Presbyterian Shadyside, Pittsburgh	61.4	5	5	90%	4,209	2.4	Yes	2	8	2.9%
20	USC Norris Cancer Hosp.-Keck Med. Ctr. of USC, Los Angeles	60.9	5	5	93%	1,169	3.3	Yes	2	8	2.4%
21	University of Chicago Medical Center	60.8	5	5	90%	2,200	2.2	Yes	2	8	2.6%
22	Perlmutter Cancer Center at NYU Langone Hospitals, New York	60.6	5	5	89%	3,198	2.2	Yes	2	8	2.7%
23	Houston Methodist Hospital	59.4	5	5	92%	1,789	2.0	No	2	8	0.3%
24	UT Southwestern Medical Center, Dallas	59.1	5	5	94%	1,873	2.1	Yes	2	8	1.0%

(CONTINUED ON PAGE 116)

Terms are explained on Page 113.

114 U.S. NEWS & WORLD REPORT

More @ usnews.com/besthospitals

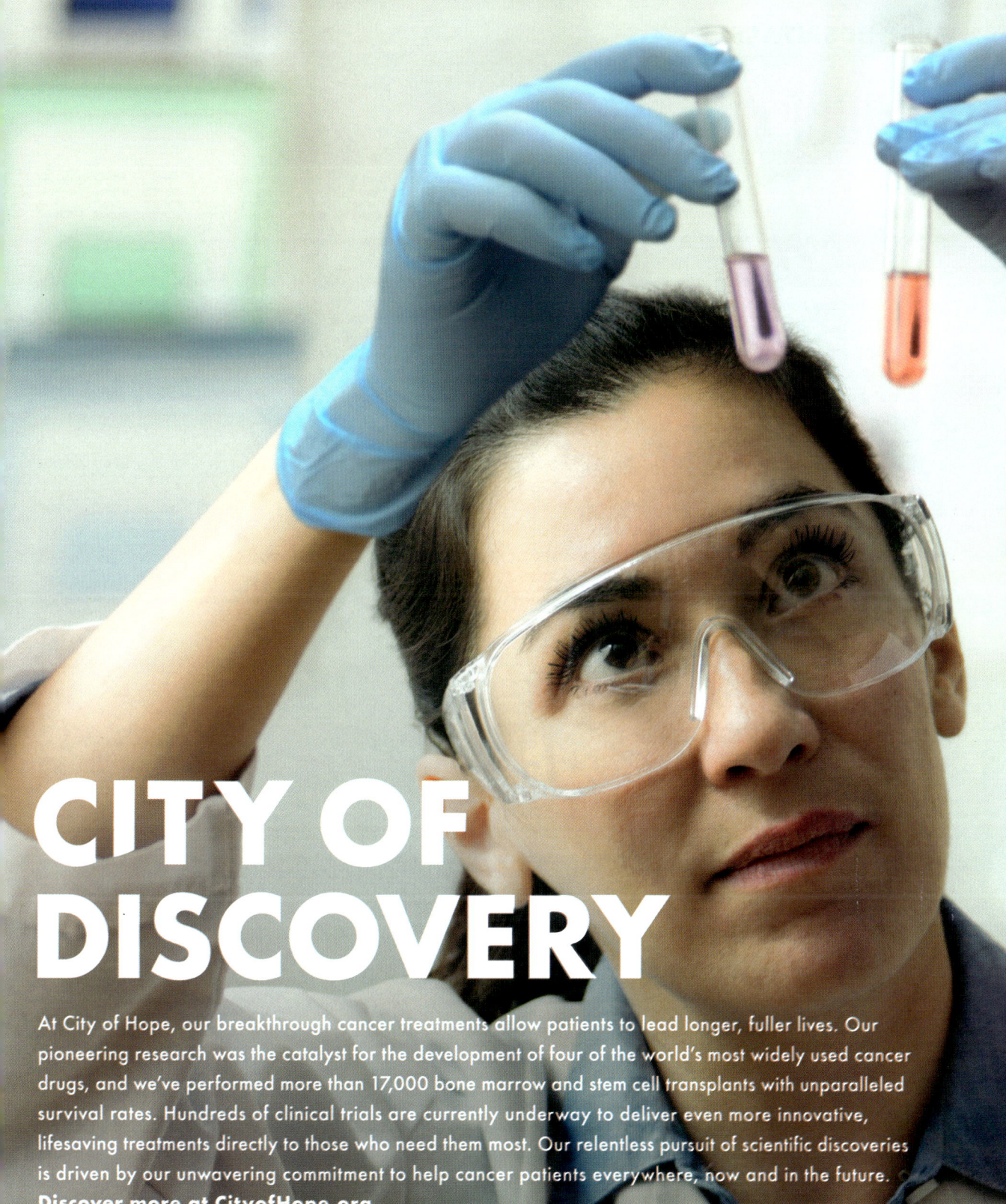

BEST HOSPITALS

Cancer (CONTINUED)

Rank	Hospital	U.S. News score	Survival score (5=best)	Discharge to home score (5=best)	Patient experience (% positive responses)	Number of patients	Nurse staffing score (higher is better)	NCI cancer center	FACT accreditation level (2=best)	Patient services score (8=best)	% of specialists recommending hospital
25	Duncan Comp. Cancer Ctr. at Baylor St. Luke's Med. Ctr., Houston	58.0	5	5	88%	810	2.0	Yes	0	8	0.4%
26	H. Lee Moffitt Cancer Center and Research Institute, Tampa	57.9	5	5	94%	2,316	1.2	Yes	2	7	6.0%
27	Ohio State University James Cancer Hospital, Columbus	57.6	5	5	95%	4,401	2.1	Yes	2	8	4.9%
27	Seattle Cancer Care Alliance/U. of Washington Medical Ctr.	57.6	5	5	93%	2,248	2.2	Yes	2	8	6.5%
27	University of Alabama at Birmingham Hospital	57.6	5	5	92%	2,230	2.2	Yes	2	8	1.1%
30	Huntsman Cancer Institute at the U. of Utah, Salt Lake City	57.3	5	5	93%	1,290	2.4	Yes	2	8	0.8%
31	Beth Israel Deaconess Medical Center, Boston	57.2	5	5	90%	2,058	1.5	Yes	2	8	2.7%
32	Jefferson Health-Thomas Jefferson U. Hospitals, Philadelphia	57.0	5	5	89%	1,877	2.0	Yes	2	8	1.2%
32	Mount Sinai Hospital, New York	57.0	5	5	87%	2,606	2.3	Yes	2	8	1.3%
34	Roswell Park Comprehensive Cancer Center, Buffalo	56.8	5	5	94%	1,625	1.8	Yes	2	8	2.1%
35	Duke University Hospital, Durham, N.C.	56.6	5	5	92%	2,794	2.0	Yes	2	8	5.6%
36	U. of Michigan Hospitals-Michigan Medicine, Ann Arbor	56.3	5	5	92%	2,744	2.6	Yes	2	8	3.4%
37	OHSU Hospital-Knight Cancer Institute, Portland, Ore.	55.7	5	5	92%	1,747	2.3	Yes	2	8	0.9%
38	University Hospitals Seidman Cancer Center, Cleveland	55.6	5	5	89%	2,009	2.5	Yes	2	8	0.6%
39	MUSC Health-University Medical Center, Charleston, S.C.	55.5	5	5	91%	1,569	2.1	Yes	2	8	0.4%
40	UC Davis Medical Center, Sacramento, Calif.	55.2	5	5	89%	1,561	2.5	Yes	2	8	1.0%
41	U. of Kentucky Albert B. Chandler Hospital, Lexington	54.3	5	5	89%	1,356	1.8	Yes	2	8	1.0%
42	Rush University Medical Center, Chicago	54.2	5	5	92%	1,618	2.0	No	2	8	0.6%
43	Emory University Hospital, Atlanta	54.0	5	5	91%	2,278	2.2	Yes	2	8	1.7%
44	Montefiore Medical Center, Bronx, N.Y.	53.7	5	5	82%	2,702	2.3	Yes	2	8	0.6%
44	Vanderbilt University Medical Center, Nashville, Tenn.	53.7	5	5	91%	2,332	2.2	Yes	2	8	2.9%
46	Mayo Clinic-Jacksonville, Fla.	53.3	5	5	95%	1,259	2.7	Yes	2	8	2.6%
47	University of Iowa Hospitals and Clinics, Iowa City	53.2	5	5	90%	1,811	1.8	Yes	2	8	0.6%
48	Queen's Medical Center, Honolulu	52.6	5	5	91%	1,708	1.6	Yes	0	8	0.0%
49	University of Kansas Hospital, Kansas City	52.5	5	5	93%	2,217	2.1	Yes	2	8	0.8%
50	UCHealth University of Colorado Hospital, Aurora	52.4	5	5	91%	1,602	2.0	Yes	2	8	1.6%

Terms are explained on Page 113.

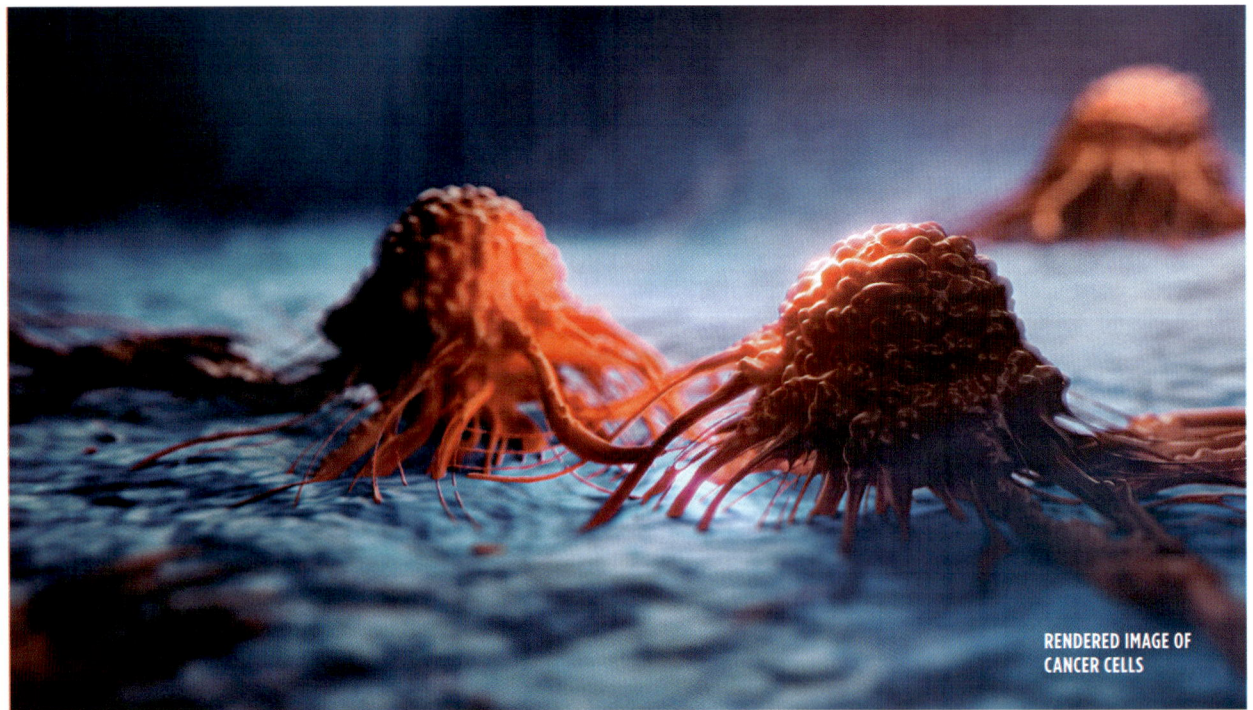

RENDERED IMAGE OF CANCER CELLS

GETTY IMAGES

Cancer won't be my last dance.

Washington Ballet, I'm back.

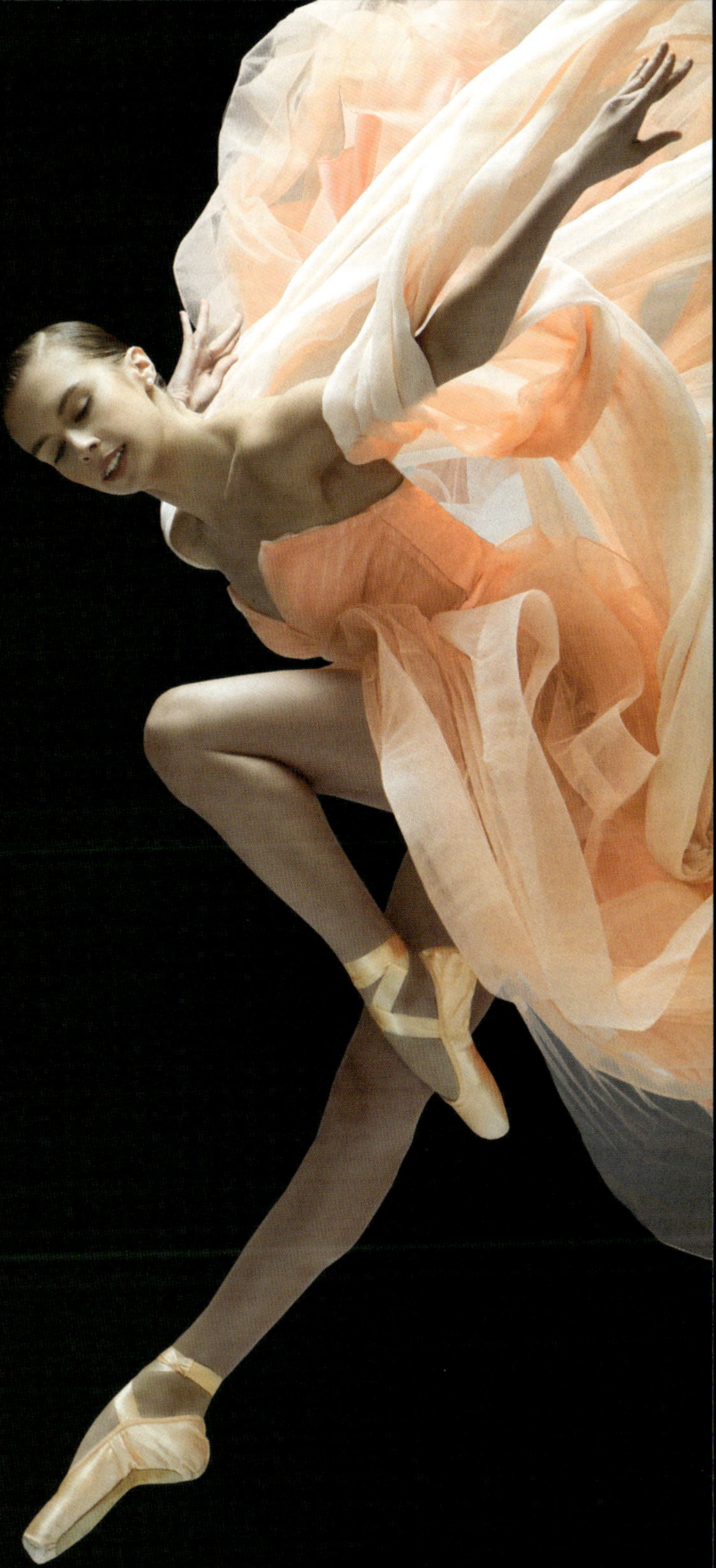

When The Washington Ballet's Chiara Valle continued to have agonizing leg pain after a previous hospital's misdiagnosis, she knew she needed a second opinion if she ever wanted to dance again. Chiara turned to Montefiore-Einstein to get back to The Washington Ballet. Everyday Montefiore-Einstein is helping passionate people keep doing what they love.

See Chiara's story at montefiore.org/chiara

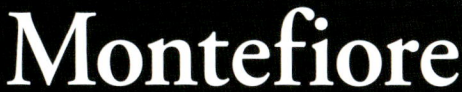
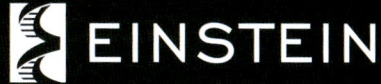
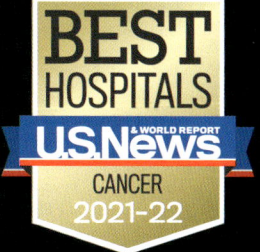

BEST HOSPITALS
Cardiology & Heart Surgery

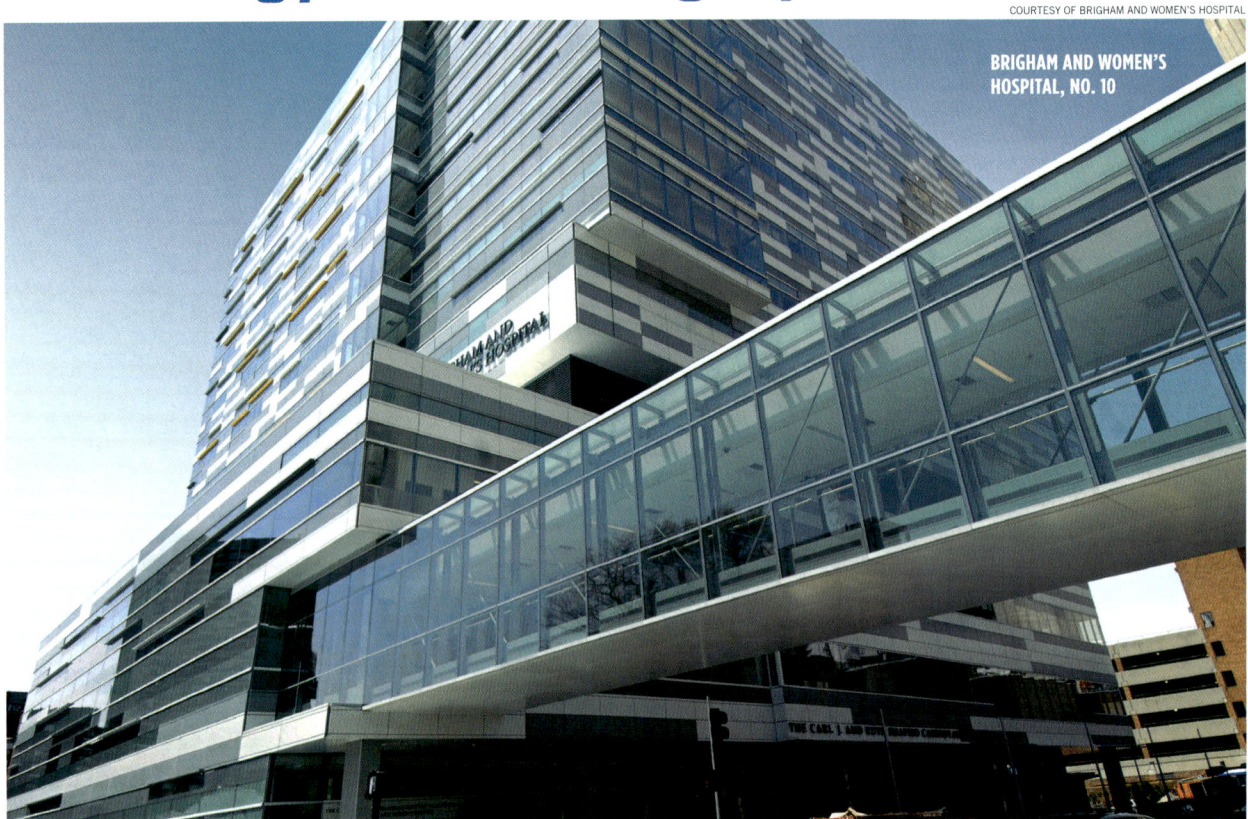

BRIGHAM AND WOMEN'S HOSPITAL, NO. 10

Rank	Hospital	U.S. News score	Survival score (5=best)	Discharge to home score (5=best)	Patient experience (% positive responses)	Trans-parency score (3=best)	Number of patients	Nurse staffing score (higher is better)	A Nurse Magnet hospital	Technology score (6=best)	Patient services score (7=best)	% of specialists recommending hospital
1	Cleveland Clinic	100.0	5	5	92%	3	17,185	2.3	Yes	6	7	36.2%
2	Mayo Clinic, Rochester, Minn.	92.0	5	5	95%	3	13,367	2.7	Yes	6	7	34.2%
3	Cedars-Sinai Medical Center, Los Angeles	88.0	5	5	91%	3	11,958	2.6	Yes	6	7	8.4%
4	New York-Presbyterian Hospital-Columbia and Cornell, N.Y.	84.7	5	5	89%	3	22,094	3.0	Yes	6	7	13.0%
5	NYU Langone Hospitals, New York, N.Y.	79.1	5	5	89%	3	19,000	2.2	Yes	6	7	5.6%
6	Mount Sinai Hospital, New York	77.9	5	5	87%	3	14,769	2.3	Yes	6	7	4.6%
7	Massachusetts General Hospital, Boston	77.7	5	5	92%	3	11,309	2.6	Yes	6	7	13.4%
8	Stanford Health Care-Stanford Hospital, Stanford, Calif.	76.9	5	5	91%	3	5,230	2.6	Yes	6	7	7.4%
9	UCLA Medical Center, Los Angeles	76.1	5	5	93%	3	5,366	3.1	Yes	6	7	4.2%
10	Brigham and Women's Hospital, Boston	73.1	5	5	92%	3	8,127	2.3	Yes	6	7	9.2%
11	UT Southwestern Medical Center, Dallas	71.2	5	5	94%	3	4,409	2.1	Yes	6	7	2.1%
12	Northwestern Memorial Hospital, Chicago	70.7	5	5	92%	3	7,056	1.9	Yes	6	6	4.1%
13	Texas Heart Inst. at Baylor St. Luke's Medical Ctr., Houston	70.2	5	5	88%	3	9,268	2.0	Yes	5	7	3.7%
14	Keck Medical Center of USC, Los Angeles	68.6	5	5	91%	3	2,436	3.3	Yes	6	7	1.1%
15	Houston Methodist Hospital	68.4	5	5	92%	3	9,768	2.0	Yes	6	7	3.0%
16	Johns Hopkins Hospital, Baltimore	68.3	5	5	93%	3	4,786	2.4	Yes	6	7	7.9%
17	Vanderbilt University Medical Center, Nashville, Tenn.	67.6	5	5	91%	3	8,022	2.2	Yes	6	7	4.1%
18	Hosps. of the U. of Pennsylvania-Penn Presby., Philadelphia	66.7	5	5	92%	3	12,179	2.5	Yes	6	7	7.0%
19	Beaumont Hospital-Royal Oak, Mich.	66.4	5	5	88%	3	11,811	2.0	Yes	5	7	1.6%
20	U. of Michigan Hospitals-Michigan Medicine, Ann Arbor	66.3	5	5	92%	3	7,931	2.6	Yes	6	7	3.7%
21	North Shore University Hospital, Manhasset, N.Y.	65.6	5	5	88%	3	12,647	2.0	Yes	6	7	1.8%
22	Mayo Clinic-Phoenix	65.2	5	5	96%	3	3,609	3.2	Yes	6	7	2.7%

(CONTINUED ON PAGE 122)

Terms are explained on Page 113.

More @ usnews.com/besthospitals

MORRISTOWN MEDICAL CENTER
#1 HOSPITAL IN NJ*

4 YEARS IN A ROW!

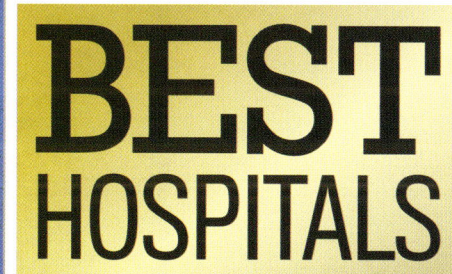

BEST HOSPITALS
U.S. News & WORLD REPORT
RANKED IN 3 SPECIALTIES
2021-22

Setting New Standards of Care with Nationally Recognized Programs

Cardiology & Heart Surgery | Gynecology | Orthopedics

*Tie, 2021-2022

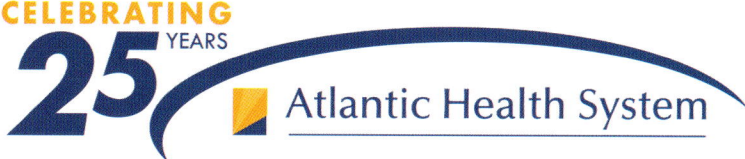

CELEBRATING 25 YEARS
Atlantic Health System

To learn more visit atlantichealth.org/usnews

Patients and clinicians **work together to decide treatment options.**

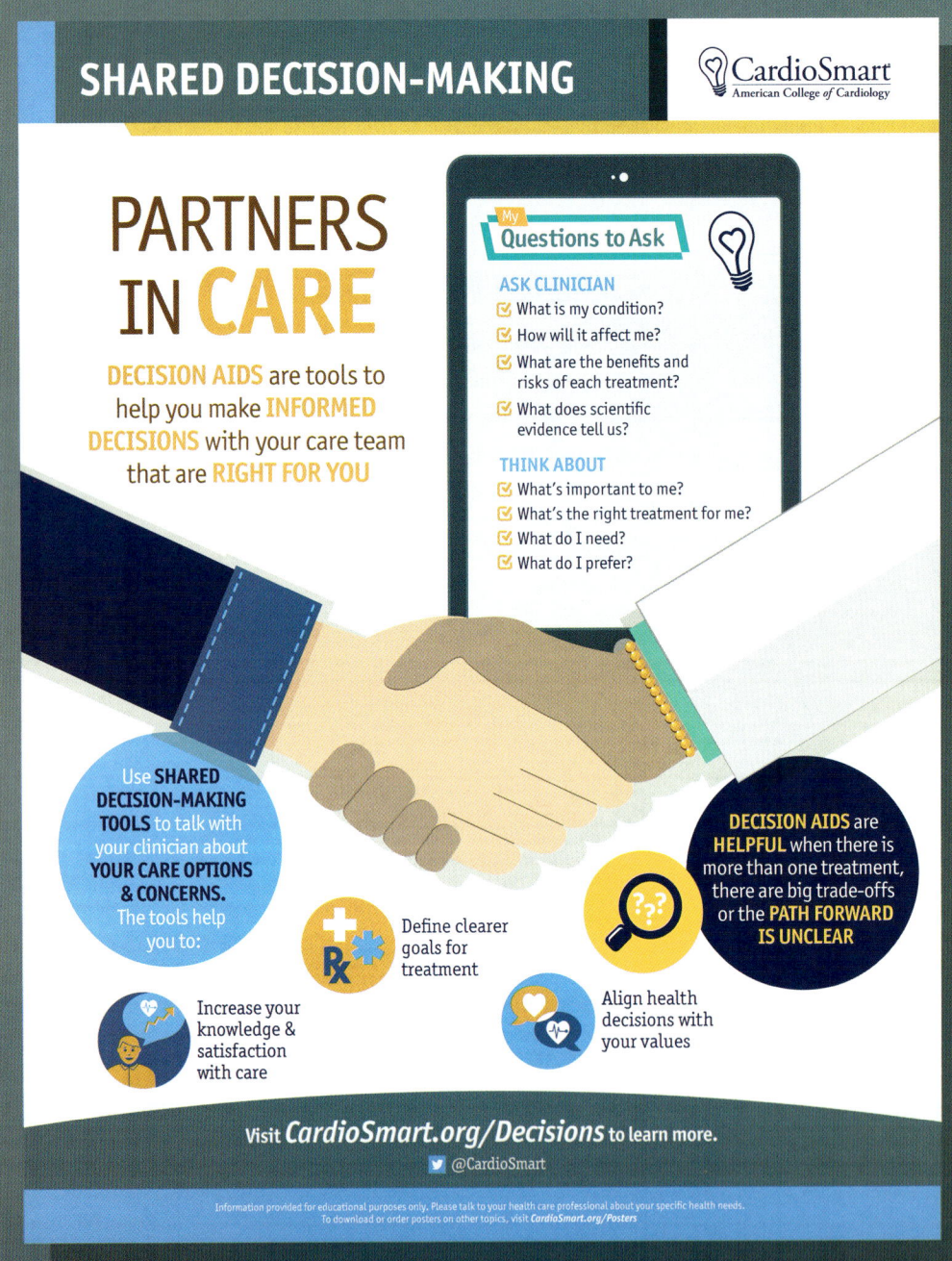

Decision aids help YOU and your HEART CARE TEAM choose the best path based on your values.

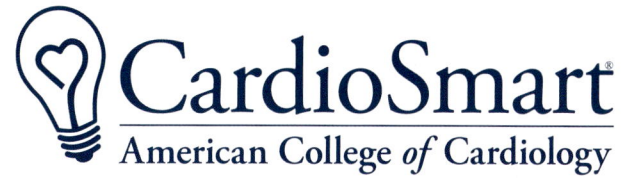

ATRIAL FIBRILLATION

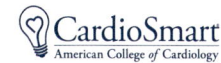

What is ATRIAL FIBRILLATION?

- Atrial Fibrillation (AFib) is a **PROBLEM** with the **RATE OR RHYTHM** of the heartbeat, causing the heart to beat quickly and irregularly.

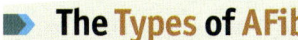

AFib affects **more than 3 million** people in the U.S.

The Types of AFib

PAROXYSMAL
- Comes and goes
- Usually stops on its own

PERSISTENT
- Lasts > 1 week
- Can become permanent

PERMANENT
- Heart cannot be restored to normal rhythm

What are the SYMPTOMS?

| Fatigue | Shortness of breath | Dizziness or light-headedness | Palpitations | Chest pain | Nothing |

How is it TREATED?

RATE CONTROL
Treatment to make sure the heart doesn't beat too quickly during AFib.

RHYTHM CONTROL
Treatment to restore the heart's rhythm to a normal state, and keep it there.

ANTICOAGULATION MEDICATION
(Blood Thinners) to reduce stroke risk.

LIFESTYLE CHANGES
Get regular exercise, eat a heart-healthy diet, don't smoke, watch alcohol and caffeine intake.

Visit **CardioSmart.org/AFib** to learn more.
@CardioSmart

Information provided for educational purposes only. Please talk to your health care professional about your specific health needs. To download or order posters on other topics, visit CardioSmart.org/Posters

©2021 American College of Cardiology Z21007

Powered by American College of Cardiology's NCDR® and CardioSmart®

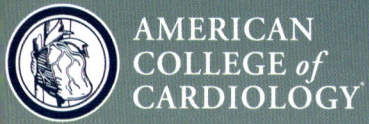

Visit **CardioSmart.org/DecisionAids** today!

Find tools to help you make treatment decisions and resources on heart health.

BEST HOSPITALS

Cardiology & Heart Surgery (CONTINUED)

Rank	Hospital	U.S. News score	Survival score (5=best)	Discharge to home score (5=best)	Patient experience (% positive responses)	Transparency score (3=best)	Number of patients	Nurse staffing score (higher is better)	A Nurse Magnet hospital	Technology score (6=best)	Patient services score (7=best)	% of specialists recommending hospital
23	UC San Diego Health-Cardiovascular Institute	64.9	5	5	91%	3	4,057	2.0	Yes	6	7	0.9%
24	St. Francis Hospital & Heart Center, Roslyn, N.Y.	64.2	5	5	95%	3	13,431	2.0	Yes	5	7	1.4%
25	St. Luke's Hospital of Kansas City, Mo.	63.4	5	5	92%	3	6,303	1.7	Yes	6	7	1.6%
26	Scripps La Jolla Hospitals, La Jolla, Calif.	63.1	5	5	92%	3	8,132	3.0	Yes	5	7	1.2%
26	UC Davis Medical Center, Sacramento, Calif.	63.1	5	5	89%	2	4,034	2.5	Yes	5	7	0.6%
28	Lenox Hill Hospital, New York	63.0	5	5	87%	3	7,037	2.6	Yes	5	7	1.1%
29	University of Alabama at Birmingham Hospital	62.9	5	5	92%	3	7,196	2.2	Yes	6	7	2.2%
30	MedStar Heart & Vascular Inst. at MedStar Washington Hosp. Ctr., D.C.	62.7	5	5	85%	3	12,139	1.9	No	6	7	1.6%
31	Montefiore Medical Center, Bronx, N.Y.	61.8	5	5	82%	3	15,272	2.3	No	6	7	0.7%
32	UCSF Medical Center, San Francisco	61.6	5	5	93%	3	3,110	2.5	Yes	6	7	1.7%
33	Rush University Medical Center, Chicago	61.5	5	5	92%	3	3,757	2.0	Yes	6	7	0.7%
34	University Hospitals Cleveland Medical Center	60.9	5	5	89%	3	6,004	2.5	Yes	6	7	1.1%
35	St. Cloud Hospital, St. Cloud, Minn.	60.7	5	5	90%	3	8,582	2.0	Yes	5	7	0.0%
36	Advocate Christ Medical Center, Oak Lawn, Ill.	60.3	5	5	87%	3	9,416	2.7	Yes	6	7	0.2%
37	Barnes-Jewish Hospital, Saint Louis	59.6	5	5	90%	3	8,220	2.3	Yes	6	7	3.2%
38	Ohio State University Wexner Medical Center, Columbus	59.4	5	5	90%	3	8,483	2.1	Yes	6	7	1.7%
39	Duke University Hospital, Durham, N.C.	59.2	5	5	92%	3	8,937	2.0	Yes	6	7	7.2%
40	Baylor Scott and White The Heart Hospital Plano, Texas	59.0	5	5	95%	3	7,352	2.5	Yes	5	7	1.9%
41	Cleveland Clinic Hillcrest Hospital	58.6	5	5	89%	3	5,753	1.6	Yes	5	7	0.4%
42	Morristown Medical Center, Morristown, N.J.	58.4	5	5	91%	3	11,853	2.1	Yes	5	7	0.9%
42	UPMC Presbyterian Shadyside, Pittsburgh	58.4	5	5	90%	3	9,774	2.4	Yes	6	7	1.8%
44	Minneapolis Heart Institute at Abbott Northwestern Hospital	58.2	5	5	91%	3	9,962	2.5	Yes	6	7	1.2%
45	Hackensack University Medical Center, Hackensack, N.J.	57.8	5	5	86%	3	6,910	2.9	Yes	5	7	0.6%
45	University of Kansas Hospital, Kansas City	57.8	5	5	93%	3	6,495	2.1	Yes	6	7	0.6%
47	Christ Hospital, Cincinnati	57.3	5	5	92%	3	6,793	1.9	Yes	5	7	0.4%
48	Memorial Hermann-Texas Medical Center, Houston	56.8	5	5	90%	3	7,055	2.1	Yes	6	7	1.5%
48	Mount Sinai Morningside & Mount Sinai West Hospitals, New York	56.8	5	5	86%	3	5,332	2.0	No	5	7	0.4%
50	UF Health Shands Hospital, Gainesville, Fla.	55.9	5	5	90%	3	6,170	2.0	Yes	6	7	2.3%

Terms are explained on Page 113.

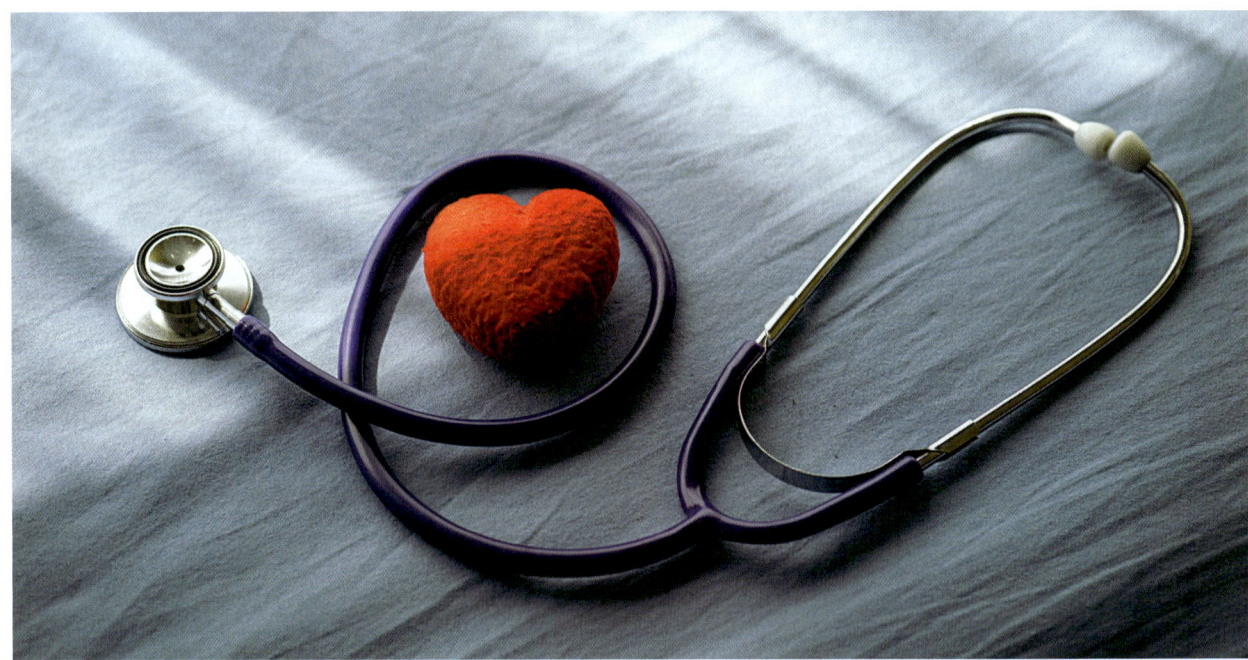

GETTY IMAGES

A high-speed heart rate can't slow me down.

Thanks to Montefiore-Einstein, Phyllis is back in the water.

Seventy-year-old Phyllis Steel is one of the most athletic retirees you'll ever meet, but when she developed an irregular beat in the upper chambers of her heart that jeopardized her active lifestyle, she looked to Montefiore-Einstein to help her get back in the water.

See Phyllis' story at montefiore.org/phyllis

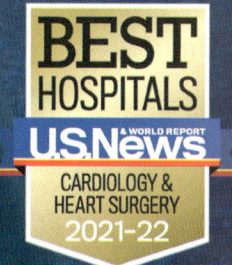

BEST HOSPITALS
U.S.News & WORLD REPORT
CARDIOLOGY & HEART SURGERY
2021-22

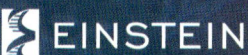

Montefiore | EINSTEIN

BEST HOSPITALS

Diabetes & Endocrinology

Rank	Hospital	U.S. News score	Survival score (5=best)	Discharge to home score (5=best)	Patient experience (% positive responses)	Number of patients	Nurse staffing score (higher is better)	A Nurse Magnet hospital	Technology score (4=best)	Patient services score (8=best)	% of specialists recommending hospital
1	Mayo Clinic, Rochester, Minn.	100.0	5	5	95%	1,056	2.7	Yes	4	8	34.0%
2	Massachusetts General Hospital, Boston	80.2	5	5	92%	1,077	2.6	Yes	4	8	24.1%
3	UCLA Medical Center, Los Angeles	75.4	5	5	93%	876	3.1	Yes	4	8	5.7%
4	NYU Langone Hospitals, New York, N.Y.	73.0	5	5	89%	1,905	2.2	Yes	4	8	6.2%
5	New York-Presbyterian Hospital-Columbia and Cornell, N.Y.	72.4	5	5	89%	2,538	3.0	Yes	4	8	8.1%
6	UCSF Medical Center, San Francisco	69.1	5	5	93%	586	2.5	Yes	4	8	7.5%
7	Barnes-Jewish Hospital, Saint Louis	67.9	5	5	90%	906	2.3	Yes	4	8	6.9%
8	Johns Hopkins Hospital, Baltimore	67.5	4	5	93%	520	2.4	Yes	4	8	12.0%
9	Montefiore Medical Center, Bronx, N.Y.	65.4	5	5	82%	2,462	2.3	No	4	8	1.2%
10	Mount Sinai Hospital, New York	64.4	5	5	87%	1,001	2.3	Yes	4	8	4.6%
10	U. of Michigan Hospitals-Michigan Medicine, Ann Arbor	64.4	5	5	92%	659	2.6	Yes	4	8	6.0%
10	University of Washington Medical Center, Seattle	64.4	5	5	91%	526	2.2	Yes	4	8	5.4%
13	Cleveland Clinic	63.6	3	5	92%	854	2.3	Yes	4	8	12.0%
14	University of Chicago Medical Center	63.1	5	5	90%	659	2.2	Yes	4	8	1.9%
15	Hosps. of the U. of Pennsylvania-Penn Presby., Philadelphia	62.5	5	5	92%	845	2.5	Yes	4	8	5.7%
16	Houston Methodist Hospital	62.4	5	5	92%	920	2.0	Yes	4	8	1.4%
17	University of Texas MD Anderson Cancer Center, Houston	62.2	5	5	95%	475	1.9	Yes	4	8	2.7%
18	Memorial Sloan Kettering Cancer Center, New York	61.9	5	5	94%	340	2.4	Yes	4	8	1.0%
19	Brigham and Women's Hospital, Boston	61.7	3	5	92%	766	2.3	Yes	4	8	9.5%
19	Ohio State University Wexner Medical Center, Columbus	61.7	5	5	90%	922	2.1	Yes	4	8	3.0%
21	Cedars-Sinai Medical Center, Los Angeles	61.6	5	5	91%	1,065	2.6	Yes	4	8	1.9%
22	Hoag Memorial Hospital Presbyterian, Newport Beach, Calif.	61.3	5	5	94%	833	2.4	Yes	4	8	0.5%
23	Beaumont Hospital-Royal Oak, Mich.	61.2	5	5	88%	1,389	2.0	Yes	4	8	0.3%
24	UPMC Presbyterian Shadyside, Pittsburgh	60.1	5	5	90%	1,034	2.4	Yes	4	8	3.1%
24	UT Southwestern Medical Center, Dallas	60.1	5	5	94%	608	2.1	Yes	4	8	2.3%
26	Mayo Clinic-Phoenix	59.6	5	5	96%	379	3.2	Yes	4	8	1.9%
27	Northwestern Memorial Hospital, Chicago	59.3	5	5	92%	663	1.9	Yes	4	7	2.3%
28	Tampa General Hospital	57.8	5	5	91%	1,151	2.6	Yes	4	8	0.5%
29	Mount Sinai Beth Israel, New York	57.3	5	5	83%	894	1.3	No	4	8	1.0%
30	Mayo Clinic-Jacksonville, Fla.	56.7	5	5	95%	419	2.7	Yes	4	8	1.6%
31	North Shore University Hospital, Manhasset, N.Y.	56.4	5	5	88%	1,043	2.0	Yes	4	8	1.1%
31	Vanderbilt University Medical Center, Nashville, Tenn.	56.4	3	5	91%	665	2.2	Yes	4	8	5.2%
33	Yale-New Haven Hospital, New Haven, Conn.	56.1	4	3	89%	1,369	1.9	Yes	4	8	4.3%
34	Beaumont Hospital-Grosse Pointe, Mich.	55.8	5	5	92%	472	2.0	Yes	4	8	0.0%
35	UCHealth University of Colorado Hospital, Aurora	55.4	3	5	91%	602	2.0	Yes	4	8	7.0%
36	Duke University Hospital, Durham, N.C.	55.3	4	5	92%	716	2.0	Yes	4	8	4.1%
36	Providence Mission Hospital-Mission Viejo & Laguna Beach, Calif.	55.3	5	5	90%	377	2.2	Yes	4	8	0.0%
38	Lenox Hill Hospital, New York	55.2	5	5	87%	582	2.6	Yes	4	8	0.9%
39	Memorial Hermann-Texas Medical Center, Houston	54.8	5	5	90%	417	2.1	Yes	4	8	0.2%
40	AdventHealth Orlando	54.7	5	5	90%	2,991	1.8	No	4	8	0.2%
41	Beth Israel Deaconess Medical Center, Boston	54.2	5	4	90%	653	1.5	No	4	8	2.5%
42	UC Davis Medical Center, Sacramento, Calif.	53.8	5	5	89%	407	2.5	Yes	4	8	0.4%
43	Mercy Hospital St. Louis, Mo.	53.4	5	5	90%	595	1.6	No	4	8	0.0%
44	John Muir Health-Walnut Creek Med. Ctr., Walnut Creek, Calif.	53.0	5	5	91%	488	2.2	Yes	4	8	0.0%
45	Emory University Hospital, Atlanta	52.9	4	5	91%	635	2.2	Yes	4	8	2.0%
46	Jefferson Health-Thomas Jefferson U. Hospitals, Philadelphia	52.7	5	5	89%	723	2.0	Yes	4	8	0.9%
47	Stanford Health Care-Stanford Hospital, Stanford, Calif.	52.6	4	5	91%	480	2.6	Yes	4	8	1.2%
48	Keck Medical Center of USC, Los Angeles	52.0	3	5	91%	191	3.3	Yes	4	8	1.7%
49	Houston Methodist Sugar Land Hospital, Houston	51.7	5	5	92%	468	1.7	Yes	4	8	0.0%
50	Froedtert Hosp. and the Medical College of Wis., Milwaukee	51.5	5	5	91%	624	1.7	Yes	4	8	0.3%

Terms are explained on Page 113.

RECOGNIZE & RESPOND
Heart Attack

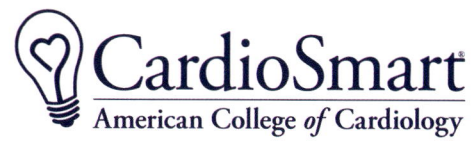

Do You Know the Signs of a Heart Attack?

Heart attacks have **beginnings.** Use CardioSmart® patient tools, including **Early Heart Attack Care™ (EHAC®),** to learn the signs so you can recognize and respond.

EARLY TREATMENT SAVES LIVES!

RECOGNIZE and RESPOND

- Chest pressure, squeezing, aching, or burning
- Pain that travels down one or both arms
- Sudden dizziness
- Excessive fatigue or weakness
- Anxiety
- Cold sweat
- Discomfort in back, neck, shoulder, or jaw
- Shortness of breath
- Nausea or vomiting

If you think you're having a heart attack, **DON'T DELAY … CALL 911!**

The American College of Cardiology (ACC), the professional home for heart care teams, works with **Accredited and Certified Chest Pain Centers** across the U.S. to improve the diagnosis and treatment of patients with heart attack symptoms.

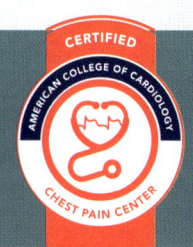
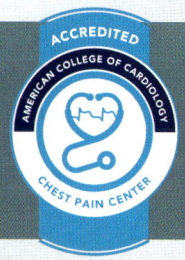

Supported by the ACC's Accreditation Foundation Committee.

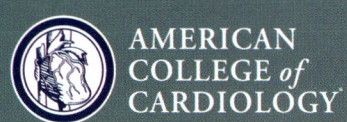

Find a center in your community and access free EHAC training videos and other resources at **CardioSmart.org/EHAC**

#EHACSavesLives

BEST HOSPITALS

Ear, Nose & Throat

Rank	Hospital	U.S. News score	Survival score (5=best)	Discharge to home score (5=best)	Patient experience (% positive responses)	Number of patients	Nurse staffing score (higher is better)	A Nurse Magnet hospital	Patient services score (8=best)	Trauma center	% of specialists recommending hospital
1	Memorial Sloan Kettering Cancer Center, New York	100.0	5	5	94%	384	2.4	Yes	8	No	2.1%
2	Massachusetts Eye & Ear Infirmary, Mass. Gen. Hosp., Boston	95.6	5	2	92%	628	2.6	Yes	8	Yes	14.1%
3	Johns Hopkins Hospital, Baltimore	92.2	4	5	93%	289	2.4	Yes	8	Yes	17.4%
4	Mayo Clinic, Rochester, Minn.	92.1	4	5	95%	564	2.7	Yes	8	Yes	11.5%
5	UCSF Medical Center, San Francisco	90.7	5	5	93%	321	2.5	Yes	8	Yes	5.9%
6	Hosps. of the U. of Pennsylvania-Penn Presby., Philadelphia	88.7	5	3	92%	532	2.5	Yes	8	Yes	9.6%
6	Mayo Clinic-Phoenix	88.7	5	5	96%	281	3.2	Yes	8	No	1.6%
8	Ohio State University Wexner Medical Center, Columbus	88.0	5	3	90%	601	2.1	Yes	8	Yes	5.9%
9	U. of Michigan Hospitals-Michigan Medicine, Ann Arbor	86.7	5	1	92%	495	2.6	Yes	8	Yes	10.0%
10	Vanderbilt University Medical Center, Nashville, Tenn.	86.0	5	5	91%	493	2.2	Yes	8	Yes	8.8%
11	University of Texas MD Anderson Cancer Center, Houston	85.7	5	5	95%	842	1.9	Yes	8	No	8.4%
12	UCLA Medical Center, Los Angeles	85.6	4	5	93%	562	3.1	Yes	8	Yes	7.5%
13	Stanford Health Care-Stanford Hospital, Stanford, Calif.	83.7	4	5	91%	364	2.6	Yes	8	Yes	8.7%
14	MUSC Health-University Medical Center, Charleston, S.C.	83.5	4	5	91%	493	2.1	Yes	8	Yes	6.1%
15	OHSU Hospital, Portland, Ore.	83.3	5	5	92%	378	2.3	Yes	8	Yes	2.2%
16	New York-Presbyterian Hospital-Columbia and Cornell, N.Y.	83.0	5	5	89%	483	3.0	Yes	8	Yes	3.9%
17	University of Kansas Hospital, Kansas City	79.0	5	4	93%	396	2.1	Yes	8	Yes	2.3%
18	Cedars-Sinai Medical Center, Los Angeles	78.2	5	5	91%	264	2.6	Yes	8	Yes	1.7%
19	Brigham and Women's Hospital, Boston	77.3	5	3	92%	298	2.3	Yes	8	Yes	2.3%
20	Barnes-Jewish Hospital, Saint Louis	75.4	4	5	90%	398	2.3	Yes	8	Yes	4.9%
21	Tampa General Hospital	75.3	4	5	91%	199	2.6	Yes	8	Yes	0.4%
22	Cleveland Clinic	75.2	4	1	92%	475	2.3	Yes	8	No	8.6%
23	University of Iowa Hospitals and Clinics, Iowa City	73.1	3	5	90%	260	1.8	Yes	8	Yes	9.4%
24	Mount Sinai Hospital, New York	72.8	4	5	87%	426	2.3	Yes	8	Yes	4.2%
25	University of Alabama at Birmingham Hospital	70.1	3	5	92%	659	2.2	Yes	8	Yes	2.3%
26	UC San Diego Health-Jacobs Medical Center	68.2	4	5	91%	176	2.0	Yes	8	Yes	2.5%
27	Manhattan Eye, Ear & Throat Hospital, New York	68.1	4	4	87%	190	2.6	Yes	8	No	1.9%
28	University of Maryland Medical Center, Baltimore	68.0	4	3	89%	318	2.7	Yes	8	Yes	0.9%
29	Emory University Hospital Midtown, Atlanta	67.8	4	5	88%	646	1.7	No	8	No	2.5%
30	UC Davis Medical Center, Sacramento, Calif.	67.3	3	5	89%	256	2.5	Yes	8	Yes	3.3%
31	University of Washington Medical Center, Seattle	66.8	3	5	91%	302	2.2	Yes	8	No	6.0%
32	UF Health Shands Hospital, Gainesville, Fla.	66.7	4	3	90%	402	2.0	Yes	8	Yes	1.2%
33	Duke University Hospital, Durham, N.C.	66.6	3	5	92%	204	2.0	Yes	8	Yes	2.8%
34	Indiana University Health Medical Center, Indianapolis	66.0	4	2	87%	309	1.9	Yes	8	Yes	1.0%
35	Keck Medical Center of USC, Los Angeles	65.3	3	3	91%	180	3.3	Yes	8	Yes	2.7%
36	University of Wisconsin Hospitals, Madison	65.1	3	5	92%	325	2.4	Yes	8	Yes	0.8%
37	Loyola University Medical Center, Maywood, Ill.	64.0	3	2	87%	323	2.7	Yes	8	Trauma	1.7%
38	UPMC Presbyterian Shadyside, Pittsburgh	63.8	3	2	90%	566	2.4	Yes	8	Yes	7.0%
39	UF Health Jacksonville, Fla.	63.7	4	5	88%	204	1.4	Yes	8	Yes	0.1%
40	Long Island Jewish Medical Center, New Hyde Park, N.Y.	62.7	3	5	85%	530	1.7	Yes	8	Yes	1.3%
41	UCHealth University of Colorado Hospital, Aurora	62.0	4	4	91%	132	2.0	Yes	8	Yes	1.6%
42	NYU Langone Hospitals, New York, N.Y.	61.7	3	4	89%	248	2.2	Yes	8	Yes	3.1%
43	Froedtert Hosp. and the Medical College of Wis., Milwaukee	61.6	4	5	91%	221	1.7	Yes	8	Yes	0.7%
44	University of Miami Hospital and Clinics-UHealth Tower, Miami	61.2	4	5	88%	415	1.3	No	8	No	2.8%
45	Rush University Medical Center, Chicago	60.9	3	5	92%	265	2.0	Yes	8	Yes	1.1%
46	University Hospitals Cleveland Medical Center	60.8	3	1	89%	448	2.5	Yes	8	Yes	1.4%
47	Yale-New Haven Hospital, New Haven, Conn.	60.2	3	3	89%	469	1.9	Yes	8	Yes	1.0%
48	Northwestern Memorial Hospital, Chicago	59.6	3	5	92%	188	1.9	Yes	7	Yes	2.1%
49	U. of Arkansas for Med. Sciences, Little Rock, Ark.	59.3	4	5	89%	282	1.9	No	7	Yes	2.0%
50	University of North Carolina Hospitals, Chapel Hill	58.9	3	5	92%	422	1.7	Yes	8	Yes	3.5%

Terms are explained on Page 113.

Financial wellness starts here.

- ✓ **Personalized Financial Plan**
- ✓ **Educational Video Lessons**
- ✓ **1-on-1 Private Coaching**
- ✓ **Progress Tracking & Accountability**

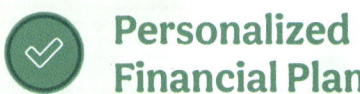

one·eleven

Reduce financial stress, elevate your relationship with money and achieve your goals.

Start now for just $1 with promo code BESTHOSPITALS

oneeleven.co

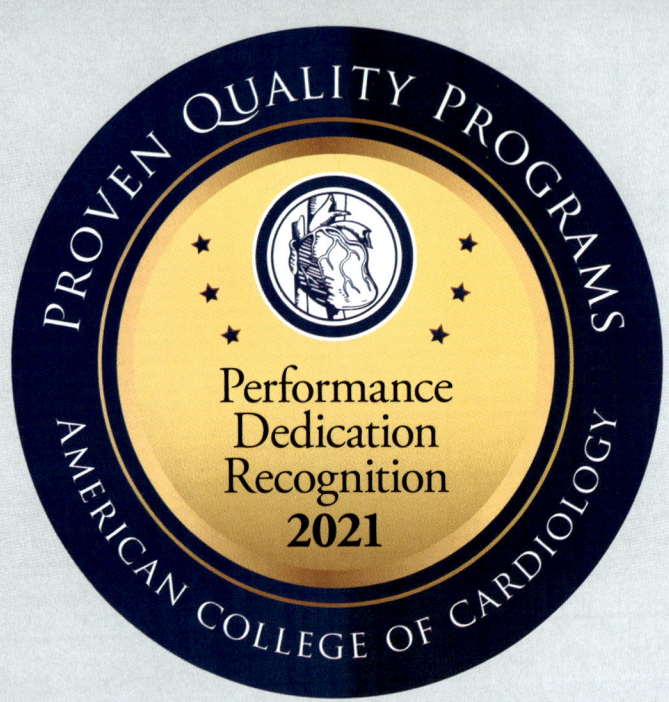

PROVEN QUALITY PROGRAMS — AMERICAN COLLEGE OF CARDIOLOGY

Performance Dedication Recognition 2021

The American College of Cardiology (ACC) recognizes these Health Systems for their commitment to drive preeminent hospital care for heart patients. Participating in the ACC's proven quality care delivery and outcomes programs demonstrates their commitment to better lives for healthier tomorrows.

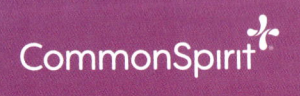 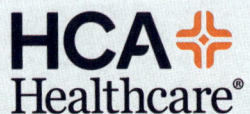 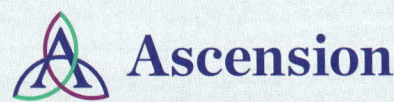

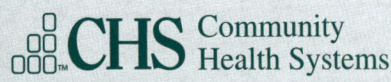 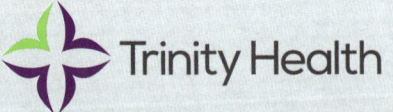 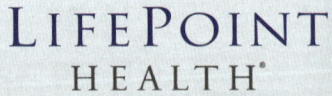

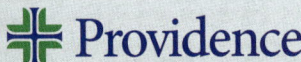 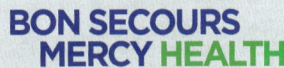 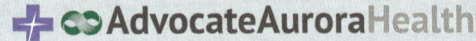

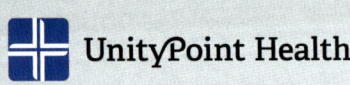 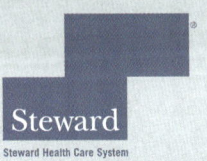 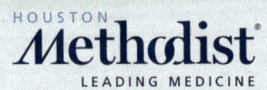 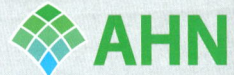

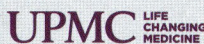 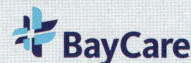 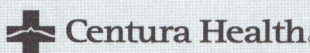 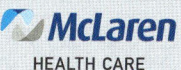 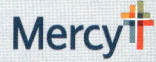
 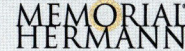 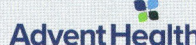 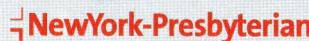
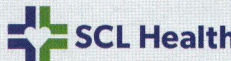 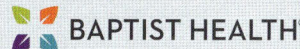 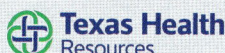 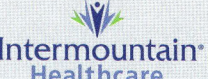
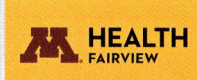 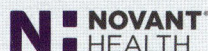 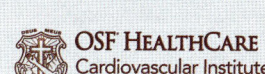
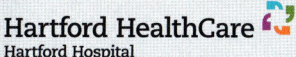 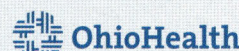 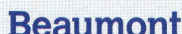 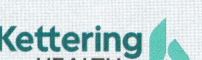 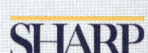
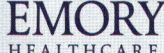 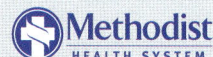 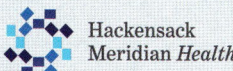 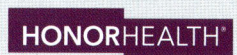 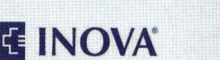
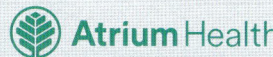 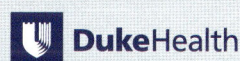 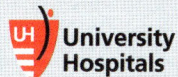 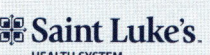
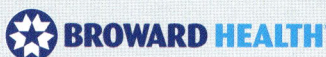 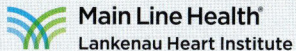 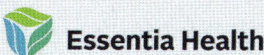
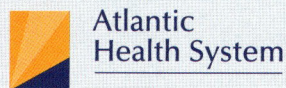 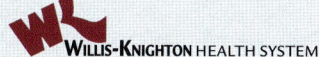 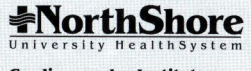

Tenet Health System
Baylor Health Care System
Sentara Healthcare
University of Pennsylvania Health System
Ballad Health System
Banner Health
Baptist Memorial Healthcare Corporation
BJC HealthCare
Christus Health System
Hendrick Health
Jackson Health System
Legacy Health

University of California Health System
Kaiser Permanente
Sutter Health
Orlando Health
Lehigh Valley Health Network
Memorial Health System of California
Methodist Healthcare
MultiCare Health System
Northside Hospital System
Northwell Health
Norton Hospitals Inc.
PeaceHealth

Yale New Haven Health
Johns Hopkins Health System
Mayo Foundation for Medical Education and Research
ProMedica Health System, Inc.
Quorum Health Corporation
Sanford Health
Singing River Health System
SSM Health Care
St. Luke's University Health Network
University of Colorado Health
University of Louisville Health, Inc.
Wellstar Health System

Visit **CVQuality.ACC.org/HealthSystems** to learn more.

©2021 American College of Cardiology B21084

BEST HOSPITALS

Gastroenterology & GI Surgery

Rank	Hospital	U.S. News score	Survival score (5=best)	Discharge to home score (5=best)	Patient experience (% positive responses)	Number of patients	Nurse staffing score (higher is better)	A Nurse Magnet hospital	Technology score (7=best)	Patient services score (8=best)	Trauma center	% of specialists recommending hospital
1	Mayo Clinic, Rochester, Minn.	100.0	5	5	95%	7,566	2.7	Yes	7	8	Yes	30.5%
2	Cedars-Sinai Medical Center, Los Angeles	93.5	5	5	91%	6,074	2.6	Yes	7	8	Yes	7.1%
3	Cleveland Clinic	90.8	5	5	92%	7,002	2.3	Yes	7	8	No	20.5%
4	UCLA Medical Center, Los Angeles	86.1	5	5	93%	3,495	3.1	Yes	7	8	Yes	7.3%
5	NYU Langone Hospitals, New York, N.Y.	85.7	5	5	89%	9,399	2.2	Yes	7	8	Yes	5.8%
6	Johns Hopkins Hospital, Baltimore	83.4	5	5	93%	3,499	2.4	Yes	7	8	Yes	13.3%
7	Mayo Clinic-Phoenix	80.6	5	5	96%	2,714	3.2	Yes	7	8	No	5.0%
8	New York-Presbyterian Hospital-Columbia and Cornell, N.Y.	80.2	5	5	89%	10,852	3.0	Yes	7	8	Yes	7.9%
9	Northwestern Memorial Hospital, Chicago	79.6	5	5	92%	3,789	1.9	Yes	7	7	Yes	5.0%
10	Houston Methodist Hospital	79.2	5	5	92%	5,469	2.0	Yes	7	8	No	1.7%
11	Massachusetts General Hospital, Boston	78.7	5	5	92%	5,825	2.6	Yes	7	8	Yes	9.7%
12	Keck Medical Center of USC, Los Angeles	78.6	5	5	91%	1,862	3.3	Yes	7	8	Yes	2.1%
13	U. of Michigan Hospitals-Michigan Medicine, Ann Arbor	78.2	5	5	92%	4,500	2.6	Yes	7	8	Yes	5.9%
14	University of Chicago Medical Center	78.1	5	5	90%	2,856	2.2	Yes	7	8	Yes	5.6%
15	Mount Sinai Hospital, New York	77.3	5	5	87%	5,267	2.3	Yes	7	8	Yes	6.4%
16	Hosps. of the U. of Pennsylvania-Penn Presby., Philadelphia	77.2	5	5	92%	4,412	2.5	Yes	7	8	Yes	6.1%
17	UPMC Presbyterian Shadyside, Pittsburgh	75.1	5	5	90%	6,817	2.4	Yes	7	8	Yes	4.3%
18	UC San Diego Health-Jacobs Medical Center	74.5	5	5	91%	2,533	2.0	Yes	7	8	Yes	2.4%
19	Beaumont Hospital-Royal Oak, Mich.	74.1	5	5	88%	6,126	2.0	Yes	7	8	Yes	0.2%
20	Barnes-Jewish Hospital, Saint Louis	73.3	5	5	90%	5,790	2.3	Yes	7	8	Yes	4.1%
21	Rush University Medical Center, Chicago	73.2	5	5	92%	2,216	2.0	Yes	7	8	Yes	0.9%
22	Memorial Sloan Kettering Cancer Center, New York	73.0	5	5	94%	5,121	2.4	Yes	6	8	No	2.5%
23	OHSU Hospital, Portland, Ore.	72.8	5	5	92%	2,509	2.3	Yes	7	8	Yes	0.8%
24	Baylor St. Luke's Medical Center, Houston	71.6	5	5	88%	3,069	2.0	Yes	7	8	No	1.3%
25	Loyola University Medical Center, Maywood, Ill.	71.4	5	5	87%	2,456	2.7	Yes	7	8	Yes	0.6%
26	Jefferson Health-Thomas Jefferson U. Hospitals, Philadelphia	71.2	5	5	89%	4,261	2.0	Yes	7	8	Yes	1.8%
26	Mayo Clinic-Jacksonville, Fla.	71.2	5	5	95%	2,727	2.7	Yes	7	8	No	5.2%
26	Tampa General Hospital	71.2	5	5	91%	2,998	2.6	Yes	7	8	Yes	0.9%
29	UCSF Medical Center, San Francisco	71.1	5	5	93%	2,859	2.5	Yes	7	8	Yes	5.9%
30	Stanford Health Care-Stanford Hospital, Stanford, Calif.	70.7	5	5	91%	3,402	2.6	Yes	7	8	Yes	2.4%
31	Brigham and Women's Hospital, Boston	70.4	5	5	92%	4,928	2.3	Yes	6	8	Yes	4.1%
32	Duke University Hospital, Durham, N.C.	69.7	5	5	92%	4,148	2.0	Yes	7	8	Yes	4.1%
33	Cleveland Clinic Weston, Fla.	69.5	5	5	92%	2,408	2.6	No	7	8	No	1.8%
34	St. Francis Hospital & Heart Center, Roslyn, N.Y.	69.4	5	5	95%	3,044	2.0	Yes	6	8	No	0.2%
35	UT Southwestern Medical Center, Dallas	69.3	5	5	94%	2,610	2.1	Yes	7	8	No	1.6%
36	Baylor University Medical Center, Dallas	69.1	5	5	93%	4,836	2.0	Yes	7	8	Yes	2.0%
37	University of Texas MD Anderson Cancer Center, Houston	69.0	5	5	95%	4,677	1.9	Yes	6	8	No	2.4%
38	UCHealth University of Colorado Hospital, Aurora	68.9	5	5	91%	2,872	2.0	Yes	7	8	Yes	1.8%
39	North Shore University Hospital, Manhasset, N.Y.	68.5	5	5	88%	5,790	2.0	Yes	6	8	Yes	1.0%
40	Beth Israel Deaconess Medical Center, Boston	68.3	5	5	90%	4,249	1.5	No	7	8	Yes	1.6%
41	DMC Harper University Hospital, Detroit	68.2	5	5	86%	934	1.4	Yes	6	8	No	0.0%
42	Loma Linda University Medical Center, Loma Linda, Calif.	67.9	5	5	90%	1,902	3.0	Yes	7	8	Yes	0.6%
43	Cleveland Clinic Hillcrest Hospital	67.7	5	5	89%	3,275	1.6	Yes	6	8	Yes	0.3%
44	Hoag Memorial Hospital Presbyterian, Newport Beach, Calif.	67.6	5	5	94%	4,408	2.4	Yes	6	8	No	0.7%
45	Yale-New Haven Hospital, New Haven, Conn.	67.4	5	5	89%	6,584	1.9	Yes	7	8	Yes	1.7%
46	Advocate Lutheran General Hospital, Park Ridge, Ill.	67.2	5	5	90%	2,737	2.2	Yes	6	8	Yes	0.1%
46	University of Wisconsin Hospitals, Madison	67.2	5	5	92%	3,624	2.4	Yes	7	8	Yes	1.1%
48	AdventHealth Orlando	67.1	5	5	90%	13,556	1.8	No	7	8	No	1.4%
48	Advocate Illinois Masonic Medical Center, Chicago	67.1	5	5	89%	1,104	2.0	Yes	6	8	Yes	0.0%
50	Ohio State University Wexner Medical Center, Columbus	66.7	5	5	90%	6,003	2.1	Yes	7	8	Yes	2.7%
50	Scripps La Jolla Hospitals, La Jolla, Calif.	66.7	5	5	92%	3,687	3.0	Yes	7	8	Yes	0.7%

Terms are explained on Page 113.

More @ usnews.com/besthospitals

Geriatrics

Rank	Hospital	U.S. News score	Survival score (5=best)	Discharge to home score (5=best)	Patient experience (% positive responses)	Number of patients	Nurse staffing score (higher is better)	A Nurse Magnet hospital	NIA Alzheimer's center	Patient services score (9=best)	% of specialists recommending hospital
1	Mount Sinai Hospital, New York	100.0	5	5	87%	29,618	2.3	Yes	Yes	9	19.0%
2	Cleveland Clinic	99.3	5	5	92%	23,522	2.3	Yes	Yes	9	8.6%
3	Mayo Clinic, Rochester, Minn.	98.1	5	5	95%	32,300	2.7	Yes	Yes	9	10.0%
4	UCLA Medical Center, Los Angeles	96.4	5	5	93%	19,273	3.1	Yes	No	9	20.0%
5	NYU Langone Hospitals, New York, N.Y.	94.8	5	5	89%	57,462	2.2	Yes	Yes	9	3.4%
6	Johns Hopkins Hospital, Baltimore	94.4	5	5	93%	10,995	2.4	Yes	Yes	9	13.7%
7	New York-Presbyterian Hospital-Columbia and Cornell, N.Y.	92.5	5	5	89%	67,784	3.0	Yes	Yes	8	4.6%
8	Northwestern Memorial Hospital, Chicago	91.4	5	5	92%	16,200	1.9	Yes	Yes	8	2.3%
9	UCSF Medical Center, San Francisco	91.3	5	5	93%	10,807	2.5	Yes	Yes	9	11.1%
10	Cedars-Sinai Medical Center, Los Angeles	88.9	5	5	91%	34,934	2.6	Yes	No	7	1.1%
11	Keck Medical Center of USC, Los Angeles	87.9	5	5	91%	5,594	3.3	Yes	Yes	9	1.0%
12	U. of Michigan Hospitals-Michigan Medicine, Ann Arbor	87.2	5	5	92%	15,702	2.6	Yes	Yes	9	5.9%
13	UC San Diego Health-Jacobs Medical Center	86.7	5	5	91%	10,777	2.0	Yes	Yes	9	3.7%
14	Massachusetts General Hospital, Boston	85.8	5	5	92%	28,453	2.6	Yes	Yes	9	6.3%
15	Stanford Health Care-Stanford Hospital, Stanford, Calif.	84.1	5	5	91%	14,479	2.6	Yes	Yes	9	1.1%
16	Rush University Medical Center, Chicago	83.8	5	5	92%	10,884	2.0	Yes	Yes	9	1.3%
17	Hosps. of the U. of Pennsylvania-Penn Presby., Philadelphia	83.5	5	5	92%	19,937	2.5	Yes	Yes	9	2.3%
18	Brigham and Women's Hospital, Boston	82.9	5	5	92%	20,402	2.3	Yes	Yes	9	1.2%
19	Barnes-Jewish Hospital, Saint Louis	81.7	5	5	90%	19,944	2.3	Yes	Yes	9	1.9%
19	UPMC Presbyterian Shadyside, Pittsburgh	81.7	5	5	90%	26,680	2.4	Yes	Yes	9	4.5%
21	Yale-New Haven Hospital, New Haven, Conn.	80.9	5	5	89%	36,744	1.9	Yes	Yes	9	4.7%
22	Houston Methodist Hospital	80.7	5	5	92%	23,836	2.0	Yes	No	9	1.2%
23	UT Southwestern Medical Center, Dallas	80.4	5	5	94%	11,350	2.1	Yes	No	9	0.5%
24	University of Kansas Hospital, Kansas City	79.8	5	5	93%	14,248	2.1	Yes	Yes	9	0.8%
25	UC Davis Medical Center, Sacramento, Calif.	79.6	5	5	89%	10,914	2.5	Yes	Yes	9	0.6%
26	University of Texas MD Anderson Cancer Center, Houston	79.5	5	5	95%	10,250	1.9	Yes	No	6	0.3%
27	Vanderbilt University Medical Center, Nashville, Tenn.	79.4	5	5	91%	15,899	2.2	Yes	Yes	9	1.7%
28	Oroville Hospital, Oroville, Calif.	79.3	5	5	79%	7,849	1.2	No	No	8	0.0%
29	North Shore University Hospital, Manhasset, N.Y.	79.2	5	5	88%	41,636	2.0	Yes	No	9	2.6%
30	Emory University Hospital at Wesley Woods, Atlanta	78.4	5	5	91%	11,994	2.2	Yes	Yes	9	1.0%
30	University of Alabama at Birmingham Hospital	78.4	5	5	92%	15,330	2.2	Yes	Yes	8	4.7%
32	OHSU Hospital, Portland, Ore.	78.2	5	5	92%	7,816	2.3	Yes	Yes	9	0.7%
33	Beaumont Hospital-Grosse Pointe, Mich.	78.1	5	5	92%	9,604	2.0	Yes	No	9	0.0%
34	Mayo Clinic-Phoenix	78.0	5	5	96%	11,616	3.2	Yes	No	7	2.0%
34	University of Wisconsin Hospitals, Madison	78.0	5	5	92%	14,393	2.4	Yes	Yes	9	2.4%
36	Beaumont Hospital-Royal Oak, Mich.	77.6	5	5	88%	37,666	2.0	Yes	No	9	0.3%
37	Mayo Clinic-Jacksonville, Fla.	77.4	5	5	95%	9,444	2.7	Yes	Yes	8	1.4%
38	St. Francis Hospital & Heart Center, Roslyn, N.Y.	77.2	5	5	95%	24,237	2.0	Yes	No	8	0.6%
39	Lenox Hill Hospital, New York	76.4	5	5	87%	18,050	2.6	Yes	No	9	0.7%
40	University Hospitals Cleveland Medical Center	75.3	5	5	89%	14,229	2.5	Yes	Yes	9	0.3%
41	Memorial Sloan Kettering Cancer Center, New York	75.1	5	5	94%	10,209	2.4	Yes	No	7	0.1%
42	Montefiore Medical Center, Bronx, N.Y.	75.0	5	5	82%	45,719	2.3	No	No	9	1.1%
42	UF Health Shands Hospital, Gainesville, Fla.	75.0	5	5	90%	18,088	2.0	Yes	Yes	9	0.7%
44	UCI Medical Center, Orange, Calif.	74.5	5	5	90%	8,506	2.0	Yes	Yes	9	1.8%
45	Mount Sinai Medical Center, Miami Beach, Fla.	73.9	5	5	88%	16,132	1.3	No	Yes	9	0.8%
46	Baylor St. Luke's Medical Center, Houston	73.8	5	5	88%	13,113	2.0	Yes	No	6	0.7%
47	Long Island Jewish Medical Center, New Hyde Park, N.Y.	73.7	5	5	85%	43,012	1.7	Yes	No	9	1.6%
48	Indiana University Health Medical Center, Indianapolis	72.9	5	5	87%	14,095	1.9	Yes	Yes	9	2.6%
49	DMC Harper University Hospital, Detroit	72.8	5	5	86%	5,291	1.4	Yes	No	8	0.1%
50	Hoag Memorial Hospital Presbyterian, Newport Beach, Calif.	72.6	5	5	94%	24,897	2.4	Yes	No	9	0.3%
50	Scripps La Jolla Hospitals, La Jolla, Calif.	72.6	5	5	92%	21,116	3.0	Yes	No	8	0.1%

Terms are explained on Page 113.

BEST HOSPITALS

Gynecology

Rank	Hospital	U.S. News score	Survival score (5=best)	Discharge to home score (5=best)	Patient experience (% positive responses)	Number of patients	Nurse staffing score (higher is better)	A Nurse Magnet hospital	Technology score (5=best)	Patient services score (9=best)	% of specialists recommending hospital
1	Mayo Clinic, Rochester, Minn.	100.0	5	5	95%	563	2.7	Yes	5	9	11.9%
2	Memorial Sloan Kettering Cancer Center, New York	94.7	5	5	94%	588	2.4	Yes	5	8	5.0%
3	Cleveland Clinic	94.0	5	3	92%	286	2.3	Yes	5	9	11.5%
4	Brigham and Women's Hospital, Boston	90.7	5	5	92%	407	2.3	Yes	5	9	7.5%
5	University of Texas MD Anderson Cancer Center, Houston	90.2	5	5	95%	502	1.9	Yes	5	9	3.3%
6	Inova Fairfax Hospital, Falls Church, Va.	86.7	5	5	91%	674	1.7	Yes	5	9	0.6%
7	University of Alabama at Birmingham Hospital	86.2	5	5	92%	417	2.2	Yes	5	9	2.0%
8	Johns Hopkins Hospital, Baltimore	84.7	4	5	93%	197	2.4	Yes	5	9	10.1%
9	Massachusetts General Hospital, Boston	81.8	5	3	92%	288	2.6	Yes	5	9	5.5%
9	Stanford Health Care-Stanford Hospital, Stanford, Calif.	81.8	5	4	91%	250	2.6	Yes	5	9	2.3%
11	New York-Presbyterian Hospital-Columbia and Cornell, N.Y.	81.0	3	5	89%	510	3.0	Yes	5	9	7.0%
12	Cedars-Sinai Medical Center, Los Angeles	78.4	5	5	91%	313	2.6	Yes	5	9	1.8%
13	University of Wisconsin Hospitals, Madison	78.3	4	5	92%	532	2.4	Yes	5	9	0.9%
14	Barnes-Jewish Hospital, Saint Louis	78.0	4	3	90%	564	2.3	Yes	5	9	4.5%
15	Long Island Jewish Medical Center, New Hyde Park, N.Y.	76.4	4	5	85%	635	1.7	Yes	5	9	2.5%
16	NYU Langone Hospitals, New York, N.Y.	75.6	3	4	89%	405	2.2	Yes	5	9	5.4%
17	MUSC Health-University Medical Center, Charleston, S.C.	75.3	4	5	91%	363	2.1	Yes	5	9	1.4%
18	Beaumont Hospital-Royal Oak, Mich.	75.0	5	5	88%	264	2.0	Yes	5	9	0.5%
19	Houston Methodist Hospital	74.7	5	3	92%	159	2.0	Yes	5	8	0.6%
20	Rush University Medical Center, Chicago	73.5	5	5	92%	237	2.0	Yes	5	9	1.1%
21	UCLA Medical Center, Los Angeles	73.4	3	3	93%	246	3.1	Yes	5	9	2.8%
22	University of Chicago Medical Center	73.2	5	3	90%	260	2.2	Yes	5	9	1.0%
23	Hosps. of the U. of Pennsylvania-Penn Presby., Philadelphia	73.0	4	3	92%	246	2.5	Yes	5	9	2.9%
24	UCI Medical Center, Orange, Calif.	72.8	4	4	90%	184	2.0	Yes	5	9	1.7%
25	Keck Medical Center of USC, Los Angeles	70.4	3	4	91%	70	3.3	Yes	5	9	1.6%
26	UC Davis Medical Center, Sacramento, Calif.	69.9	4	3	89%	168	2.5	Yes	5	9	1.0%
27	Mayo Clinic-Phoenix	69.6	3	5	96%	73	3.2	Yes	5	8	1.9%
28	Morristown Medical Center, Morristown, N.J.	69.2	4	2	91%	373	2.1	Yes	5	9	0.3%
29	UC San Diego Health-Jacobs Medical Center	69.1	3	5	91%	203	2.0	Yes	5	9	2.2%
30	Northside Hospital Atlanta	68.8	3	5	92%	321	3.9	No	5	7	1.0%
31	Lenox Hill Hospital, New York	68.4	3	5	87%	176	2.6	Yes	5	9	3.2%
31	Scripps La Jolla Hospitals, La Jolla, Calif.	68.4	3	3	92%	284	3.0	Yes	5	9	0.9%
31	Vanderbilt University Medical Center, Nashville, Tenn.	68.4	3	3	91%	170	2.2	Yes	5	9	4.2%
34	UCSF Medical Center, San Francisco	68.3	3	3	93%	157	2.5	Yes	5	9	3.7%
34	University of North Carolina Hospitals, Chapel Hill	68.3	3	5	92%	327	1.7	Yes	5	9	5.0%
36	MemorialCare Long Beach Medical Center, Long Beach, Calif.	68.1	3	4	89%	289	2.0	Yes	5	9	0.1%
37	Beth Israel Deaconess Medical Center, Boston	68.0	5	3	90%	248	1.5	No	5	9	0.7%
37	John Muir Health-Walnut Creek Med. Ctr., Walnut Creek, Calif.	68.0	3	5	91%	293	2.2	Yes	5	8	0.0%
39	University of Washington Medical Center, Seattle	67.3	3	3	91%	368	2.2	Yes	5	9	2.8%
40	U. of Michigan Hospitals-Michigan Medicine, Ann Arbor	67.1	3	4	92%	290	2.6	Yes	5	9	3.9%
41	Baylor University Medical Center, Dallas	66.7	3	3	93%	324	2.0	Yes	5	9	0.9%
41	University of Iowa Hospitals and Clinics, Iowa City	66.7	3	2	90%	385	1.8	Yes	5	9	1.5%
43	Montefiore Medical Center, Bronx, N.Y.	66.5	4	3	82%	359	2.3	No	5	9	0.3%
44	Duke University Hospital, Durham, N.C.	66.1	3	5	92%	293	2.0	Yes	5	8	5.7%
45	UF Health Shands Hospital, Gainesville, Fla.	65.6	4	3	90%	222	2.0	Yes	5	9	1.0%
46	Ohio State University Wexner Medical Center, Columbus	65.5	3	1	90%	448	2.1	Yes	5	9	1.9%
47	Yale-New Haven Hospital, New Haven, Conn.	65.4	3	3	89%	437	1.9	Yes	5	9	2.4%
48	Advocate Lutheran General Hospital, Park Ridge, Ill.	65.3	4	2	90%	167	2.2	Yes	5	9	0.2%
49	Advocate Christ Medical Center, Oak Lawn, Ill.	65.2	3	3	87%	429	2.7	Yes	5	9	0.2%
49	Greater Baltimore Medical Center	65.2	5	3	88%	137	2.6	No	5	7	0.8%

Terms are explained on Page 113.

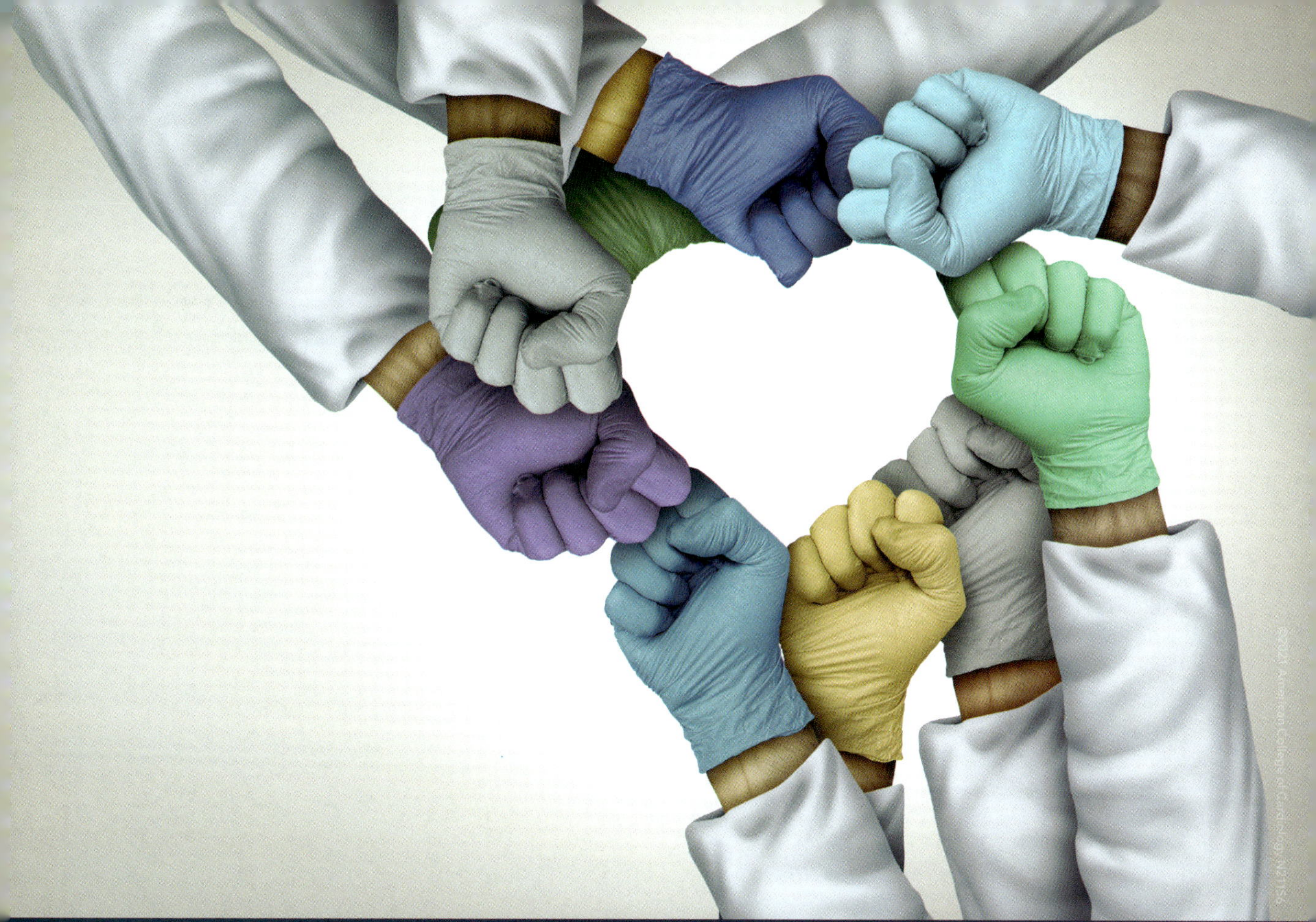

THANK YOU TO HEALTH CARE HEROES EVERYWHERE

The American College of Cardiology is deeply grateful for health care workers around the world who have worked tirelessly and courageously to help and heal patients.

Compassionate care has always been at the heart of what you do.

We thank you for all the unflagging sacrifices you have made and continue to make in the lives of your patients, their families and your communities. Your commitment, persistence and dedication deserve our unending admiration and we thank you.

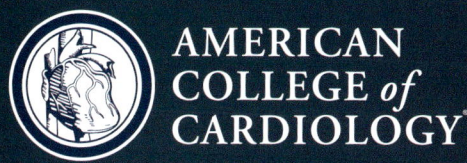

Advancing Heart Care Worldwide

ACC is working to provide resources to help health care workers to look after their mental and physical well-being while on the front lines of the COVID-19 pandemic.

Please visit ACC's Resources For Clinician Well-Being for tools and resources specific to these unprecedented times at **www.acc.org/clinicianwellbeing**.

BEST HOSPITALS

Neurology & Neurosurgery

Rank	Hospital	U.S. News score	Survival score (5=best)	Discharge to home score (5=best)	Patient experience (% positive responses)	Number of patients	Nurse staffing score (higher is better)	Public transparency	NAEC epilepsy center	Technology score (5=best)	Patient services score (9=best)	% of specialists recommending hospital
1	UCSF Medical Center, San Francisco	100.0	5	5	93%	2,628	2.5	Yes	Yes	5	9	20.3%
2	New York-Presbyterian Hospital-Columbia and Cornell, N.Y.	91.5	5	5	89%	9,392	3.0	Yes	Yes	5	9	11.8%
3	Rush University Medical Center, Chicago	91.3	5	5	92%	2,961	2.0	Yes	Yes	5	9	3.4%
4	Johns Hopkins Hospital, Baltimore	91.1	5	5	93%	2,960	2.4	Yes	Yes	5	9	22.9%
5	NYU Langone Hospitals, New York, N.Y.	90.2	5	5	89%	7,071	2.2	Yes	Yes	5	9	6.2%
6	Mayo Clinic, Rochester, Minn.	89.7	5	5	95%	4,914	2.7	Yes	Yes	5	9	26.8%
7	Cleveland Clinic	84.2	5	5	92%	4,147	2.3	Yes	Yes	5	9	13.6%
8	UCLA Medical Center, Los Angeles	83.0	5	5	93%	2,938	3.1	Yes	Yes	5	9	7.6%
9	Northwestern Memorial Hospital, Chicago	82.8	5	5	92%	3,028	1.9	Yes	Yes	5	8	4.1%
10	Mount Sinai Hospital, New York	81.7	5	5	87%	3,479	2.3	Yes	Yes	5	9	2.6%
11	Cedars-Sinai Medical Center, Los Angeles	81.3	5	5	91%	4,085	2.6	Yes	Yes	5	8	1.6%
12	Massachusetts General Hospital, Boston	77.4	4	5	92%	5,143	2.6	Yes	Yes	5	9	17.8%
13	Stanford Health Care-Stanford Hospital, Stanford, Calif.	76.2	5	5	91%	2,570	2.6	Yes	Yes	5	9	5.6%
14	Hosps. of the U. of Pennsylvania-Penn Presby., Philadelphia	75.3	5	1	92%	3,967	2.5	Yes	Yes	5	9	7.1%
15	U. of Michigan Hospitals-Michigan Medicine, Ann Arbor	75.2	5	5	92%	2,793	2.6	Yes	Yes	5	9	3.5%
16	Mayo Clinic-Jacksonville, Fla.	74.5	5	5	95%	2,120	2.7	Yes	Yes	5	9	4.1%
17	Barnes-Jewish Hospital, Saint Louis	74.3	5	5	90%	5,079	2.3	Yes	Yes	5	9	6.3%
18	Brigham and Women's Hospital, Boston	73.0	5	5	92%	4,505	2.3	Yes	Yes	5	9	4.7%
19	UT Southwestern Medical Center, Dallas	71.7	5	5	94%	2,596	2.1	Yes	Yes	5	9	2.1%
20	Long Island Jewish Medical Center, New Hyde Park, N.Y.	71.4	5	5	85%	4,712	1.7	Yes	Yes	5	9	0.8%
21	Houston Methodist Hospital	71.3	5	5	92%	4,298	2.0	Yes	Yes	5	9	1.0%
22	Emory University Hospital, Atlanta	69.9	5	5	91%	2,879	2.2	Yes	Yes	5	9	3.7%
23	Beaumont Hospital-Grosse Pointe, Mich.	69.6	5	5	92%	843	2.0	Yes	No	5	9	0.0%
23	Lenox Hill Hospital, New York	69.6	5	5	87%	1,914	2.6	Yes	Yes	5	9	1.0%
23	UPMC Presbyterian Shadyside, Pittsburgh	69.6	5	4	90%	7,357	2.4	Yes	Yes	5	9	3.1%
26	UC San Diego Health-Jacobs Medical Center	68.7	5	5	91%	1,982	2.0	Yes	Yes	5	9	2.0%
27	Barrow Neurological Institute, Phoenix	68.0	5	5	89%	6,476	2.1	Yes	Yes	5	9	5.9%
28	Ohio State University Wexner Medical Center, Columbus	66.6	5	5	90%	5,087	2.1	Yes	Yes	5	9	1.6%
29	OHSU Hospital, Portland, Ore.	66.2	5	5	92%	2,348	2.3	Yes	Yes	5	9	0.6%
30	University of Kansas Hospital, Kansas City	65.9	5	5	93%	3,448	2.1	Yes	Yes	5	9	0.8%
31	Duke University Hospital, Durham, N.C.	65.6	5	5	92%	3,884	2.0	Yes	Yes	5	9	5.3%
31	Ochsner Medical Center, New Orleans	65.6	5	5	89%	4,366	1.8	Yes	Yes	5	9	0.7%
33	Baylor St. Luke's Medical Center, Houston	65.4	5	5	88%	2,816	2.0	Yes	Yes	5	8	0.5%
34	St. Francis Hospital & Heart Center, Roslyn, N.Y.	65.2	5	5	95%	1,803	2.0	Yes	No	5	8	0.2%
35	University of Miami Hospital and Clinics-UHealth Tower, Miami	65.1	5	5	88%	1,082	1.3	Yes	Yes	5	9	1.8%
36	Keck Medical Center of USC, Los Angeles	65.0	3	5	91%	990	3.3	Yes	Yes	5	9	2.2%
37	Abbott Northwestern Hospital, Minneapolis	64.9	5	5	91%	3,225	2.5	Public	Yes	5	9	0.1%
38	Montefiore Medical Center, Bronx, N.Y.	64.4	5	5	82%	5,933	2.3	Yes	Yes	5	9	0.7%
39	University Hospitals Cleveland Medical Center	64.0	5	2	89%	3,481	2.5	Yes	Yes	5	9	1.0%
40	Cleveland Clinic Fairview Hospital, Cleveland	63.8	5	4	91%	1,871	1.7	Yes	No	5	9	0.4%
41	Inova Loudoun Hospital, Leesburg, Va.	63.7	5	5	89%	796	1.3	Yes	No	5	9	0.0%
42	Yale-New Haven Hospital, New Haven, Conn.	63.6	5	5	89%	5,542	1.9	Yes	Yes	5	9	1.8%
43	Cleveland Clinic Hillcrest Hospital	63.4	5	3	89%	2,097	1.6	Yes	No	5	9	0.4%
43	University of Wisconsin Hospitals, Madison	63.4	5	5	92%	3,322	2.4	Yes	Yes	5	9	1.1%
45	UC Davis Medical Center, Sacramento, Calif.	63.1	4	5	89%	2,008	2.5	Yes	Yes	5	9	0.6%
46	North Shore University Hospital, Manhasset, N.Y.	63.0	5	5	88%	4,809	2.0	Yes	Yes	5	9	1.2%
47	AdventHealth Orlando	62.9	5	5	90%	10,177	1.8	Yes	Yes	5	9	0.3%
48	Providence St. John's Health Center, Santa Monica, Calif.	62.7	5	5	89%	1,309	3.4	Yes	No	5	9	0.1%
48	Vanderbilt University Medical Center, Nashville, Tenn.	62.7	3	5	91%	4,792	2.2	Yes	Yes	5	9	1.8%
50	Hackensack University Medical Center, Hackensack, N.J.	62.4	5	5	86%	2,921	2.9	Yes	Yes	5	9	0.3%

Terms are explained on Page 113.

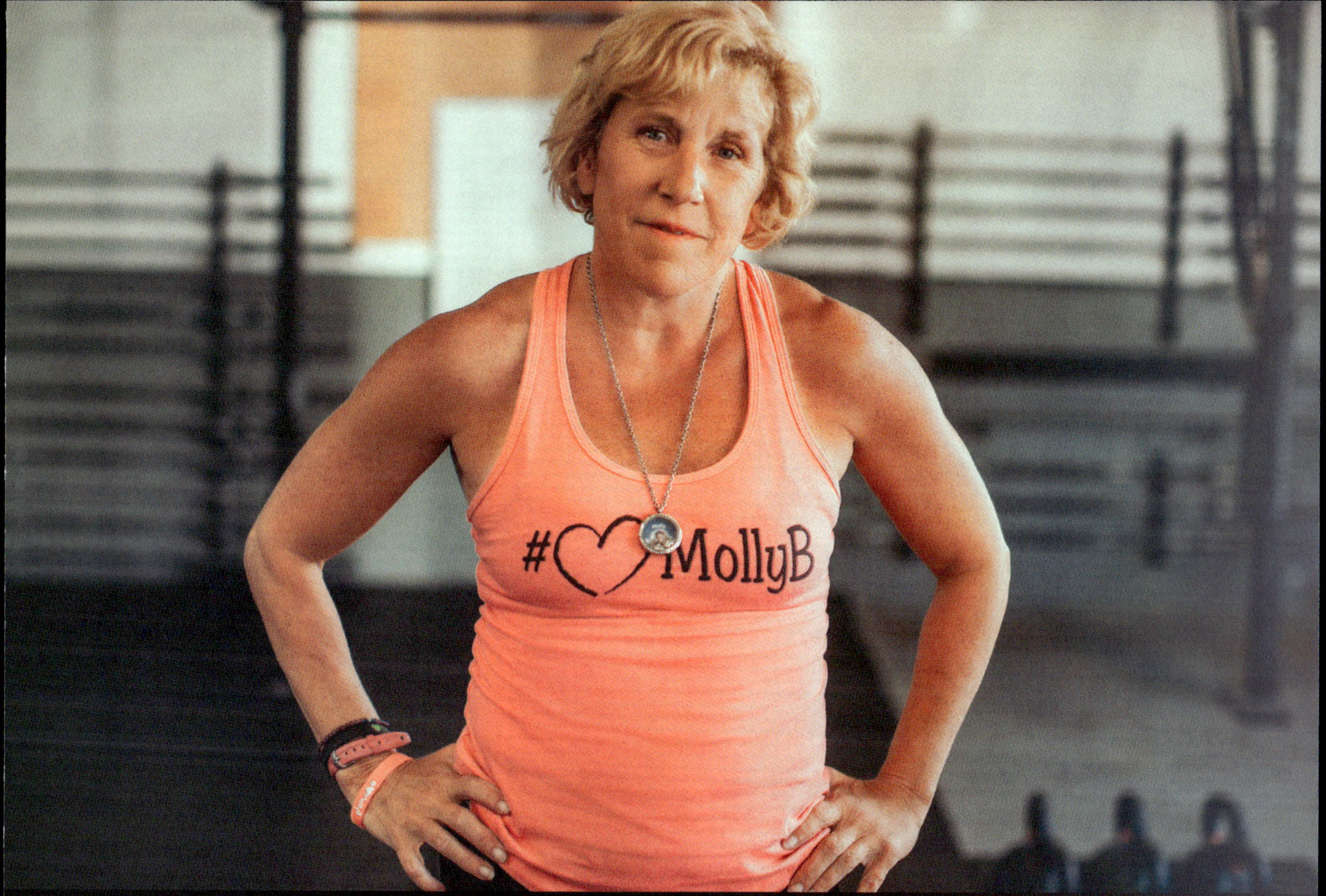

Diagnosed with 3 brain tumors, Barbara got a second act.

Barbara's daughter, Molly, died of a ruptured brain tumor that doctors had missed. So when she was diagnosed a year later with three brain tumors, she was terrified. That's when a friend recommended Dr. Eskandar, the Chair of Neurosurgery at Montefiore-Einstein.

See Barbara's story at montefiore.org/barbara

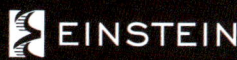 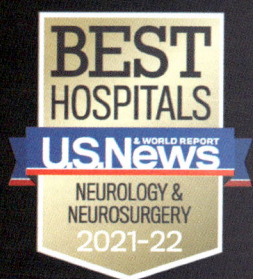

BEST HOSPITALS

Orthopedics

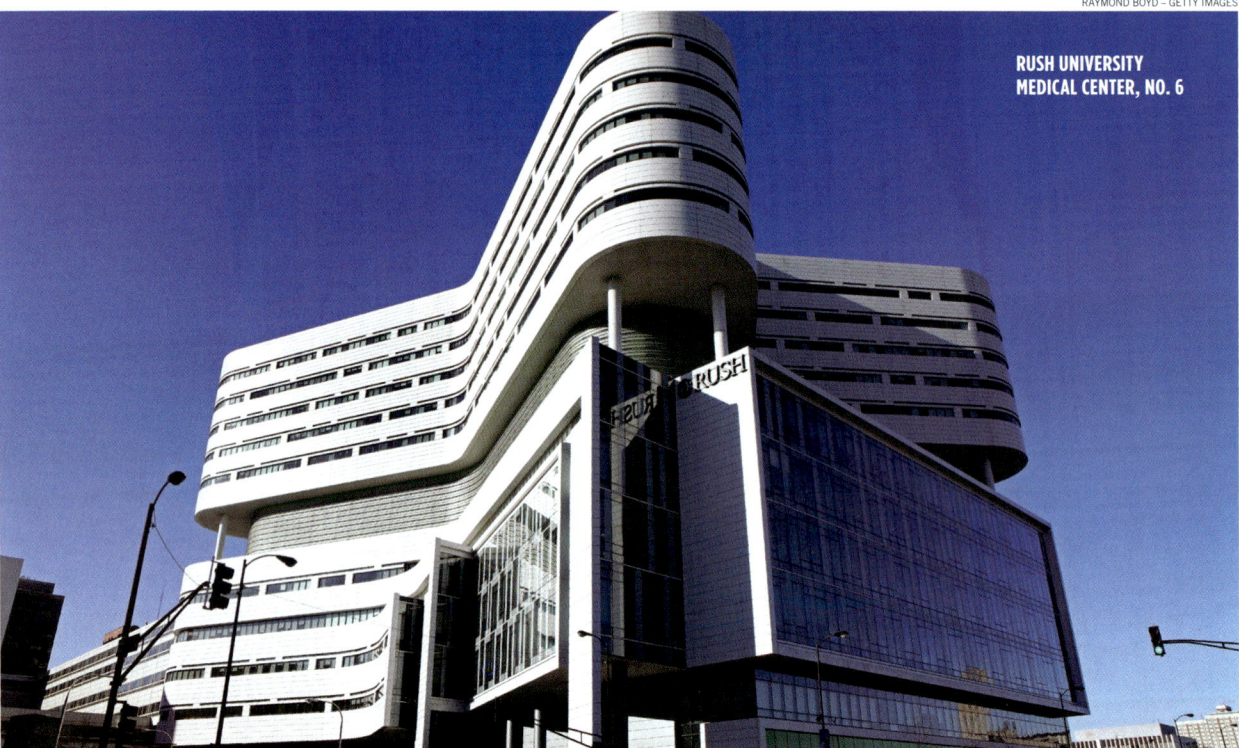

RUSH UNIVERSITY MEDICAL CENTER, NO. 6

RAYMOND BOYD – GETTY IMAGES

Rank	Hospital	U.S. News score	Survival score (5=best)	Discharge to home score (5=best)	Patient experience (% positive responses)	Number of patients	Nurse staffing score (higher is better)	A Nurse Magnet hospital	Technology score (2=best)	Patient services score (7=best)	% of specialists recommending hospital
1	Hospital for Special Surgery, New York	100.0	5	5	95%	6,973	3.7	Yes	2	7	21.9%
2	Mayo Clinic, Rochester, Minn.	80.8	5	5	95%	6,516	2.7	Yes	2	7	22.2%
3	Cedars-Sinai Medical Center, Los Angeles	78.5	5	5	91%	4,896	2.6	Yes	2	7	3.0%
4	NYU Langone Orthopedic Hospital, New York	76.0	5	5	89%	7,085	2.2	Yes	2	7	6.6%
5	UCLA Medical Center, Los Angeles	71.2	5	5	93%	2,040	3.1	Yes	2	7	2.9%
6	Rush University Medical Center, Chicago	70.6	5	5	92%	3,038	2.0	Yes	2	7	5.8%
7	Cleveland Clinic	66.8	5	3	92%	3,876	2.3	Yes	2	7	13.3%
8	Massachusetts General Hospital, Boston	66.0	5	1	92%	3,707	2.6	Yes	2	7	7.3%
9	New York-Presbyterian Hospital-Columbia and Cornell, N.Y.	65.0	5	1	89%	6,339	3.0	Yes	2	6	2.6%
10	Jefferson Health-Thomas Jefferson U. Hospitals, Philadelphia	64.0	5	3	89%	5,598	2.0	Yes	2	7	7.9%
11	Scripps La Jolla Hospitals, La Jolla, Calif.	63.9	5	5	92%	4,540	3.0	Yes	2	7	1.4%
12	Houston Methodist Hospital	63.2	5	5	92%	3,683	2.0	Yes	2	7	1.1%
13	Stanford Health Care-Stanford Hospital, Stanford, Calif.	62.8	5	5	91%	3,408	2.6	Yes	2	7	2.8%
14	Mount Sinai Hospital, New York	61.0	5	5	87%	2,694	2.3	Yes	2	7	0.6%
15	University of Wisconsin Hospitals, Madison	60.6	5	5	92%	2,629	2.4	Yes	2	7	0.5%
16	UCSF Medical Center, San Francisco	60.3	5	1	93%	3,107	2.5	Yes	2	7	3.0%
17	New England Baptist Hospital, Boston	60.2	5	1	95%	3,617	2.9	Yes	2	4	1.4%
18	Beaumont Hospital-Royal Oak, Mich.	59.8	5	5	88%	5,124	2.0	Yes	2	7	0.8%
19	Northwestern Memorial Hospital, Chicago	59.7	5	5	92%	2,080	1.9	Yes	2	6	2.4%
20	U. of Michigan Hospitals-Michigan Medicine, Ann Arbor	59.5	5	1	92%	1,972	2.6	Yes	2	7	1.8%
21	Beaumont Hospital-Troy, Mich.	59.4	5	4	90%	3,937	1.7	Yes	2	7	0.2%
22	Duke University Hospital, Durham, N.C.	59.1	4	5	92%	3,016	2.0	Yes	2	7	7.0%
23	Tampa General Hospital	58.6	5	5	91%	2,583	2.6	Yes	2	7	1.6%
24	North Shore University Hospital, Manhasset, N.Y.	58.5	5	1	88%	3,846	2.0	Yes	2	7	0.6%

(CONTINUED ON PAGE 138)

Terms are explained on Page 113.

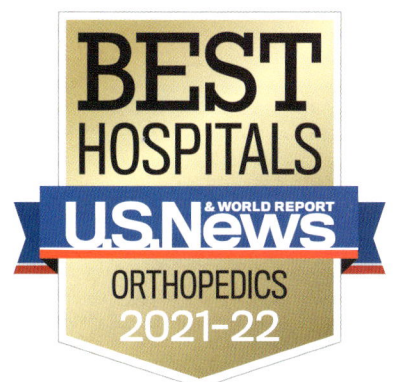

WHAT DO YOU DO WHEN YOU'VE WON BEST ORTHO 11 TIMES?
EARN IT AGAIN.

CHOOSE BETTER. MOVE BETTER.

As the U.S. #1 in Orthopedics for 12 years in a row, our team of experts continuously delivers the highest-quality musculoskeletal care available. We accept most major insurance plans, so you can choose better care and get back to doing what you love.

Learn more at **HSS.edu**

NY • NJ • CT

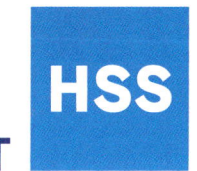

BEST HOSPITALS

Orthopedics (CONTINUED)

Rank	Hospital	U.S. News score	Survival score (5=best)	Discharge to home score (5=best)	Patient experience (% positive responses)	Number of patients	Nurse staffing score (higher is better)	A Nurse Magnet hospital	Technology score (2=best)	Patient services score (7=best)	% of specialists recommending hospital
25	Lenox Hill Hospital, New York	57.2	5	5	87%	1,958	2.6	Yes	2	7	1.0%
26	UPMC Presbyterian Shadyside, Pittsburgh	57.1	5	5	90%	4,523	2.4	Yes	2	7	2.5%
27	Hoag Orthopedic Institute, Irvine, Calif.	56.5	5	5	94%	4,420	2.4	Yes	2	7	1.3%
28	Memorial Hermann Memorial City Medical Center, Houston	56.4	5	5	91%	1,601	1.3	Yes	2	7	0.0%
29	Hosps. of the U. of Pennsylvania-Penn Presby., Philadelphia	56.2	5	1	92%	2,657	2.5	Yes	2	7	4.5%
30	Morristown Medical Center, Morristown, N.J.	56.0	5	1	91%	3,519	2.1	Yes	2	7	1.3%
31	Barnes-Jewish Hospital, Saint Louis	55.9	3	5	90%	4,051	2.3	Yes	2	7	4.7%
31	Cleveland Clinic Fairview Hospital, Cleveland	55.9	5	1	91%	1,164	1.7	Yes	2	7	0.2%
31	John Muir Health-Walnut Creek Med. Ctr., Walnut Creek, Calif.	55.9	5	5	91%	2,221	2.2	Yes	2	6	0.1%
34	Keck Medical Center of USC, Los Angeles	55.7	4	5	91%	1,481	3.3	Yes	2	7	2.3%
35	Mayo Clinic-Jacksonville, Fla.	55.0	5	5	95%	1,451	2.7	Yes	2	7	2.1%
36	UC Davis Medical Center, Sacramento, Calif.	54.9	5	5	89%	1,920	2.5	Yes	2	7	1.4%
37	Penn State Health Milton S. Hershey Medical Center, Hershey, Pa.	54.7	5	5	90%	2,028	2.2	Yes	2	7	0.7%
37	University of Washington Medical Center, Seattle	54.7	5	5	91%	2,160	2.2	Yes	2	7	2.1%
39	Huntington Hospital, Pasadena, Calif.	54.5	5	5	92%	2,394	1.7	Yes	1	7	0.0%
39	Mayo Clinic-Phoenix	54.5	5	5	96%	1,896	3.2	Yes	2	7	2.4%
41	Johns Hopkins Hospital, Baltimore	54.4	3	3	93%	1,864	2.4	Yes	2	7	4.9%
41	Mount Sinai Morningside & Mount Sinai West Hospitals, New York	54.4	5	1	86%	2,277	2.0	No	2	7	0.4%
43	St. Francis Hospital & Heart Center, Roslyn, N.Y.	54.3	5	1	95%	1,470	2.0	Yes	2	7	0.2%
44	Huntington Hospital, Huntington, N.Y.	54.2	5	3	90%	1,529	1.8	Yes	2	7	0.2%
45	UC San Diego Health-Jacobs Medical Center	54.1	5	5	91%	1,695	2.0	Yes	2	7	2.0%
46	UCHealth Poudre Valley Hospital, Fort Collins, Colo.	53.8	5	5	90%	2,417	1.6	Yes	2	7	0.0%
47	Baylor University Medical Center, Dallas	53.6	5	1	93%	3,639	2.0	Yes	2	6	0.8%
48	Lancaster General Hospital, Lancaster, Pa.	53.5	5	5	92%	3,930	1.6	Yes	2	7	0.1%
48	NorthShore University HealthSystem-Metro Chicago	53.5	5	1	90%	4,443	2.0	Yes	1	7	0.2%
48	Providence Mission Hospital-Mission Viejo & Laguna Beach, Calif.	53.5	5	5	90%	2,380	2.2	Yes	2	7	0.4%

Terms are explained on Page 113.

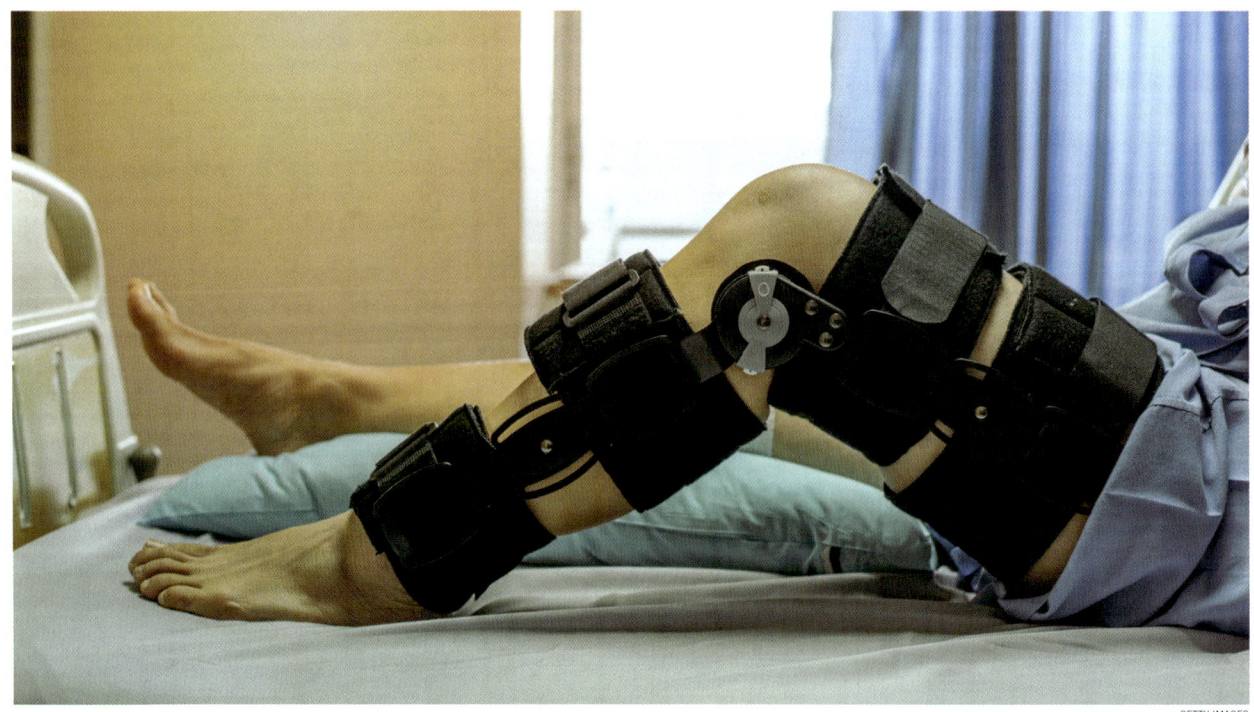

GETTY IMAGES

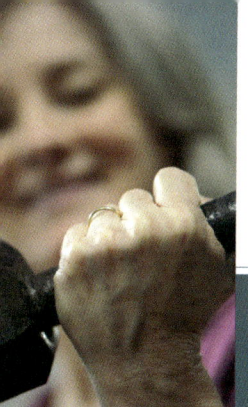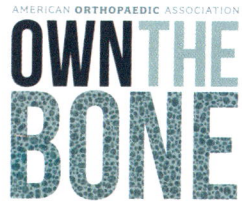

OUTSTANDING HOSPITALS DON'T SIMPLY TREAT FRAGILITY FRACTURES—
THEY PREVENT FRACTURES FROM RECURRING

THE BEST HOSPITALS AND PRACTICES OWN THE BONE

The American Orthopaedic Association applauds the following institutions for their achievements and participation in the Own the Bone® quality improvement program:

STAR PERFORMERS

Institutions are recognized for at least 75% compliance on at least 5 of the 10 recommended secondary fracture prevention measures over the last year.

^Advanced Orthopedics of Oklahoma - Tulsa, OK
AdventHealth Orthopedic Institute, Central Florida Division - Winter Park, FL
Allegheny Health Network (AHN) - Jefferson Hospital - Pittsburgh, PA
Anne Arundel Medical Group Orthopedic Specialists - Annapolis, MD
Ascension Sacred Heart - Pensacola, FL
**AtlantiCare Regional Medical Center - Pomona, NJ
*Atrium Health CMC Orthopaedics - Charlotte, NC
Baptist Orthopedic Hospital at Mission Trail - San Antonio, TX
Berkshire Medical Center - Pittsfield, MA
Bryan Medical Center - Lincoln, NE
**Cedars-Sinai Medical Center - Los Angeles, CA
^ChristianaCare, Christiana Hospital - Greenville, DE
^ChristianaCare, Wilmington Hospital - Wilmington, DE
CHRISTUS Mother Frances Hospital - Tyler - Tyler, TX
**Clark Memorial Health - Jeffersonville, IN
Concord Hospital - Concord, NH
Eastern Maine Medical Center - Bangor, ME
Froedtert & the Medical College of Wisconsin - Milwaukee, WI
Greater Baltimore Medical Center - Baltimore, MD
Hartford HealthCare Bone and Joint Institute - Hartford, CT
Henry Ford Hospital - Detroit, MI
Hoag Orthopedic Institute - Irvine, CA
Huntington Hospital - Northwell Health - Huntington, NY
JPS Health Network - Fort Worth, TX
Lahey Hospital and Medical Center - Burlington, MA

LewisGale Medical Center - Salem, VA
*Lexington Medical Center - West Columbia, SC
MaineGeneral Orthopaedics - Augusta, ME
Marshfield Clinic Health System - Marshfield, WI
Medical City Arlington - Arlington, TX
Medical University of South Carolina - Charleston, SC
Memorial Regional Hospital - Hollywood, FL
Mendelson Kornblum Orthopedic & Spine Specialists - Livonia, MI
*Mid-Maryland Musculoskeletal Institute - Frederick, MD
Michigan Neurosurgical Institute, PC - Grand Blanc, MI
Mission Hospital - Asheville, NC
**Mount Sinai South Nassau - Oceanside, NY
NMC Health - Newton, KS
North Central Baptist Hospital - San Antonio, TX
^NorthShore University Health System - Evanston, IL
Norton Women's and Children's Hospital - Louisville, KY
NYU Langone Orthopedic Hospital - New York, NY
NYU Winthrop Hospital - Mineola, NY
*OhioHealth Orthopedic & Sports Medicine Physicians- Mansfield Hospital - Columbus, OH
OHSU Department of Orthopaedics & Rehabilitation - Portland, OR
^Orthopedic Associates of SW Ohio - Dayton, OH
Overlake Medical Center & Clinics - Bellevue, WA
Paramount Care, Inc. - Maumee, OH
^Park Nicollet Methodist Hospital/TRIA Orthopaedic Center - Minneapolis, MN
Penn Medicine Princeton Medical Center - Plainsboro, NJ
^Penrose-St. Francis Health Services - Colorado Springs, CO

^Prisma Health - Upstate - Greenville, SC
ProMedica Toledo Hospital - Toledo, OH
**Resolute Health Hospital - New Braunfels, TX
^Sanford Medical Center - Fargo - Fargo, ND
South Texas Fracture Prevention Clinic - San Antonio, TX
Southeast Georgia Health System - Brunswick, GA
Southern Illinois Healthcare Herrin Hospital - Herrin, IL
*Springfield Orthopaedic & Sports Medicine - Springfield, OH
Tahoe Forest Health System - Truckee, CA
Tallahassee Memorial HealthCare - Tallahassee, FL
The Bone and Joint Center at AdventHealth Zephyrhills - Zephyrhills, FL
*The Bone and Joint Center- Capital Region Orthopaedic Associates - Albany, NY
The Methodist Hospitals, Ortho Spine Center - Merrillville, IN
UnityPoint Health Endocrinology and Midwest Orthopedics - Des Moines, IA
University Hospital - San Antonio, TX
University of Iowa Hospitals & Clinics - Iowa City, IA
University of Wisconsin Hospitals and Clinics - Madison, WI
VCU Health - Richmond, VA
Wake Forest Baptist Medical Center - Winston-Salem, NC
**West Coast Bone Health & Wellness Center - Camarillo, CA
**Wooster Community Hospital - Wooster, OH
^WVU Medicine Department of Orthopaedics - Morgantown, WV
^Yale New Haven Hospital Fragility Hip Fracture Program - New Haven, CT

^first in state to enroll in Own the Bone® | *recognized as a newly enrolled institution | **newly enrolled and Star Performer institution

Own the Bone is a national quality improvement initiative that provides tools and a web-based registry to ensure fragility fracture patients receive bone health care to prevent future fractures.

www.ownthebone.org

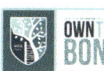

The AOA recognizes **Amgen** for its 2021 Educational Alliance support.

BEST HOSPITALS

Pulmonology & Lung Surgery

Rank	Hospital	U.S. News score	Survival score (5=best)	Discharge to home score (5=best)	Patient experience (% positive responses)	Number of patients	Nurse staffing score (higher is better)	A Nurse Magnet hospital	Technology score (6=best)	Patient services score (8=best)	% of specialists recommending hospital
1	Mayo Clinic, Rochester, Minn.	100.0	5	5	95%	8,264	2.7	Yes	6	8	21.5%
2	National Jewish Health, Denver-U. of Colorado Hosp., Aurora	94.3	5	5	91%	4,035	2.0	Yes	6	8	29.6%
3	Cedars-Sinai Medical Center, Los Angeles	92.1	5	5	91%	9,578	2.6	Yes	6	8	3.3%
4	UCLA Medical Center, Los Angeles	90.0	5	5	93%	7,009	3.1	Yes	6	8	6.0%
5	Cleveland Clinic	89.1	5	5	92%	5,798	2.3	Yes	6	8	15.3%
6	NYU Langone Hospitals, New York, N.Y.	88.6	5	5	89%	16,751	2.2	Yes	6	8	5.7%
7	Johns Hopkins Hospital, Baltimore	85.7	5	5	93%	3,160	2.4	Yes	6	8	17.4%
8	Hosps. of the U. of Pennsylvania-Penn Presby., Philadelphia	84.3	5	5	92%	6,631	2.5	Yes	6	8	9.1%
9	UC San Diego Health-Jacobs Medical Center	83.0	5	5	91%	4,183	2.0	Yes	6	8	5.6%
10	New York-Presbyterian Hospital-Columbia and Cornell, N.Y.	81.2	5	5	89%	17,475	3.0	Yes	6	8	7.8%
11	UCSF Medical Center, San Francisco	80.5	5	5	93%	3,540	2.5	Yes	6	8	10.5%
12	Mayo Clinic-Phoenix	80.4	5	5	96%	4,165	3.2	Yes	5	8	3.0%
12	Stanford Health Care-Stanford Hospital, Stanford, Calif.	80.4	5	5	91%	4,226	2.6	Yes	6	8	3.3%
14	Northwestern Memorial Hospital, Chicago	80.0	5	5	92%	4,806	1.9	Yes	6	7	1.8%
15	U. of Michigan Hospitals-Michigan Medicine, Ann Arbor	79.7	5	5	92%	4,968	2.6	Yes	6	8	5.5%
16	Massachusetts General Hospital, Boston	78.0	5	5	92%	7,710	2.6	Yes	6	8	8.5%
17	North Shore University Hospital, Manhasset, N.Y.	77.5	5	5	88%	11,054	2.0	Yes	5	8	1.8%
17	Vanderbilt University Medical Center, Nashville, Tenn.	77.5	5	5	91%	4,880	2.2	Yes	6	8	6.8%
19	Houston Methodist Hospital	76.9	5	5	92%	7,173	2.0	Yes	6	8	0.5%
20	Mount Sinai Hospital, New York	76.5	5	5	87%	8,138	2.3	Yes	5	8	4.0%
21	Keck Medical Center of USC, Los Angeles	75.5	5	5	91%	1,112	3.3	Yes	6	8	1.7%
22	UT Southwestern Medical Center, Dallas	74.5	5	5	94%	4,322	2.1	Yes	6	8	1.5%
23	Brigham and Women's Hospital, Boston	74.3	5	5	92%	5,858	2.3	Yes	6	8	5.9%
24	Memorial Sloan Kettering Cancer Center, New York	74.1	5	5	94%	4,785	2.4	Yes	6	8	1.3%
25	Barnes-Jewish Hospital, Saint Louis	73.1	5	5	90%	5,974	2.3	Yes	6	8	5.4%
26	Beaumont Hospital-Royal Oak, Mich.	72.7	5	5	88%	10,162	2.0	Yes	5	8	0.1%
27	Yale-New Haven Hospital, New Haven, Conn.	72.0	5	5	89%	12,244	1.9	Yes	5	8	3.0%
28	Rush University Medical Center, Chicago	71.4	5	5	92%	3,034	2.0	Yes	5	8	0.8%
29	Ohio State University Wexner Medical Center, Columbus	71.3	5	5	90%	7,740	2.1	Yes	6	8	2.1%
30	UC Davis Medical Center, Sacramento, Calif.	71.2	5	5	89%	4,038	2.5	Yes	5	8	0.7%
31	University of Alabama at Birmingham Hospital	70.6	5	5	92%	5,432	2.2	Yes	6	8	2.7%
32	Hoag Memorial Hospital Presbyterian, Newport Beach, Calif.	70.3	5	5	94%	8,409	2.4	Yes	5	8	1.3%
33	University of Kansas Hospital, Kansas City	70.2	5	5	93%	4,879	2.1	Yes	5	8	1.5%
34	John Muir Health-Walnut Creek Med. Ctr., Walnut Creek, Calif.	70.0	5	5	91%	5,007	2.2	Yes	5	8	0.1%
35	Duke University Hospital, Durham, N.C.	69.8	5	5	92%	5,634	2.0	Yes	6	8	7.7%
36	Northwestern Lake Forest Hospital, Lake Forest, Ill.	69.7	5	5	92%	1,843	1.8	A	5	7	0.0%
37	UF Health Shands Hospital, Gainesville, Fla.	69.3	5	5	90%	6,752	2.0	Yes	6	8	1.5%
38	Advocate Lutheran General Hospital, Park Ridge, Ill.	69.1	5	5	90%	6,387	2.2	Yes	5	8	0.0%
39	Jefferson Health-Thomas Jefferson U. Hospitals, Philadelphia	69.0	5	5	89%	5,101	2.0	Yes	5	8	1.7%
39	St. Cloud Hospital, St. Cloud, Minn.	69.0	5	5	90%	5,809	2.0	Yes	5	8	0.0%
41	UPMC Presbyterian Shadyside, Pittsburgh	68.8	5	5	90%	7,579	2.4	Yes	5	8	5.3%
42	OHSU Hospital, Portland, Ore.	68.7	5	5	92%	2,257	2.3	Yes	5	8	0.4%
43	Loyola University Medical Center, Maywood, Ill.	68.5	5	5	87%	3,249	2.7	Yes	6	8	1.1%
44	Beaumont Hospital-Grosse Pointe, Mich.	68.4	5	5	92%	3,082	2.0	Yes	5	8	0.0%
45	Sharp Memorial Hospital, San Diego	68.3	5	5	93%	4,734	2.3	Yes	5	8	0.1%
45	University of Chicago Medical Center	68.3	5	5	90%	3,230	2.2	Yes	6	8	2.2%
47	Huntington Hospital, Huntington, N.Y.	68.1	5	5	90%	5,196	1.8	Yes	5	8	0.1%
48	Avera McKennan Hosp. and U. Hlth. Ctr., Sioux Falls, S.D.	67.7	5	5	89%	4,167	2.3	Yes	5	8	0.0%
49	Carle Foundation Hospital, Urbana, Ill.	67.6	5	5	88%	4,978	1.5	Yes	5	8	0.0%
50	Reading Hospital, West Reading, Pa.	67.5	5	5	89%	7,496	1.9	Yes	5	8	0.0%

Terms are explained on Page 113.

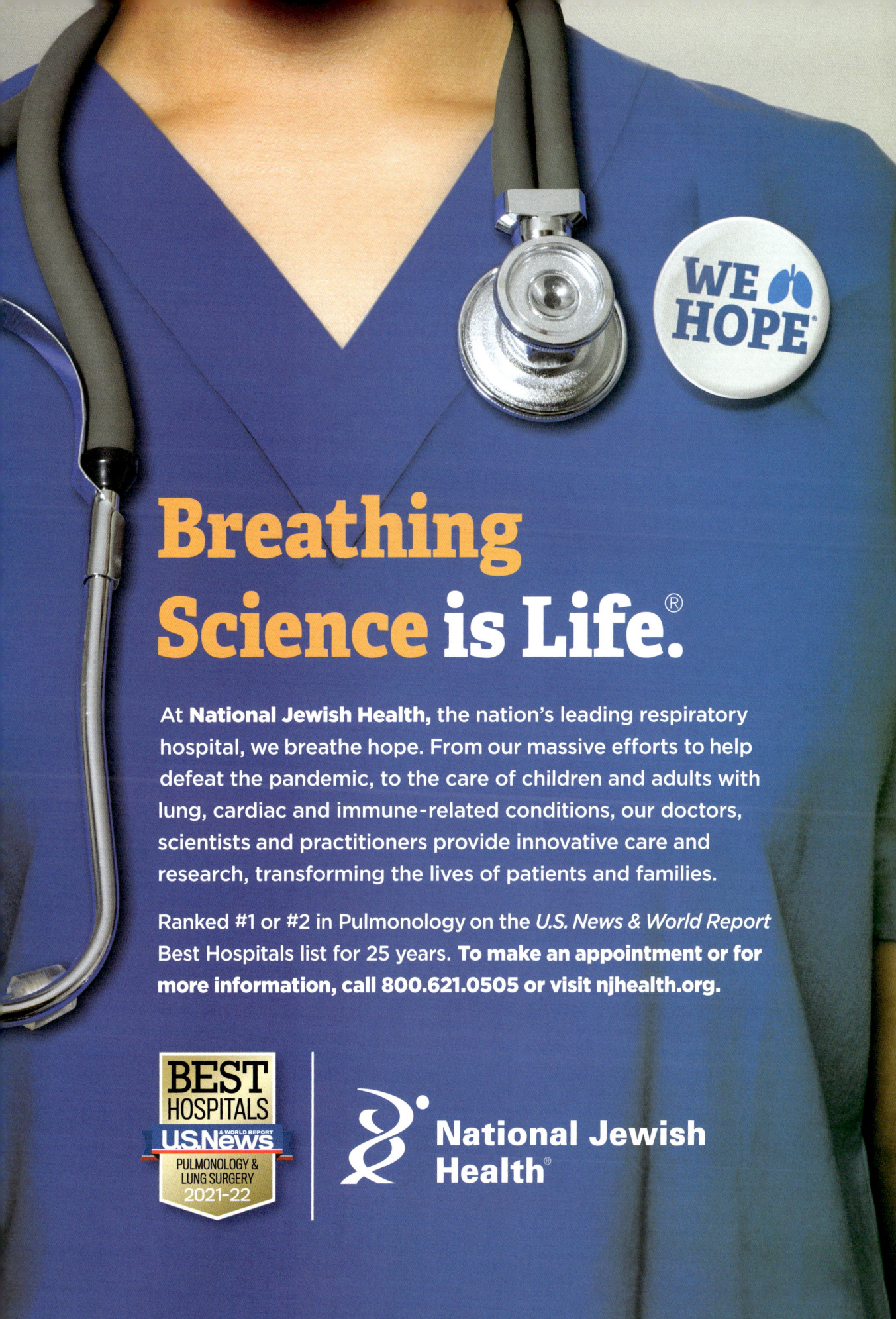

BEST HOSPITALS

Rehabilitation

Rank	Hospital	U.S. News score	Readmission prevention rate (%)	Completion of care rate (%)	Successful discharge rate	Flu vaccination rate	Number of patients	Technology score (7=best)	Patient services score (16=best)	Accredited by CARF	% of specialists recommending hospital
1	Shirley Ryan AbilityLab, Chicago	100.0	94%	59%	95%	79%	Very High	7	16	No	28.0%
2	TIRR Memorial Hermann, Houston	90.0	94%	60%	96%	98%	Very High	7	16	Yes	16.1%
3	Spaulding Rehabilitation Hospital, Charlestown, Mass.	85.4	94%	51%	95%	95%	Very High	7	16	Yes	18.6%
4	Kessler Institute for Rehabilitation, West Orange, N.J.	84.8	94%	60%	94%	81%	Very High	6	12	Yes	15.6%
5	University of Washington Medical Center, Seattle	78.0	93%	65%	96%	100%	Low	7	16	Yes	13.8%
6	Mayo Clinic, Rochester, Minn.	73.1	93%	63%	96%	88%	Average	7	16	Yes	12.0%
7	Shepherd Center, Atlanta	72.8	NA	NA	NA	NA	NA	7	16	Yes	8.2%
8	Rusk Rehabilitation at NYU Langone Hospitals, New York	70.9	93%	59%	96%	97%	Very High	7	16	Yes	9.0%
9	MossRehab, Elkins Park, Pa.	69.1	93%	62%	95%	89%	Very High	6	16	Yes	7.0%
10	Craig Hospital, Englewood, Colo.	67.6	NA	NA	NA	NA	NA	6	14	No	8.2%
11	UPMC Mercy, Pittsburgh	67.3	94%	60%	95%	98%	Very High	7	16	No	5.8%
12	New York-Presbyterian Hospital-Columbia and Cornell, N.Y.	64.8	94%	63%	96%	90%	Average	6	16	Yes	7.9%
13	Baylor Scott and White Institute for Rehabilitation-Dallas	64.1	94%	64%	96%	96%	Very High	7	15	Yes	2.2%
14	Mount Sinai Hospital, New York	62.7	94%	57%	96%	95%	Very High	7	16	Yes	4.5%
15	Carolinas Rehabilitation, Charlotte, N.C.	61.8	93%	65%	96%	95%	Very High	7	16	Yes	3.2%
16	Santa Clara Valley Medical Center, San Jose, Calif.	59.1	94%	71%	96%	91%	High	7	15	Yes	3.7%
17	Mary Free Bed Rehabilitation Hospital, Grand Rapids, Mich.	59.0	94%	68%	96%	98%	Very High	6	15	Yes	1.7%
17	UT Southwestern Medical Center, Dallas	59.0	94%	67%	96%	86%	High	7	15	Yes	2.2%
19	WakeMed Health and Hospitals, Raleigh Campus, N.C.	58.0	94%	71%	97%	99%	Very High	7	15	Yes	0.6%
20	MedStar National Rehabilitation Hospital, Washington, D.C.	57.7	94%	56%	96%	99%	Very High	7	16	Yes	3.0%
21	Magee Rehabilitation Hospital-Jefferson Health, Philadelphia	57.4	94%	55%	94%	100%	Very High	7	15	Yes	4.6%
22	University of Alabama at Birmingham Hospital	57.3	94%	69%	96%	95%	Very High	7	16	No	1.1%
23	Johns Hopkins Hospital, Baltimore	54.5	NA	NA	NA	NA	NA	7	16	Yes	2.7%
24	MetroHealth Medical Center, Cleveland	54.4	94%	57%	96%	100%	High	7	16	Yes	2.0%
25	U. of Michigan Hospitals-Michigan Medicine, Ann Arbor	53.8	94%	59%	95%	97%	High	7	15	No	4.2%
26	Banner Del E. Webb Medical Center, Sun City West, Ariz.	53.5	94%	80%	97%	94%	High	6	15	No	0.0%
26	Emory Rehabilitation Hospital, Atlanta	53.5	94%	67%	96%	90%	Very High	7	16	Yes	1.8%
26	Legacy Good Samaritan Hosp. and Health Ctr., Portland, Ore.	53.5	94%	72%	96%	93%	Very High	6	15	Yes	0.0%
29	Kaiser Permanente Vallejo Medical Center, Vallejo, Calif.	53.4	93%	77%	96%	69%	Very High	6	15	Yes	2.0%
30	JFK Johnson Rehab. Inst. at Hackensack Meridian Hlth., Edison, N.J.	52.9	93%	50%	95%	89%	Very High	7	16	Yes	2.6%
31	Ohio State University Wexner Medical Center, Columbus	52.5	93%	57%	92%	97%	Very High	7	16	Yes	5.5%
32	UW Medicine/Harborview Medical Center, Seattle	52.3	93%	58%	96%	91%	Low	7	16	Yes	2.4%
33	St. David's Medical Center, Austin	51.6	94%	68%	97%	90%	Very High	7	15	No	0.1%
34	Banner Boswell Medical Center, Sun City, Ariz.	51.5	94%	85%	97%	90%	High	6	15	No	0.0%
34	OhioHealth Rehabilitation Hospital, Columbus, Ohio	51.5	94%	63%	96%	93%	Very High	7	15	Yes	0.2%
36	Brooks Rehabilitation Hospital, Jacksonville, Fla.	51.4	94%	57%	95%	86%	Very High	6	16	Yes	0.6%
36	Tampa General Hospital	51.4	93%	70%	96%	93%	Very High	7	16	Yes	0.3%
38	WellStar Kennestone Hospital, Marietta, Ga.	51.3	93%	79%	97%	80%	High	7	15	Yes	0.0%
39	Sarasota Memorial Hospital, Fla.	50.9	94%	66%	96%	95%	Very High	7	15	Yes	0.0%
40	Providence St. Jude Medical Center, Fullerton, Calif.	50.7	94%	69%	96%	83%	High	7	16	Yes	0.7%
41	Swedish Medical Center-Cherry Hill, Seattle	50.6	94%	73%	96%	98%	High	6	14	Yes	0.0%
41	UCHealth University of Colorado Hospital, Aurora	50.6	94%	67%	96%	100%	Very Low	6	16	No	1.7%
43	Atrium Medical Center-Middletown, Ohio	50.5	94%	72%	96%	99%	Average	7	16	Yes	0.0%
44	Froedtert Hosp. and the Medical College of Wis., Milwaukee	50.4	94%	67%	96%	98%	Low	7	16	Yes	0.5%
44	Hosps. of the U. of Pennsylvania-Penn Presby., Philadelphia	50.4	94%	62%	95%	97%	High	7	15	Yes	1.7%
46	Sunnyview Rehabilitation Hospital, Schenectady, N.Y.	50.3	94%	64%	96%	88%	Very High	6	16	Yes	0.1%
47	St. David's North Austin Medical Center, Austin	50.1	94%	75%	96%	89%	Low	7	15	No	0.1%
48	CarolinaEast Medical Center, New Bern, N.C.	50.0	94%	72%	96%	100%	Very Low	6	13	Yes	0.0%
48	Texas Health Presbyterian Hospital Dallas	50.0	94%	63%	96%	100%	High	7	15	Yes	0.1%
48	University of North Carolina Hospitals, Chapel Hill	50.0	94%	73%	96%	96%	High	5	16	Yes	0.4%

NA=not applicable. Terms are explained on Page 113.

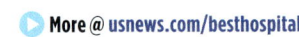

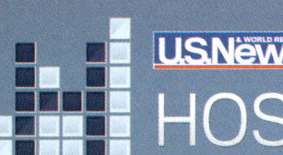

HOSPITAL DATA INSIGHTS | ADULTS

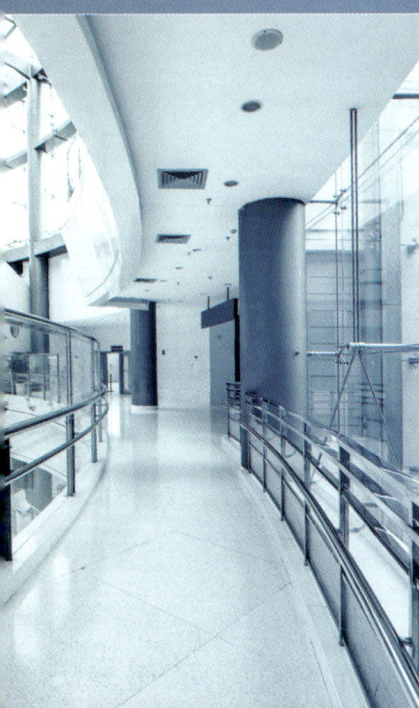

Your Hospital by the Numbers

U.S. News Hospital Data Insights is a new analytics platform from U.S. News & World Report based on the data underpinning the Best Hospitals rankings.

Why Hospital Data Insights?

- Best-in-class analytics
- Superior peer benchmarking
- Extract charts and graphs easily for detailed analysis
- Study year on year data trends to drive clinical improvements

2,900+ HOSPITALS

2,000+ METRICS

45+ MILLION DATA POINTS

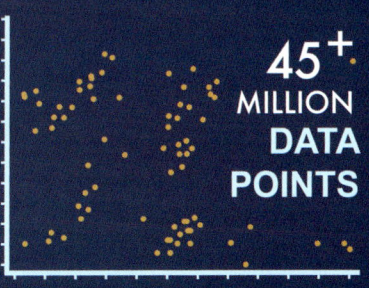

EXCLUSIVE, UNPUBLISHED DATA POINTS & RANKINGS

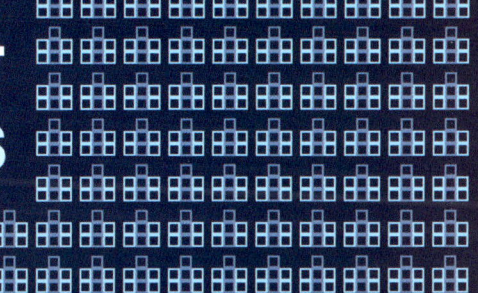

23 YEARS OF DATA
1998 — 2021

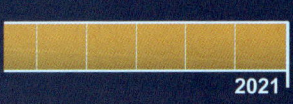

UNLIMITED PEER GROUPS

 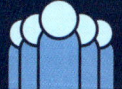 

To request a demo, contact us **hdi.usnews.com** ✉ hdi@usnews.com ☏ 202.955.2171

BEST HOSPITALS

Urology

Rank	Hospital	U.S. News score	Survival score (5=best)	Discharge to home score (5=best)	Patient experience (% positive responses)	Number of patients	Nurse staffing score (higher is better)	A Nurse Magnet hospital	Technology score (6=best)	Patient services score (9=best)	% of specialists recommending hospital
1	Mayo Clinic, Rochester, Minn.	100.0	5	5	95%	1,424	2.7	Yes	6	9	24.2%
2	Cleveland Clinic	93.1	5	5	92%	1,538	2.3	Yes	6	9	29.7%
3	Memorial Sloan Kettering Cancer Center, New York	86.2	5	5	94%	918	2.4	Yes	6	8	8.4%
4	University of Texas MD Anderson Cancer Center, Houston	84.2	5	5	95%	1,732	1.9	Yes	6	9	9.8%
5	Johns Hopkins Hospital, Baltimore	82.8	5	5	93%	1,049	2.4	Yes	6	9	19.9%
6	New York-Presbyterian Hospital-Columbia and Cornell, N.Y.	81.4	5	5	89%	2,111	3.0	Yes	6	9	6.2%
7	Cedars-Sinai Medical Center, Los Angeles	80.3	5	5	91%	1,063	2.6	Yes	6	9	1.2%
8	UCLA Medical Center, Los Angeles	79.8	5	5	93%	783	3.1	Yes	6	9	10.5%
9	NYU Langone Hospitals, New York, N.Y.	78.7	5	5	89%	1,783	2.2	Yes	6	9	5.6%
10	Keck Medical Center of USC, Los Angeles	77.0	5	5	91%	1,026	3.3	Yes	6	9	6.8%
11	Northwestern Memorial Hospital, Chicago	76.7	5	5	92%	1,389	1.9	Yes	6	8	3.0%
12	UCSF Medical Center, San Francisco	75.4	5	5	93%	738	2.5	Yes	6	9	9.1%
13	U. of Michigan Hospitals-Michigan Medicine, Ann Arbor	74.9	5	5	92%	954	2.6	Yes	6	9	7.1%
14	Vanderbilt University Medical Center, Nashville, Tenn.	73.0	5	5	91%	1,089	2.2	Yes	6	9	8.3%
15	Mayo Clinic-Phoenix	70.7	5	5	96%	714	3.2	Yes	6	8	3.5%
16	Mount Sinai Hospital, New York	69.6	5	5	87%	1,385	2.3	Yes	6	9	4.2%
17	Hosps. of the U. of Pennsylvania-Penn Presby., Philadelphia	69.0	5	5	92%	1,060	2.5	Yes	6	9	3.2%
17	UT Southwestern Medical Center, Dallas	69.0	5	5	94%	1,160	2.1	Yes	6	9	3.7%
19	Brigham and Women's Hospital, Boston	67.5	5	5	92%	884	2.3	Yes	6	9	2.2%
20	Stanford Health Care-Stanford Hospital, Stanford, Calif.	66.5	4	5	91%	660	2.6	Yes	6	9	3.6%
21	Fox Chase Cancer Center, Philadelphia	65.7	5	5	92%	633	1.3	Yes	6	9	0.5%
22	Beaumont Hospital-Royal Oak, Mich.	65.6	5	5	88%	975	2.0	Yes	6	9	1.5%
22	Long Island Jewish Medical Center, New Hyde Park, N.Y.	65.6	5	5	85%	1,619	1.7	Yes	6	9	1.3%
24	Scripps La Jolla Hospitals, La Jolla, Calif.	65.4	5	5	92%	435	3.0	Yes	6	9	0.2%
25	North Shore University Hospital, Manhasset, N.Y.	65.2	5	5	88%	861	2.0	Yes	6	9	1.1%
26	Beaumont Hospital-Troy, Mich.	65.0	5	5	90%	805	1.7	Yes	6	9	0.4%
27	University of Kansas Hospital, Kansas City	64.9	5	5	93%	833	2.1	Yes	6	9	2.3%
28	New York-Presbyterian Brooklyn Methodist Hospital, Brooklyn	64.6	5	4	88%	501	1.4	No	6	9	0.1%
29	Houston Methodist Hospital	64.3	5	5	92%	943	2.0	Yes	6	8	1.8%
30	Beaumont Hospital-Grosse Pointe, Mich.	64.2	5	5	92%	299	2.0	Yes	6	9	0.0%
31	Ohio State University Wexner Medical Center, Columbus	64.0	5	5	90%	841	2.1	Yes	6	9	1.6%
32	UF Health Shands Hospital, Gainesville, Fla.	63.9	5	5	90%	687	2.0	Yes	6	9	1.4%
33	St. Cloud Hospital, St. Cloud, Minn.	63.7	5	5	90%	624	2.0	Yes	6	9	0.1%
34	Emory University Hospital, Atlanta	63.6	5	5	91%	688	2.2	Yes	6	9	1.6%
35	University of Chicago Medical Center	63.3	5	5	90%	835	2.2	Yes	6	9	3.1%
36	Lancaster General Hospital, Lancaster, Pa.	63.1	5	4	92%	754	1.6	Yes	6	9	0.0%
37	UPMC Presbyterian Shadyside, Pittsburgh	62.8	4	4	90%	1,176	2.4	Yes	6	9	1.9%
38	Massachusetts General Hospital, Boston	62.5	4	5	92%	1,198	2.6	Yes	6	9	3.3%
39	UC San Diego Health-Jacobs Medical Center	62.3	4	5	91%	639	2.0	Yes	6	9	1.7%
40	Oroville Hospital, Oroville, Calif.	61.8	5	5	79%	384	1.2	No	6	9	0.2%
40	Sentara Norfolk General Hospital, Norfolk, Va.	61.8	5	5	90%	571	1.6	Yes	6	9	1.0%
42	Duke University Hospital, Durham, N.C.	61.5	3	5	92%	952	2.0	Yes	6	8	6.2%
43	Barnes-Jewish Hospital, Saint Louis	60.9	4	5	90%	742	2.3	Yes	6	9	1.9%
44	UCHealth University of Colorado Hospital, Aurora	60.8	5	5	91%	559	2.0	Yes	6	9	0.6%
45	University of North Carolina Hospitals, Chapel Hill	60.6	4	5	92%	797	1.7	Yes	6	9	2.3%
46	University of Wisconsin Hospitals, Madison	60.5	4	5	92%	749	2.4	Yes	6	9	2.1%
47	Mayo Clinic-Jacksonville, Fla.	60.4	4	5	95%	508	2.7	Yes	6	8	2.6%
48	Hackensack University Medical Center, Hackensack, N.J.	60.3	4	5	86%	907	2.9	Yes	6	9	2.0%
48	Providence Alaska Medical Center, Anchorage	60.3	4	5	90%	191	1.5	Yes	6	8	0.0%
50	Montefiore Medical Center, Bronx, N.Y.	60.2	5	5	82%	1,224	2.3	No	6	9	0.4%

Terms are explained on Page 113.

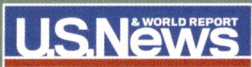

Connect with Patients Seeking the Right Specialists

U.S. News and Doximity have joined together to provide Patient Connect, a tool to reach consumers seeking a new healthcare provider during the critical decision-making process. With patients connected to existing scheduling channels, Patient Connect is a quick, turnkey solution.

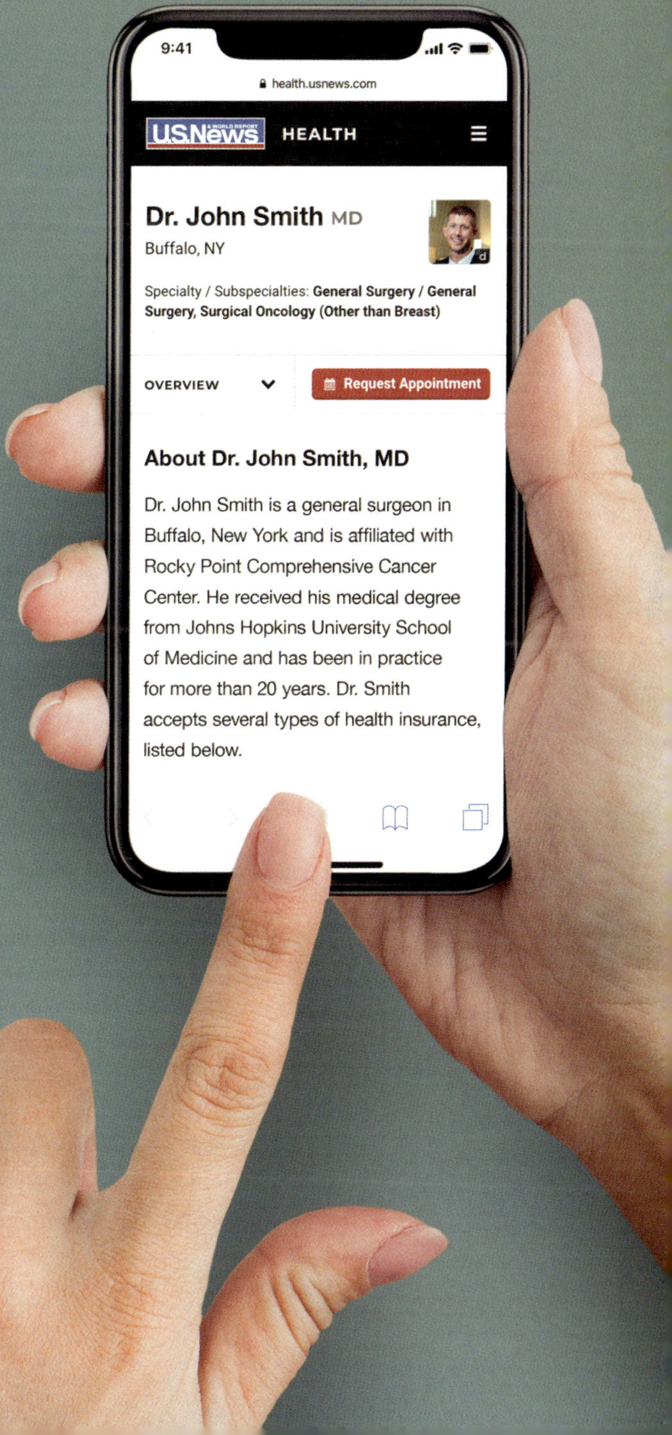

7M+
Visitors per month

77%
Visitors are looking for a specialist

8%
Click or call to schedule an appointment

To learn more about Patient Connect, email:
patientconnect@doximity.com

BEST HOSPITALS

These hospitals are among the best in their specialty

for particularly challenging patients, in the view of at least 5% of medical specialists surveyed by U.S. News over the past three years.

Ophthalmology

Rank	Hospital	% of specialists recommending hospital
1	Bascom Palmer Eye Institute-U. of Miami Hosp. and Clinics, Miami	46.0%
2	Jefferson Health-Thomas Jefferson U. Hospitals, Philadelphia	41.2%
3	Wilmer Eye Institute, Johns Hopkins Hospital, Baltimore	31.4%
4	Massachusetts Eye & Ear Infirmary, Mass. Gen. Hosp., Boston	25.3%
5	Stein and Doheny Eye Institutes, UCLA Med. Ctr., Los Angeles	20.4%
6	Duke University Hospital, Durham, N.C.	11.4%
7	University of Iowa Hospitals and Clinics, Iowa City	11.3%
8	U. of Michigan Hospitals-Michigan Medicine, Ann Arbor	8.3%
9	UCSF Medical Center, San Francisco	7.3%
10	Cole Eye Institute, Cleveland Clinic	6.5%
11	John A. Moran Eye Ctr., U. of Utah Hosps. & Clinics, Salt Lake City	6.0%
12	New York Eye and Ear Infirmary of Mount Sinai, N.Y.	5.5%
13	USC Roski Eye Institute, Los Angeles	5.0%

Psychiatry

Rank	Hospital	% of specialists recommending hospital
1	Johns Hopkins Hospital, Baltimore	20.2%
2	McLean Hospital, Belmont, Mass.	19.8%
3	Massachusetts General Hospital, Boston	19.0%
4	New York-Presbyterian Hospital-Columbia and Cornell, N.Y.	14.6%
5	Resnick Neuropsychiatric Hospital at UCLA, Los Angeles	9.0%
6	UCSF Medical Center, San Francisco	8.5%
7	Sheppard Pratt Hospital, Baltimore	7.2%
8	Menninger Clinic, Houston	7.1%
9	Mayo Clinic, Rochester, Minn.	6.6%
10	NYU Langone Hospitals, New York, N.Y.	6.2%
11	Yale-New Haven Hospital, New Haven, Conn.	5.9%

Rheumatology

Rank	Hospital	% of specialists recommending hospital
1	Johns Hopkins Hospital, Baltimore	40.6%
2	Cleveland Clinic	31.3%
3	Mayo Clinic, Rochester, Minn.	25.3%
4	Hosp. for Special Surgery, New York-Presbyterian Hosp., N.Y.	24.3%
5	Brigham and Women's Hospital, Boston	15.4%
6	Massachusetts General Hospital, Boston	14.2%
7	UCSF Medical Center, San Francisco	12.2%
8	NYU Langone Hospitals, New York	12.1%
9	UCLA Medical Center, Los Angeles	10.6%
10	University of Alabama at Birmingham Hospital	6.8%
11	UCHealth University of Colorado Hospital, Aurora	5.5%

More @ usnews.com/besthospitals

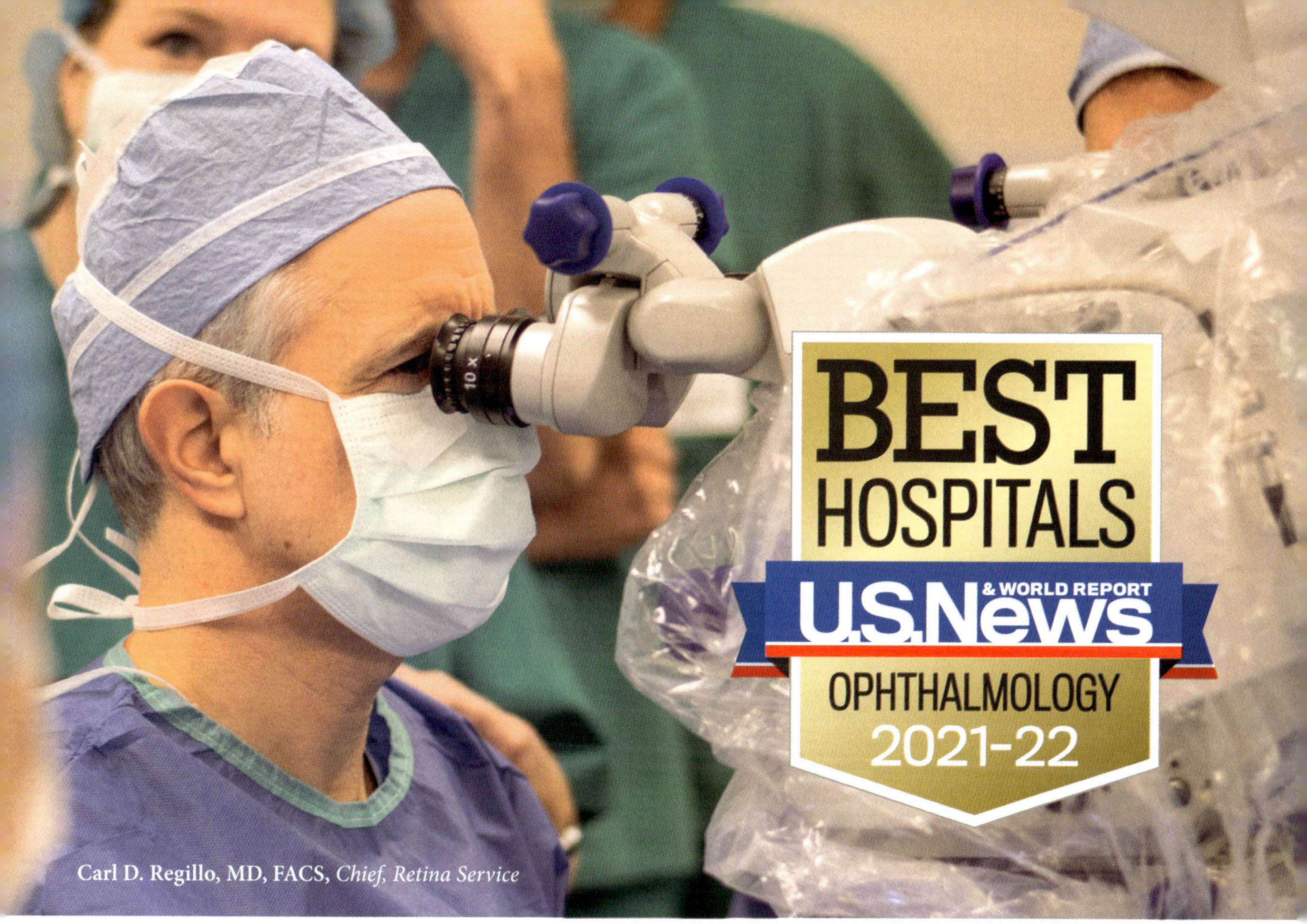

Carl D. Regillo, MD, FACS, *Chief, Retina Service*

Once again, ranked in the top tier of the best eye hospitals in the nation.

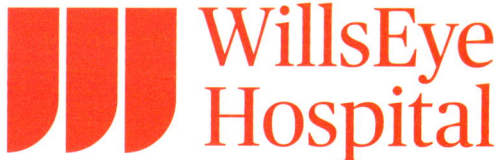

840 Walnut Street, Philadelphia, PA 19107 | www.willseye.org | 877.289.4557

Once again, proudly ranked as a top 10 children's hospital in the nation

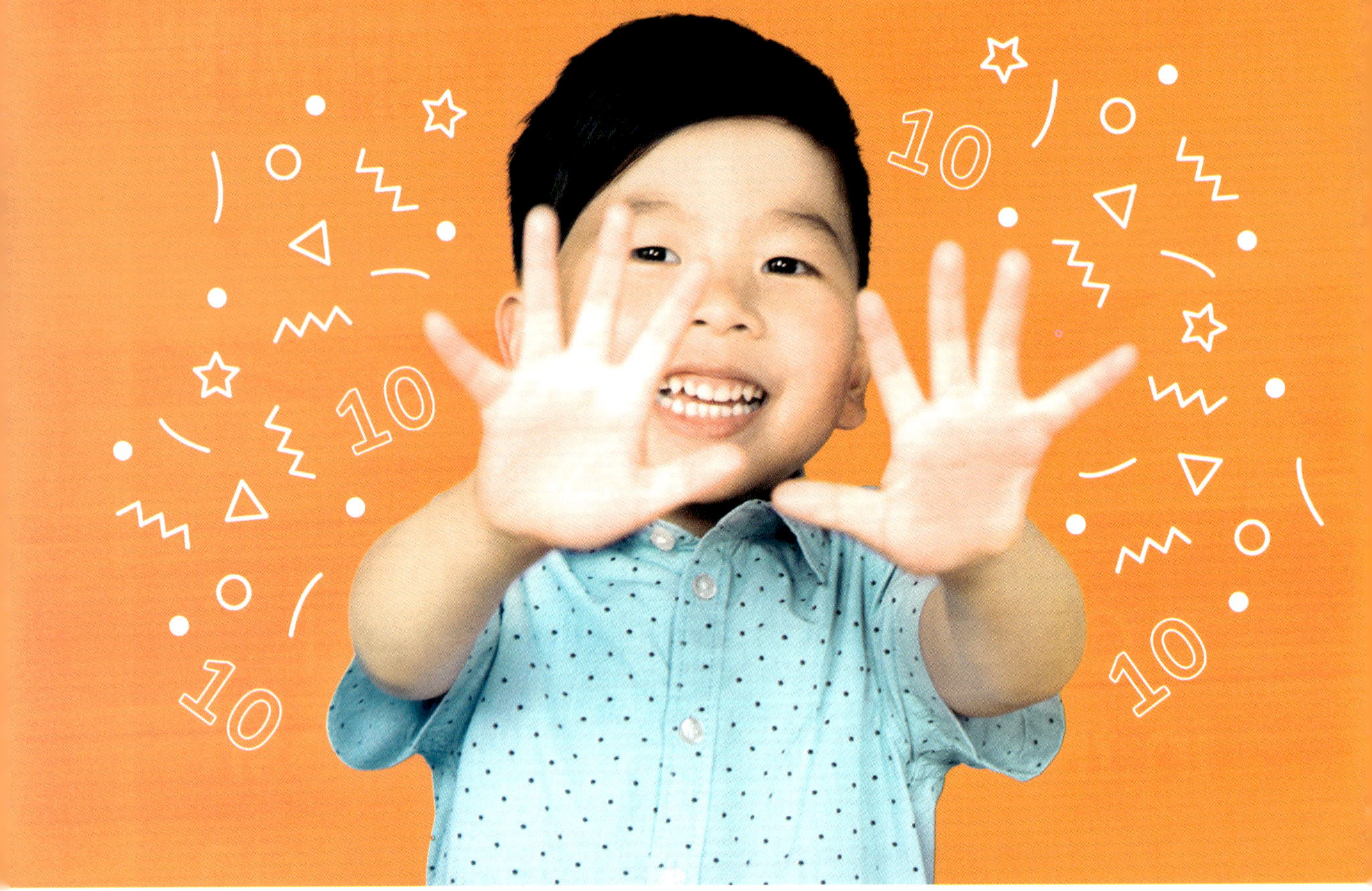

For the second year in a row, we're honored to be named one of just 10 children's hospitals nationwide on the 2021–22 *U.S. News & World Report* Best Children's Hospitals Honor Roll. Stanford Children's Health is also ranked as a top two children's hospital in the Pacific region and top-ranked in Northern California. This distinction affirms our faculty, physicians, and staff's enduring pursuit of excellence and the exceptional quality they provide to patients and families. With our network of 65+ Bay Area locations, our patients can access this same great care close to home.

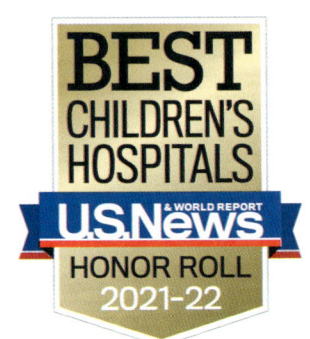

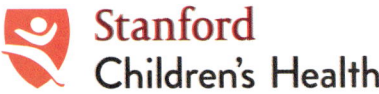

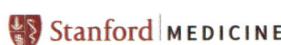

CHAPTER 4

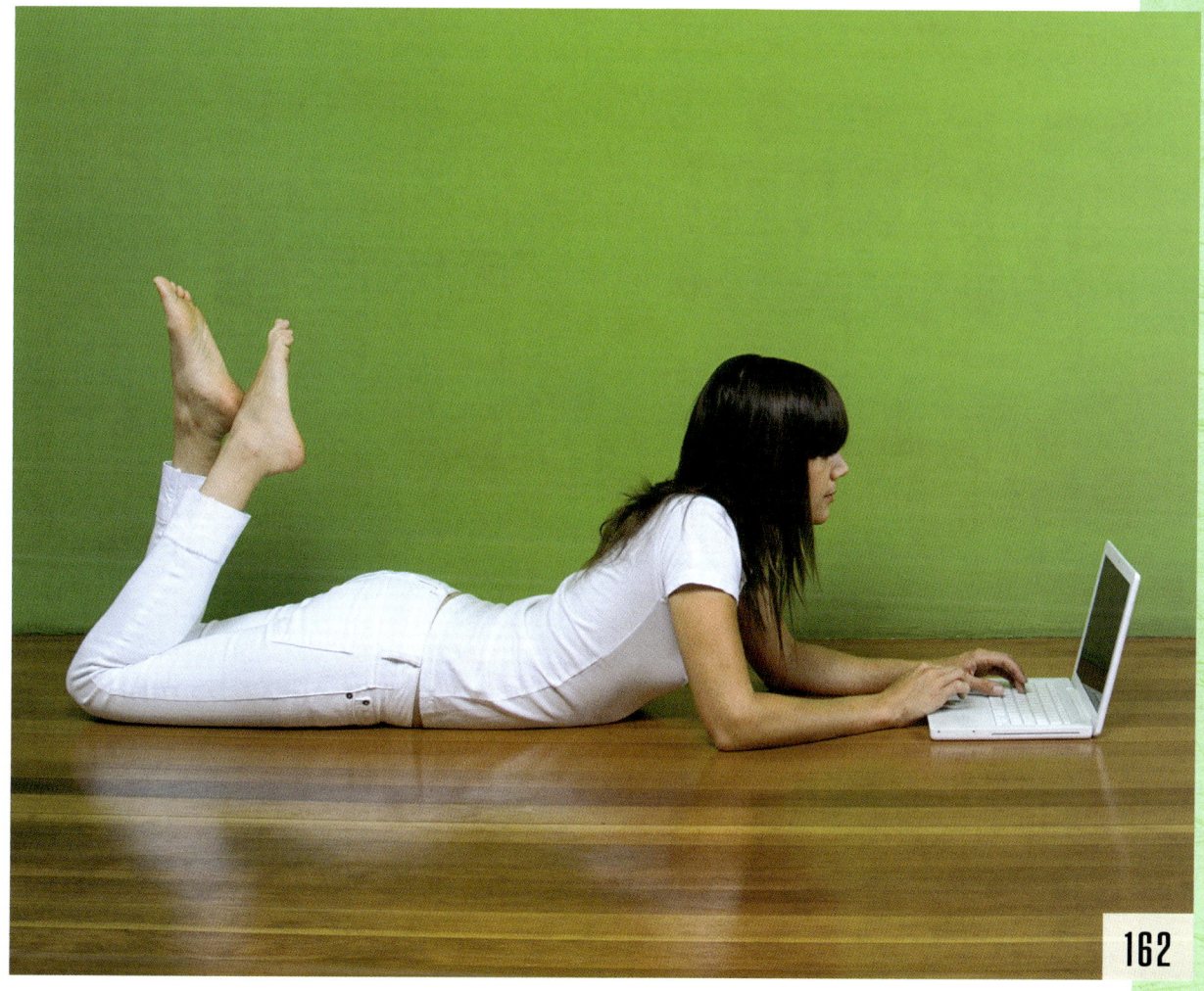

162

Children's Health

Pediatric Priority: Kids' Mental Health — 150

Why Your Child's Weight Matters — 158

The Health Effects of So Much Screen Time — 162

CHILDREN'S HEALTH

A Focus on Mental Health

Children's hospitals are stepping up to improve access to treatment

by **Lisa Esposito**

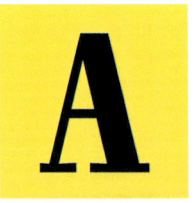

A **RISE IN SERIOUS** mental health problems – and suicide – in children and adolescents already had experts plenty worried. And then the pandemic put more strain on kids' emotional stability. Given the trends of the past 10 years or so, the situation today is "kind of a crisis on top of a crisis," says Dr. C.J. Glawe, co-medical director of the psychiatric crisis department at Nationwide Children's Hospital in Ohio.

The proportion of children ages 6 to 17 ever diagnosed with anxiety or depression increased from less than 5.5% in 2003 to nearly 8.5% in 2011-2012, according to the Centers for Disease Control and Prevention. One in 6 students had enough emotional or behavioral impairment to be diagnosed with a childhood mental health disorder in a separate CDC study conducted in four school districts from 2014 to 2018. In late 2019, the CDC reported that the suicide rate for teens ages 15 to 19 had risen 76% between 2007 and

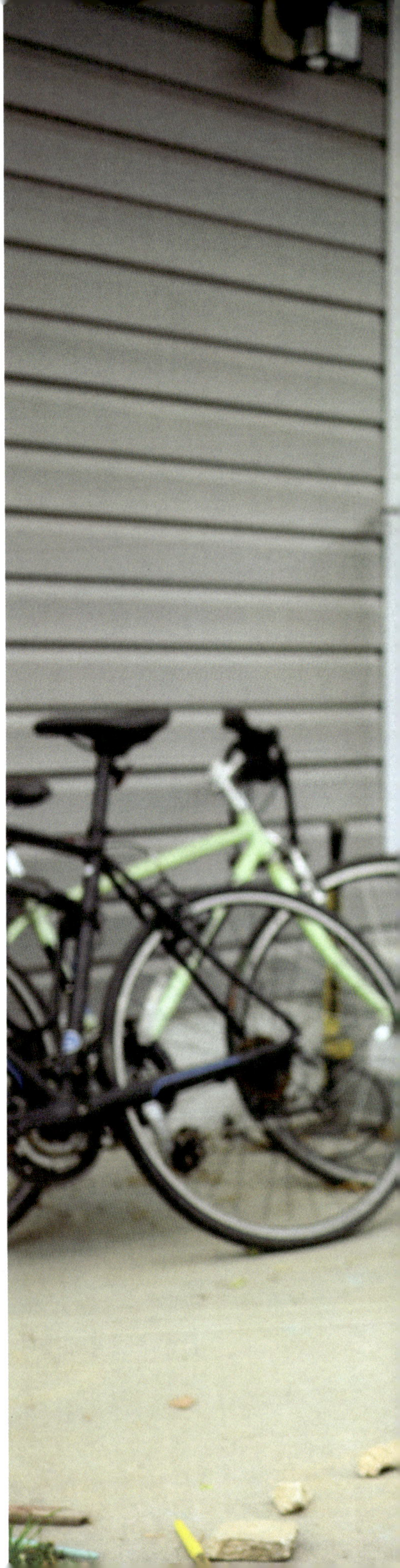

THERAPY AT CHILDREN'S NATIONAL HOSPITAL HAS "MADE A HUGE DIFFERENCE" FOR BERINNA DOGGETT'S SON.

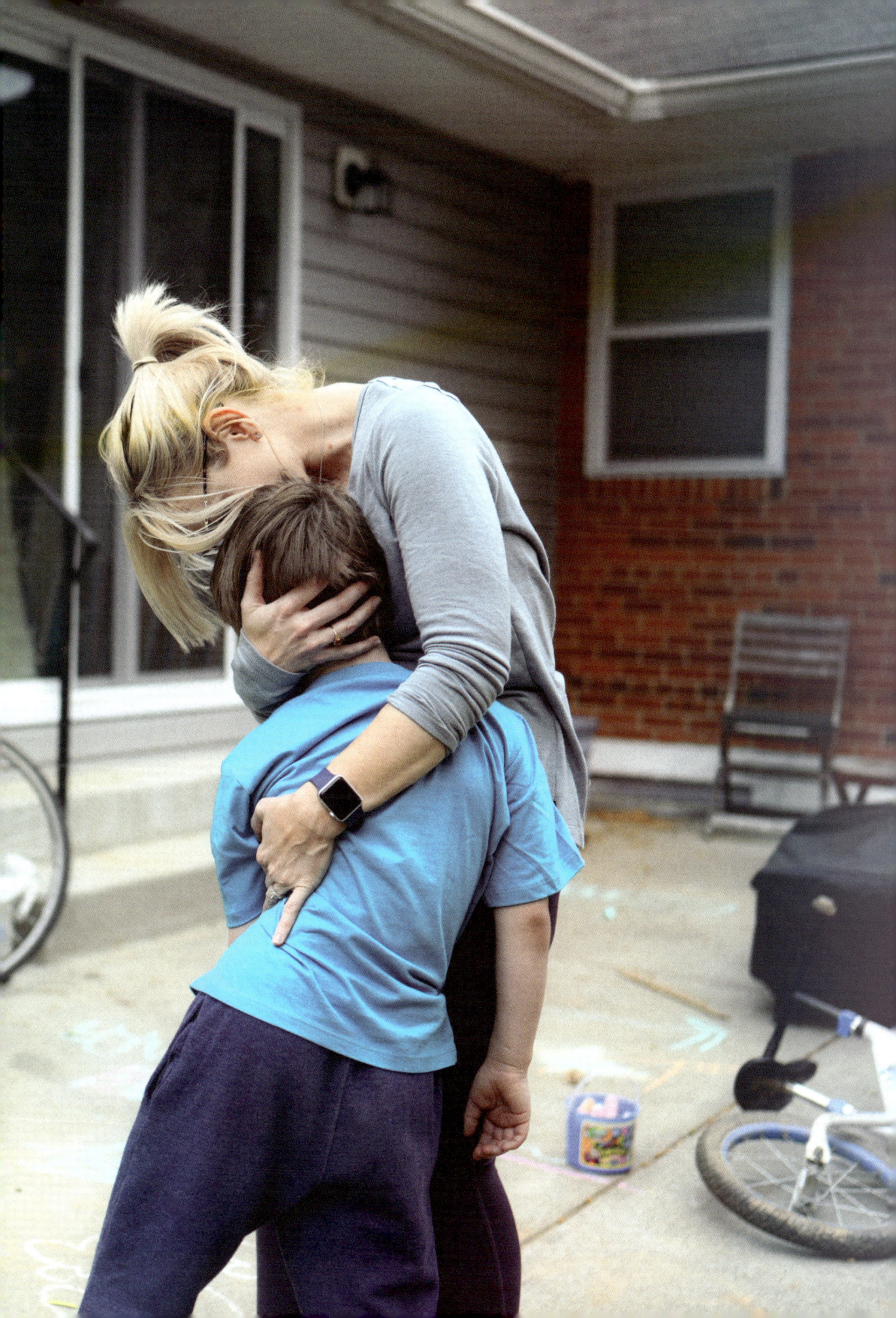

CHILDREN'S HEALTH

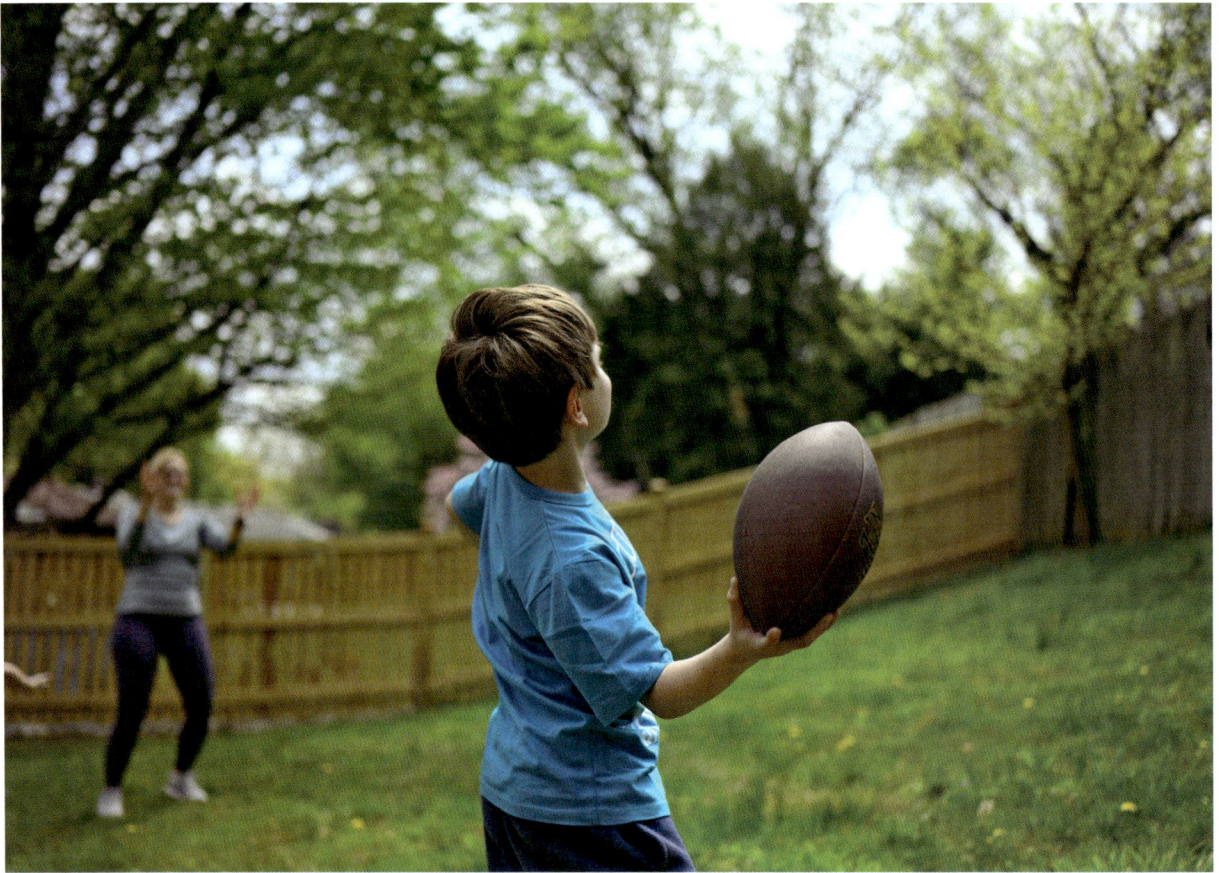

2017 and nearly tripled for children 10 to 14.

The COVID-19 pandemic exacted a mental health toll of its own. For American kids ages 13 to 18, private mental health insurance claims roughly doubled as a proportion of all medical claims in March and April 2020 compared to the same period in the previous year, according to a recent report by the nonprofit FAIR Health. Claims for intentional self-harm rose by more than 90% in that age group, with similar increases in generalized anxiety and major depressive disorders.

At the same time, the U.S. health system struggles with a dearth of pediatric mental health specialists. "Not a single state in the country has an adequate supply of child psychiatrists, and 43 states are considered to have a severe shortage," noted a March 2017 Milbank Memorial Fund report. General medical facilities must fill the void for families with nowhere else to go. "Pediatric emergency departments face higher volumes of patients presenting with psychiatric concerns," warned a February 2020 letter in JAMA Pediatrics. "Many patients who require psychiatric hospitalization board in the ED despite needing treatment that extends beyond the scope of most EDs." According to the Milbank report, only an estimated 15% to 25% of children with psychiatric disorders receive specialty care.

DOGGETT OPTED TO HAVE HER SON BEGIN VIRTUAL THERAPY WHEN THE PANDEMIC INTENSIFIED HIS SYMPTOMS.

In response, children's hospitals are ramping up their commitment to providing that care. In early 2020, for example, Nationwide Children's opened a new state-of-the-art pavilion devoted to kids' mental and behavioral health that offers multiple dimensions of care. In addition to the psychiatric crisis department, services include a youth crisis stabilization unit, family-based intensive therapy, a critical assessment and treatment clinic, a mood and anxiety program, a general psychiatry program and the Center for Suicide Prevention and Research.

Kids in distress may be referred to the emergency service by schools or police departments, or brought in by family members. Sometimes, they come in on their own. The issue with kids referred from school is typically a mood or anxiety disorder expressed to a counselor, or indications of self-harm or suicidal thoughts, Glawe says. Sometimes, it's a behavioral problem such as outbursts or aggression.

Added adversity. Similarly, mood and anxiety disorders and disruptive behaviors and conflicts at home are frequent reasons families bring a child in for treatment. Bipolar disorder, psychosis – including first-episode psychosis – are among other diagnoses. "We see a good number of autism and development disorders," Glawe

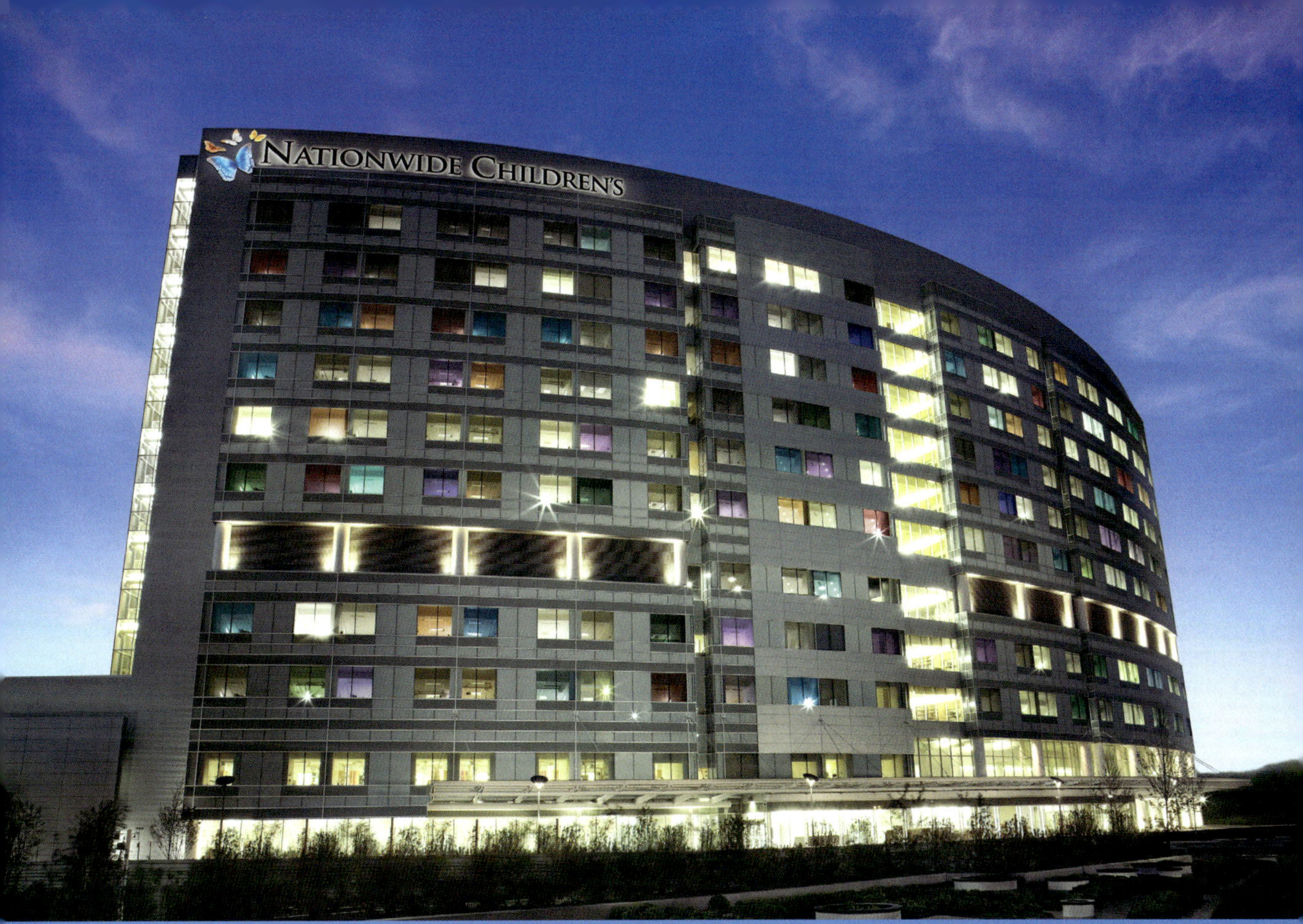

The Destination for Pediatric Neuro-Oncology Care.

Defining the future of pediatric brain tumor survival: what does it take? It takes clinicians and researchers who have dedicated their lives to finding solutions for children. It takes a forward-thinking team of experts who specialize in every aspect of care–not just treatment of disease, but also the quality of life after treatment. It takes the trust of the global community and a commitment to a single focus: the health of children.

And it all has to be built at an institution with the vision to provide life-saving treatment for children from around the world. Nationwide Children's Hospital knows what it takes. And that's what we've built. This is the destination for pediatric Neuro-Oncology care.

To learn more or to speak to a specialist, visit NationwideChildrens.org/Specialties/Neuro-Oncology.

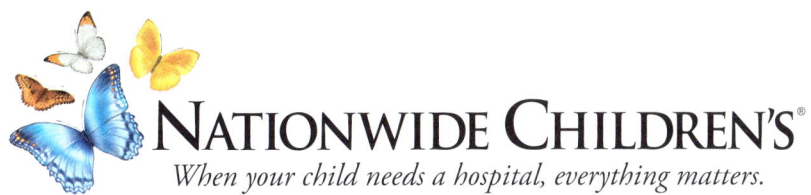

CHILDREN'S HEALTH

says, along with "smatterings" of other issues such as substance abuse or catatonia. The pandemic added a new dimension of stress, as families faced adversity and kids lost their routines and ability to play and socialize freely. Changes in structure have been particularly difficult for kids with autism and intellectual disabilities who rely on school programs and other services for their treatment and education, he says.

Community outpatient clinics and resources, as well as in-hospital services, are striving to meet growing demand. "Right now, the need has become so great that even though we are opening a new program and working on staffing as fast as we can," Glawe says, "the need is so outstripping the access."

That reality, coupled with the shortage of specialists, has put pediatricians and family practitioners on the front line. "I had one pediatrician say to me that recently they've seen more kids with mental health concerns than with ear infections," says Dr. Lee Beers, medical director of community health and advocacy at Children's National Hospital in the District of Columbia and president of the American Academy of Pediatrics.

Arming pediatricians. Beers leads an innovative project called DC MAP (for Mental Health Access in Pediatrics) that aims to arm physicians citywide with the support they need to help suffering children. Launched in September 2015, DC MAP is staffed in a collaboration between Children's National Hospital and MedStar Georgetown University Hospital. Psychiatrists, psychologists, social workers and case managers from both health systems comprise DC MAP teams. In the community, primary care pediatricians can consult with these specialists whenever they identify a young patient with a mental health concern – for instance, while doing a routine screening during a wellness visit.

DC MAP represents part of a larger nationwide movement. Established in 2011, the National Network of Child Psychiatry Access Programs supports child psychiatry consultation initiatives to help integrate pediatric mental health and primary care and make it easier for families to overcome barriers to getting treatment. "Many mental health providers don't take insurance and require out-of-pocket pay-

> 'Virtual learning has made it easier to miss the signs of trouble.'

ment," putting care out of reach for many families, Beers says. Language and transportation can pose other challenges.

During the pandemic, it's been important to recognize that "kids who are likely hardest hit are also likely to have the least equitable access to mental health resources, Beers says. The DC MAP teams help families get supports they need.

Early access to mental health care gives developing children an immense advantage, experts say. Berinna Doggett's young son, now 7 and a second-grader, first connected with Children's National Hospital in 2018 through its clinic for celiac disease. The autoimmune condition primarily affects the digestive system but can cause complications including childhood behavioral issues and attention deficit hyperactivity disorder. Every year, he would undergo a comprehensive evaluation, meeting with a mental health specialist, gastroenterologist and other team members. "We had started seeing some behavioral issues and just some anxiety, focus and attention issues" during preschool, says Doggett, a clinical social worker in the District of Columbia.

For nearly a year, the child worked with a psychologist at Children's National. "We saw a lot of improvement – he was doing really well," Doggett says. As kindergarten approached, the parents and psychologist paused therapy.

Then, just a couple months into the pandemic, Doggett says, some of those behaviors returned. Some new ones appeared as well, such as biting or sucking on his arm, leaving marks. Temper tantrums were frequent.

A huge difference. The family decided to resume therapy virtually, and the child's therapist gave him "the tools and language to help him share his feelings," Doggett says. For example, he learned to name colors to indicate his emotions, like red for "angry." During one-on-one time with his psychologist, she says, he would take his computer to his room, and "show her where he would go to be calm, and they could talk about it." After "graduating" from therapy in March, "he's doing excellent now," his mother says. "It made a huge difference."

Comprehensive mental health care

takes place on a continuum, says Jason Williams, a child psychologist and director of operations for the Pediatric Mental Health Institute at Children's Hospital Colorado in Aurora. Outpatient, partial hospitalization, inpatient and emergency services are available for kids depending on their needs at any given time.

"We can really care for a kid in acute crisis coming to our emergency department, help stabilize them in our inpatient unit, and actually work to get them – in a step-down way – back to their community and provide care ongoing at a lower level of need," Williams says. "And the reverse is true."

For kids whose psychiatric issues disrupt their ability to function, the partial hospitalization program allows them to receive intensive treatment five days a week and then go home at night. They're able to practice their skills with their families as well as within the program's classroom-like setting.

Suicide scare. Right now, the emergency department is exceptionally busy, Williams says, and at times he's finding that "the No. 1 reason" for seeking treatment is suicidal ideation. "I have never seen that before," he says. A roughly 10% increase started in March 2020, and kids are coming in with more serious physical injuries from suicide attempts than in the past. Self-harm is also increasing. Kids as young as 11 are coming in after suicide attempts, and kids as young as 6 are coming in with suicidal ideation, he says.

"That tells me we're not getting to them earlier on, when these symptoms start to show," Williams says. In a typical school setting, a teacher or peer might pick up on red flags and alert parents or a school counselor, and distressed kids could be identified. But virtual learning has made it easier to miss the signs of trouble.

Bailey Shelden, 17, is a Denver high school student who advocates with peers from area schools to raise awareness of – and reduce the stigma of – mental illness, including by creating and appearing in a video for school faculty on reaching out to troubled kids. Bailey speaks from experience, as she has coped with several serious mental health issues herself, including anxiety and depression, an eating disorder and several suicide attempts.

Her speaking out started with a ninth-grade English class discussion in which a student made a "backwards" comment about a young character in "The Kite Runner" who attempted suicide. "What does a Gen Z'er do if faced with a situation like that?" Bailey says. "I took it to Twitter, and I just made a tweet about how I was amazed that this ignorance still exists."

The tweet caught the eye of a Youth Action Board member for Children's Hospital Colorado Pediatric Mental Health Institute, where Bailey has received care. The YAB advises hospital faculty and staff on better ways to treat kids and teens with mental health issues, and raises community awareness through projects to support change. "Basically, I and several other ambassadors help to advise the school on ways that we can better the community and kind of better teach mental health to students every day," she says.

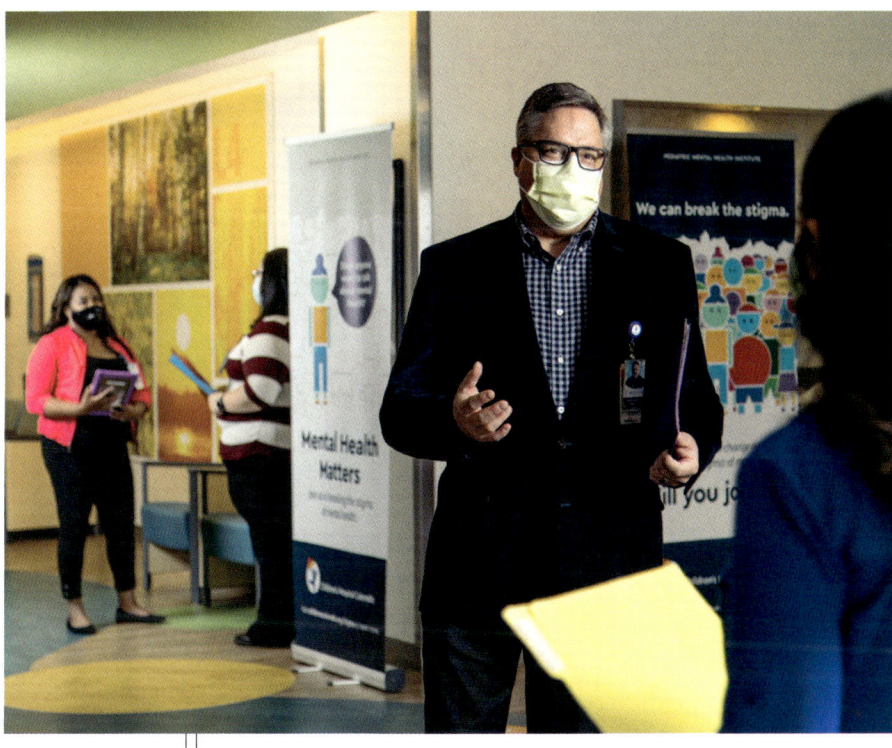

CHILD PSYCHOLOGIST JASON WILLIAMS, IN THE PEDIATRIC MENTAL HEALTH INSTITUTE AT CHILDREN'S COLORADO

Bailey is also dealing with just being a teen. She pushes herself in school, taking tough classes in the international baccalaureate program. In therapy, what she finds most helpful is an emphasis on mental health education and skills to help her cope, such as a calming method called box breathing. "It's kind of a technique to center me and force me out of what my therapist and I like to call 'anxiety brain,'" she says. "Or if I'm about to have a panic attack."

Here's what Bailey wants everyone to understand: "Young people and mentally ill people – we just want more support, through all the highs and the lows, and the productivity and the nonproductivity. Just through all of it, we really want your support." •

FROM DIAGNOSTIC ODYSSEY TO DIAGNOSTIC DISCOVERY

A new flagship program of the Children's Mercy Research Institute is accelerating answers for pediatric rare disease

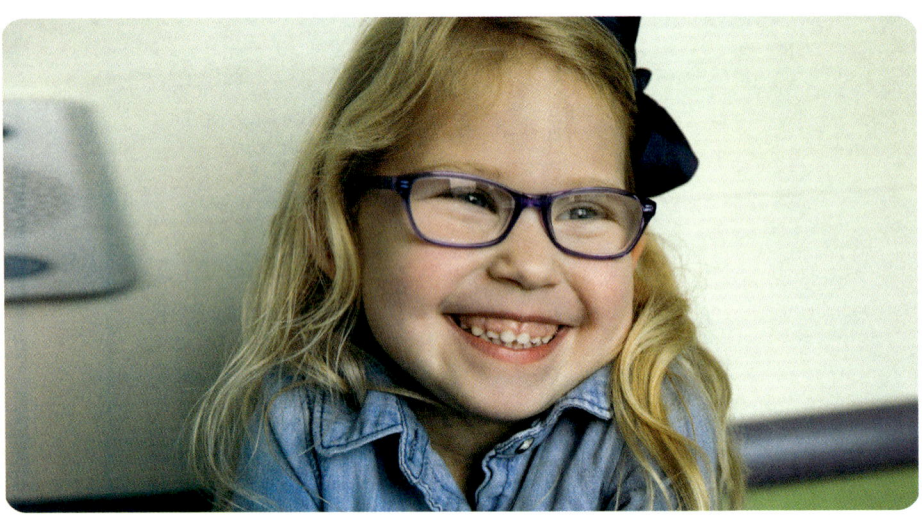
June received a diagnosis through Genomic Answers for Kids in three short months.

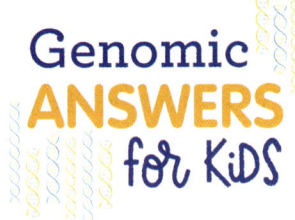

KANSAS CITY — **A six-year wait. An average of three misdiagnoses. All while living with challenging medical conditions, robbing kids of a healthy childhood.**

That's the typical experience of a family with a child fighting rare disease. A long, painful diagnostic odyssey, full of hospital stays, doctor visits and lots of tests. And waiting. Waiting for answers.

Waiting to understand the answers to fundamental questions like, "What is wrong?" "What is my child's diagnosis?" "What is causing this array of medical needs?"

But the Children's Mercy Research Institute in Kansas City is changing this diagnostic odyssey through a flagship program called Genomic Answers for Kids.

Genomic Answers for Kids is a first-of-its-kind pediatric data repository to facilitate the search for answers and novel treatments for pediatric genetic conditions. Thanks to early investments in one of the very few pediatric genome centers in the world carrying out clinical whole genome sequencing, advanced long-read and single-cell genomics performed in patients, Genomic Answers for Kids is leading the world in diagnosis rates for rare disease. This program, combined with having one of the largest pediatric clinical pharmacology programs in the nation in-house, means Children's Mercy will provide the highest rate of genetically targeted therapeutic dosing regimens for kids.

Philanthropic support has allowed Children's Mercy to rapidly expand this program, accelerating a 20-year project to an anticipated seven short years. In the first two years of the program, Genomic Answers for Kids has already enrolled nearly 2,650 families, analyzed more than 12,000 genomes and established 415 DNA diagnoses, using the world's most advanced system for finding reasons for missed diagnoses, transforming future clinical diagnostics. This is an astonishing achievement for families who would otherwise wait more than six years for a correct diagnosis, and often receive the wrong diagnosis. Families like June's.

THE PHONE CALL THAT CHANGED EVERYTHING

Genomic Answers for Kids provides hope for kids like June. June was born with several health challenges, including a congenital diaphragmatic hernia, pulmonary hypertension, a heart arrythmia and other complications. After many years of trying to understand how to best treat June, her parents desperately wanted more answers.

"Not having a diagnosis, you kind of feel helpless. It always makes you question. You want to know what happened," Megan, June's mom, said.

After waiting more than five years for a diagnosis, Megan received an unexpected phone call. Through the Genomic Answers for Kids project, researchers were able to diagnose June with a MYRF-related disorder (myelin regulatory factor gene) in just three short months.

"We were very happy to hear that there is a name for it. It's rare, but there are other kids [who have it]. Without research and Genomic Answers for Kids, June would still be stuck in a world with no hope. We now have the hope and answers we need to give her the best quality of life possible," Megan said.

RARE IS COMMON

While individually rare, collectively rare disease is very common. One in 10 Americans has a rare disease. Fifty percent of people with rare diseases are children, and 30% of those children won't live to see their fifth birthday. Only 5% of rare diseases have an FDA-approved treatment, leaving families without hope.

Rare disease places a heavy burden on the families who are navigating them, and on hospital systems nationwide. One in six hospital admissions of children are due to rare disease.

Often, rare disease isn't diagnosed quickly because of lack of access to next-generation whole genome sequencing, and the molecular knowledge to identify and classify rare disease and then pursue treatment options.

Tom Curran, PhD, FRS, Senior Vice President, Executive Director and Chief Scientific Officer, Children's Mercy Research Institute, said studying the genetics of thousands of children will help make rapid progress against unknown diseases, "We are one of the first organizations, indeed anywhere in the world, to be doing this."

SHARING THE KNOWLEDGE

Genomic Answers for Kids will be a rich resource for researchers studying genetic conditions and will lead to answers and new treatments for children.

The data collected for Genomic Answers for Kids will also be openly shared with the wider international rare disease research community to hopefully lead to the discovery of unconventional genetic variants. The Children's Mercy Research Institute is also uploading sequencing information to the National Institutes of Health's database of Genotypes and Phenotypes.

"Clinician-scientists, anywhere in the world, can compare the genetic makeup of their patients against individual cases that have already been sequenced, to help discover more relevant diagnoses," said Tomi Pastinen, MD, PhD, Director, Genomic Medicine Center.

ACCELERATED BY PHILANTHROPY

"Normally to get a project of this magnitude up and running would take years, but thanks to generous donations from the community we're investing in thousands of families

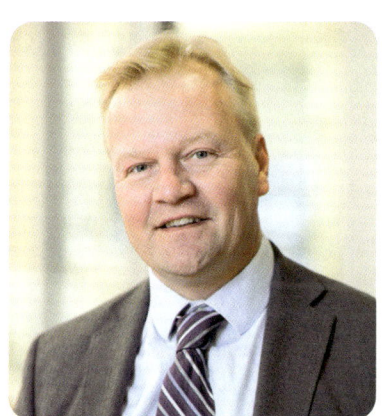

here in the Kansas City region and beyond to give families the answers they deserve," said Pastinen.

Donors generously gave nearly $20M to get this program off the ground and accelerate answers for children everywhere. These forward-thinking, community-minded friends of Children's Mercy understood the potential for a project like this and helped pioneer rapid advancement in rare disease diagnosis and research.

THE CHILDREN'S MERCY RESEARCH INSTITUTE

The Children's Mercy Research Institute opened a new research center in early 2021. After three years of design and planning and 32 months of construction, the nine-story, 375,000-square-foot structure is located on the hospital's downtown Kansas City, Missouri, campus.

The Children's Mercy Research Institute is centered around four Areas of Emphasis: genomic medicine, precision therapeutics, health care innovation and population health.

The support and resources provided by these Areas of Emphasis are driven by the value of bringing science to the bedside to meet the specific needs of the children and families – it is research with a purpose.

LEFT: Tomi Pastinen, MD, PhD, Director, Genomic Medicine Center.
BELOW: Children's Mercy Research Institute

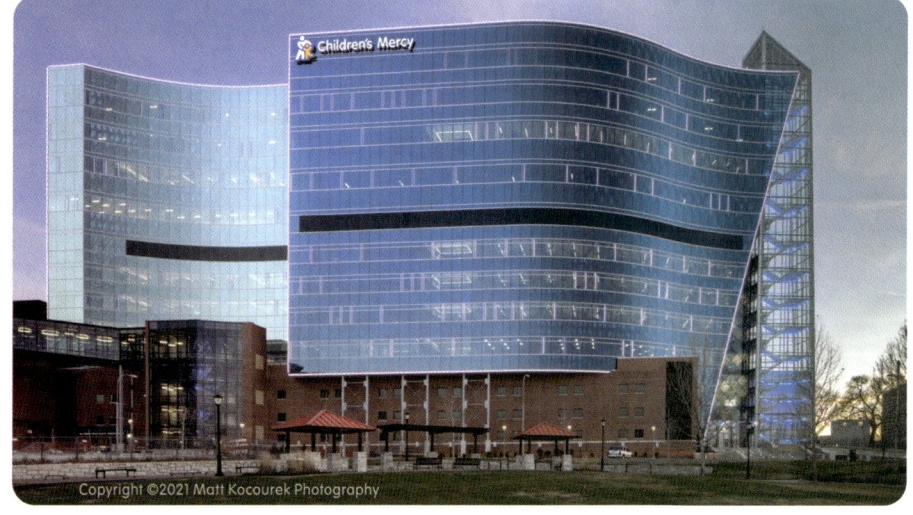

CHILDREN'S HEALTH

Why Your Child's Weight Matters

Addressing excess weight gain early can help prevent serious conditions in adulthood

by **Kadakkal Radhakrishnan, M.D.**

OBESITY IN CHILDREN is a growing problem in the United States, one that could lead to serious conditions such as Type 2 diabetes, high cholesterol, high blood pressure and heart problems as these children become adults. Kids with obesity are also at high risk of developing low self-esteem and depression. According to data from the Centers for Disease Control and Prevention, about 19.3% of children ages 2 to 19 meet the definition of obesity. That's a nearly 30% increase over a 15-year period. Across different age groups, the rate is: 13.4% among children ages 2 to 5; 20.3% among those ages 6 to 11; and 21.2% among kids ages 12 to 19. There is also a noticeable disparity among different population groups, with Black and Hispanic children being most affected, followed by Caucasians and Asians.

The good news: There's growing evidence that addressing the issue early promotes better health in adulthood. Tackling obesity requires a concerted and persistent effort that involves the entire family and entails creating healthy eating habits and choices as well as promoting regular physical activity. Seeking help from a team of professionals that includes your child's pediatrician and other specialists can help ensure that your child works toward appropriate weight-loss goals while receiving medical supervision.

Effects of childhood obesity

These conditions are common – and preventable – outcomes:

Type 2 diabetes. This chronic problem results in elevated blood sugar, secondary to a less-than-ideal response to insulin, the hormone that regulates sugar. Being less active physically and gaining excess weight are risk factors for developing Type 2 diabetes with long-term morbidities like higher risk of infections, stroke and kidney failure and conditions associated with it, such as cardiovascular disease.

Elevated cholesterol. Poor diet leading to excess weight gain is a risk factor for elevated cholesterol. A family history of high cholesterol also increases risk. High cholesterol levels can lead to thickening in the blood vessels, called plaques, and ultimately heighten the likelihood of heart attacks and stroke.

High blood pressure. Having high blood pressure for a long time increases the risk of plaque formation in the arteries, upping the odds of heart attack and strokes. It can also lead to kidney damage.

Nonalcoholic fatty liver disease. Obesity is associated with excess fat accumulation in the liver. This can lead to inflammation in the liver, scarring and liver failure.

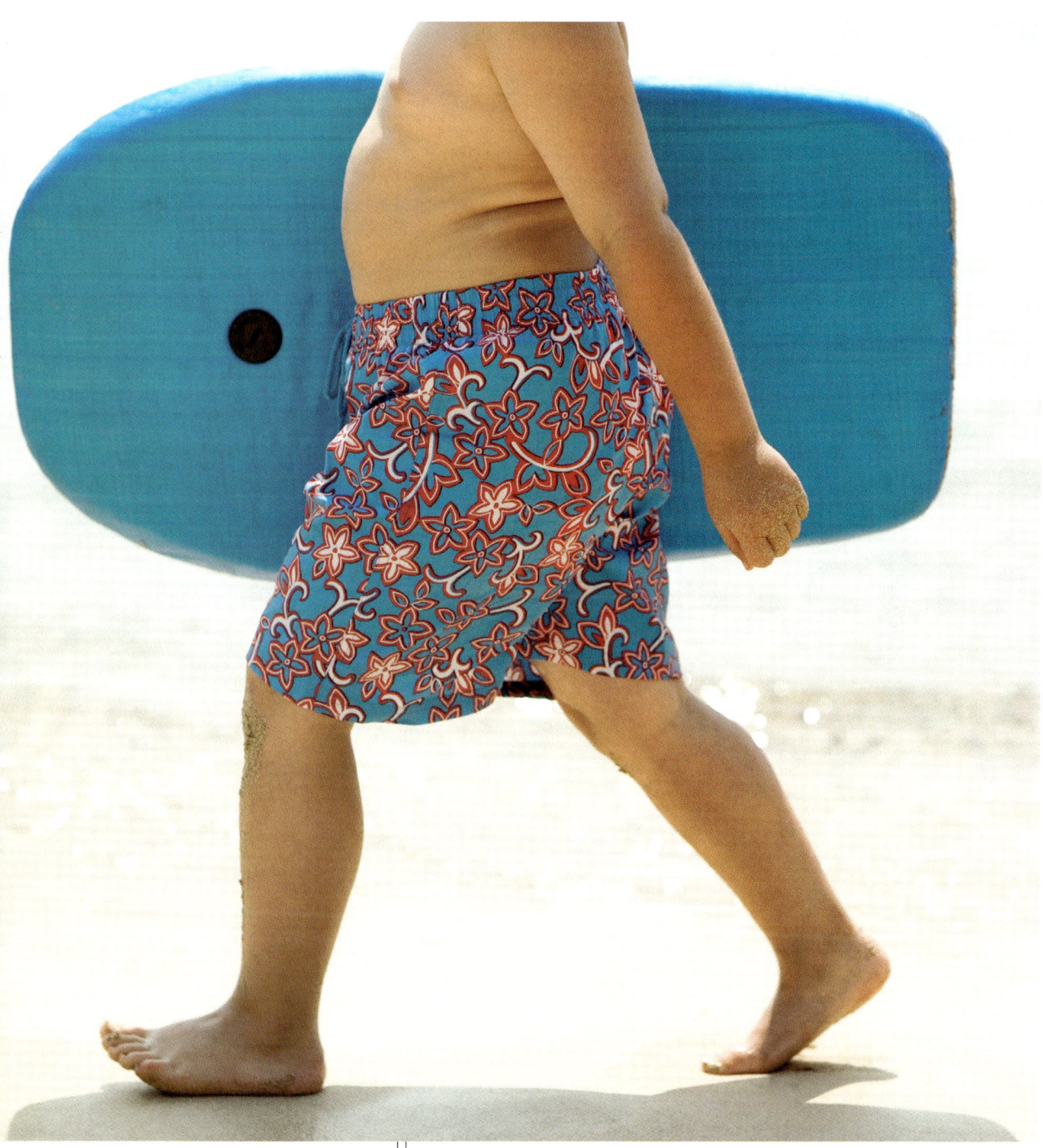

Breathing issues. Obstructive sleep apnea is a potentially serious health issue that leads to interrupted breathing during sleep and is more common in children with obesity. It can cause excess fatigue and sleepiness during the day, as well as an inability to focus at school.

Joint problems. Excess weight gain can place stress on the joints of the back, hips, knees and ankles, affecting mobility and leading to a more sedentary lifestyle. Rarely, kids may develop a problem with a hip joint that causes abnormalities at the top end of the femur bone requiring surgery.

Emotional problems. Poor self-esteem is frequently observed in children with obesity. This can be compounded by a higher risk of bullying, and it raises the odds of developing anxiety and depression.

It's always best to seek help from your child's physician if you're concerned about his or her weight. Your kid's doctor may use the body mass index to help assess the level of weight gain. A child with greater muscle mass and a larger body frame may have a higher BMI, and the doctor will take that into account.

Your child's eating habits, activity level, other health problems, psychological issues and family history of weight issues will help provide insight

> A WEIGHT-MAINTENANCE PROGRAM CAN HELP KIDS GROW WHILE EASING INTO NORMAL BMI RANGES.

CHILDREN'S HEALTH

and guide treatment plans. Doctors can also check sugar and cholesterol levels and monitor thyroid function, which might be a contributing factor to weight gain.

How obesity in children can be managed

It's important to consider and identify whether your child may be at risk of developing obesity, and to then be proactive about preventing excess weight gain. This starts with setting healthy eating habits as a family and encouraging physical activity. Healthy eating habits may include limiting carbohydrates – mainly simple sugars like juice and soda – and adding more fruits and vegetables and ensuring an adequate amount of fat. Other tips:

- Children affected by obesity would be best served by a multidisciplinary team that includes a pediatrician, registered dietitian, physical therapist and specialists such as a pediatric gastroenterologist, pediatric endocrinologist, and sometimes a psychologist.
- A weight-maintenance program, rather than a weight-loss plan, can help children continue to grow while easing into normal BMI ranges.
- Children between ages 6 and 11 may be placed on a diet plan and physical activity schedule to encourage weight loss of no more

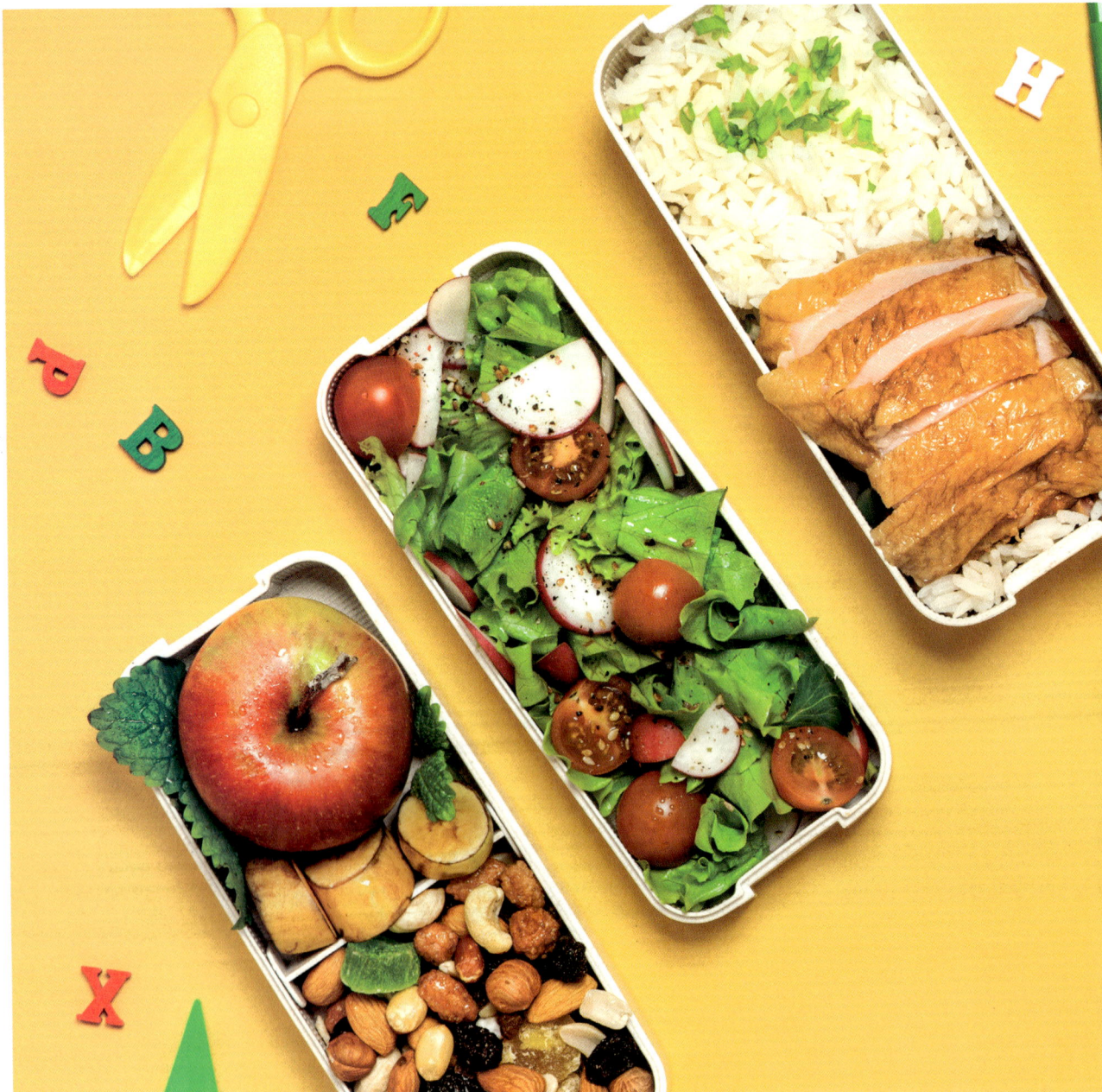

than 1 pound per month. For older children, a weight-loss goal of 2 pounds per week is typically reasonable.
- Support and commitment from the child's family is required.
- Creating healthy eating habits involves limiting highly processed foods such as cookies and crackers, and discouraging consumption of sweetened beverages.

Weight-loss medications are hardly ever used in children, but weight-loss surgery is sometimes recommended for adolescent patients who have been unable to lose weight through lifestyle changes. The doctor might recommend this option if your child's heath risk from obesity poses a bigger risk than the potential problems related to surgery.

It's important that a child being evaluated for weight-loss surgery be seen by a team of providers with experience managing children with obesity. The surgery may not always result in weight loss. And it requires both a diet and a real commitment to physical activity to yield an optimal outcome. ●

Dr. Kadakkal Radhakrishnan is a pediatric gastroenterologist and hepatologist at Cleveland Clinic Children's.

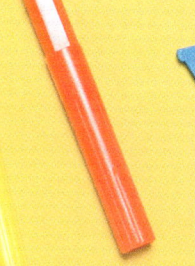

Lunch That Packs a Punch

LUNCH HAS looked a bit different this past year for a lot of families. Not having the school cafeteria to rely on gave parents the hat of lunchtime chef as well as homeschool teacher and trusty employee. Hanging on to that hat even when a lunchbox is again required gives parents a lot of power to affect their kids' health – and weight. Here's how:

Focus on the food groups
The goal is to create a balanced lunch that fuels your child throughout the day. To do this, make sure the meal has adequate protein, fiber and some healthy fats. I find too often that lunches consist of high-carb, high-sugar snack foods. Because of this, kids get a blood sugar spike and often crash in the early afternoon. If you include something from each food group, you can achieve a blood sugar balance without having to overthink it.

My suggestion is to make a fun chart of the food groups that kids can use to select choices from each group each day. There are many sample templates online. You can mix and match foods from each group; it doesn't have to be as boring as a sandwich and sides (though it can be). It's important to have variety.

Choices include:
Proteins: leftover chicken, hard-boiled eggs, tuna packets, lunch meat, beans or chickpeas, frozen meatballs, chicken sausages, vegetarian options (veggie burgers, tofu).
Grains: whole-grain bread or wraps, brown rice, quinoa, potatoes or sweet potatoes, crackers, pretzels, granola bar, popcorn, chips or tortilla chips.
Fruits: any whole fruit (apples, pears, peaches), berries, raisins, unsweetened applesauce.
Vegetables: raw veggies (carrots, cucumbers, bell peppers, baby tomatoes), leftover veggies from dinner, frozen veggies (including veggie spirals), salad, kale chips.
Dairy: white milk, unsweetened milk alternatives (soy, almond, pea protein) Greek yogurt, string cheese, cottage cheese.
Fats, dips: avocado/guacamole, hummus, ranch dressing, Italian dressing, olives, nuts and nut butters.

If you take a little extra time on the weekend, it can make the weekdays much easier. Consider preparing a pasta salad, crockpot meal or another mixed dish that you can keep in the refrigerator for three to four days and dish out as needed. You'll get your protein, fiber and healthy fats all in one. Then add a fruit and veggie on the side, and you're good to go.

Using leftovers? The trick is to serve what you ate the night before to the kiddos in a different way. If you had grilled chicken for dinner, put it in a wrap or chop it up to make a chicken salad. If you have spaghetti and meatballs in the fridge, put the extra meatballs on a flatbread and turn it into pizza. And anything "build your own" offers an added bonus: The kids will be more likely to eat it. *–Jennifer Hyland*

Jennifer Hyland is a registered dietitian at Cleveland Clinic Children's.

CHILDREN'S HEALTH

The Costs of So Much Screen Time

Migraines, eye strain and sleep issues are a few of them

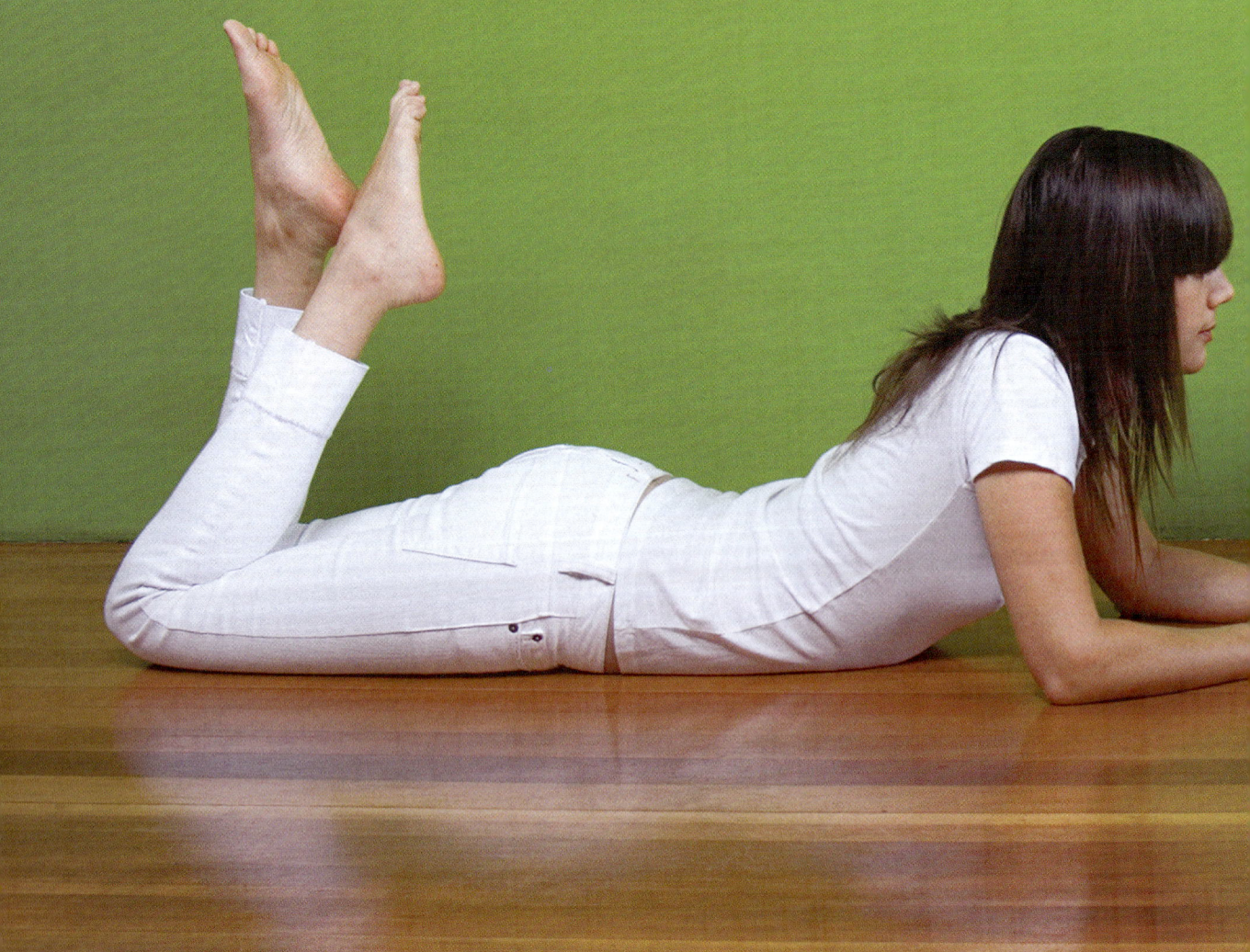

by **Stacey Colino**

REMEMBER WHEN the American Academy of Pediatrics recommended limiting kids' screen time to a maximum of two hours per day? Looking back, those guidelines seem almost quaint. With most schools moving entirely or mostly to online learning this past year and kids' ability to socialize limited to video-chatting, time spent in front of computer screens and other electronic devices has risen exponentially. And doctors suspect they're now seeing the negative impacts on kids' health.

"We've seen an increase in eye strain and eye fatigue, headaches and sleep issues among kids," says Dr. Hina Talib, a pediatrician and adolescent medicine specialist at Children's Hospital at Montefiore in New York City. "I'm seeing more new-onset migraine and more migraine attacks in kids, teens and adults," says Dr. Lauren R. Natbony, a neurologist and headache specialist at the Icahn School of Medicine at Mount Sinai, also in New York. Screen time, she says, "can be a trigger for an increase in the frequency and severity of symptoms."

While it's difficult to prove direct cause and effect, experts think there are too many parallels for the upswing to be coincidental. A study appearing in January in JAMA Ophthalmology found a significant increase (ranging from 1.4 to 3 times higher) in the prevalence of nearsightedness among kids ages 6 through 8 during the pandemic; the researchers believe this was due to more time staring at screens and less spent outdoors. A survey by researchers at Children's National Hospital in Washington, D.C., found that 42 percent of kids reported having a constant headache, compared to 18 percent before the pandemic; 41 percent said they've experienced worsening headaches since the pandemic began, and 42 percent believe that spending more time on their devices is making their headaches worse. Meanwhile, during the early lockdown in Italy, researchers noted a significant increase in the prevalence of seizures among kids ages 4 to 14 who went to the ER, and speculated that this may have stemmed from the increase in screen time and changes in sleep.

Need for a neurologist. Karen Feldman, a mother of three in New York City, has seen these effects firsthand. "She refuses to go off screen when she has a headache or to get off the computer until the assignments are done," she says of her daughter Noa, 13. With the pandemic in full swing, Noa's previously occasional headaches began arriving every few days, sometimes accompanied by nausea, and lasted longer. She has also experienced eyestrain. The headaches became a big enough concern

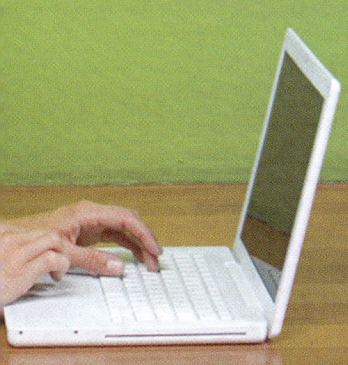

CHILDREN'S HEALTH

that their pediatrician referred them to a neurologist, who diagnosed adolescent migraines and prescribed a triptan medication to ease the pain when it strikes.

"On the one hand, I love seeing her work ethic. On the other hand, she needs to know how much screen time she can deal with. I'm definitely worried about the long-term health effects this is going to have," says Feldman, a 7th and 8th grade American history and Holocaust studies teacher who is in front of the computer herself from 7:50 a.m. until late in the evening. Not surprisingly, Feldman has experienced an uptick in headaches herself as well as changes in her vision, making her reliant on stronger reading glasses.

Meanwhile, some experts are concerned about possible long-term effects on kids' developing brains. Spending so much time on computers and other electronic devices alters attention levels, leading kids and adults to expect something new to happen every seven to 10 seconds, notes Keith Humphreys, a professor of psychiatry and behavioral sciences at Stanford University. As in-person activities resume, "there will be a period of epic withdrawal," he predicts, as young people have to sustain their attention in normal interactions once again.

What's more, that unmet expectation that things will happen quickly can decrease cognitive controls and the ability to regulate emotions, says Jane Timmons-Mitchell, a senior research associate and an associate clinical professor of psychology at Case Western Reserve University School of Medicine. In a study published in a 2018 issue of Preventive Medicine Reports, researchers examined the use of cell phones, computers, electronic devices, electronic games and TV along with measures of psychological well-being among 40,337 kids ages 2 to 17.

Overall, kids who used devices for seven or more hours a day were significantly more likely to exhibit poor emotion regulation (such as not being able to stay calm or being difficult to get along with), an inability to complete tasks and lower curiosity than those who used them for just an hour a day. High-school students who were high users were more than

> 'Some experts worry about long-term effects on kids' brains.'

twice as likely to have been diagnosed with depression or anxiety.

What can worried parents do? Experts advise taking the following steps to mitigate these health risks for your kids:

Encourage kids to moisten their eyes. "The average person blinks 15 times a minute, but when using digital devices, people blink half to a third as often," says Dr. Laura B. Enyedi, a clinical spokesperson for the American Academy of Ophthalmology and an ophthalmologist at Duke Eye Center. "Blinking is important for keeping the eyes' surface moisturized." To prevent dry eyes, eye strain and headaches, it can help to use lubricating drops (a.k.a. artificial tears) regularly; avoid the get-the-red-out kind of eye drops. Also, you might set a timer to go off every 20 minutes and have your child blink a few times then refocus on something at least 20 feet away for 20 seconds.

Adjust the ergonomic set-up. The goal is to prevent eye strain and neck and upper back pain. The computer monitor should be at eye level and the keyboard at a height so that the arms are relaxed, Natbony says. Encourage kids to keep their computer screen 24 inches away from their faces, their mobile phone one foot away, and the TV 10 feet away, adds Talib.

Set a digital curfew. After looking at blue-light-emitting devices all day, kids are often not getting a sufficiently restorative sleep, Humphreys notes. The remedy: Power down electronic devices at least an hour or two before bedtime; if that's not possible, have your child use a blue-light filter on the computer and place a mobile phone on a nighttime setting to reduce blue-light exposure, Enyedi advises.

Make time for movement. Instead of sitting like a statue at a desk for hours, get your child up for some exercise, such as a short bike ride, an impromptu dance party in your living room, or shooting baskets in the driveway. Besides giving your eyes and brain a break and potentially preventing a headache, the movement can help set the stage for a better night's sleep, Natbony says. Plus, regular physical activity is a boon for kids' mental, physical and emotional health, during a pandemic or not. •

After 20 years of caring for children, we've got a lot of causes to celebrate.

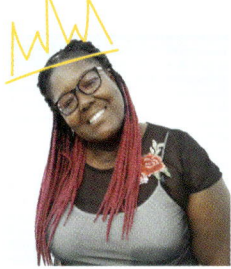
Khara B. age: 20
Rare inflammatory GI disorder

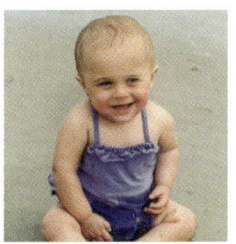
Eva C. age: Preemie
Born at 25 weeks

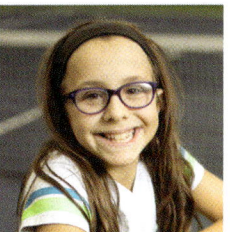
Elli P. age: 10
Brain surgery

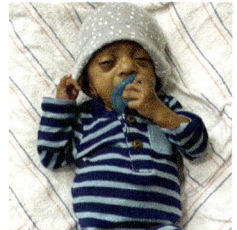
Kiaan D. age: Preemie
GI disorder

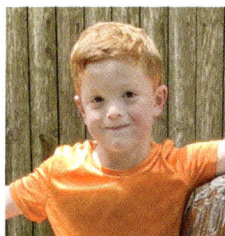
Ryan M. age: Preemie
Necrotizing Enterocolitis

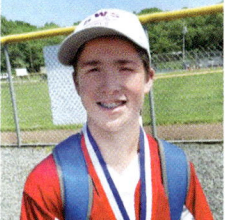
Jacob L. age: Newborn
Cystic Fibrosis & Lymphoma

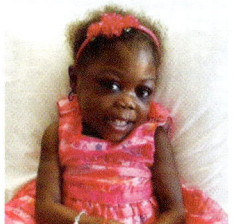
Armoni S. age: 5
Multiple GI disorders

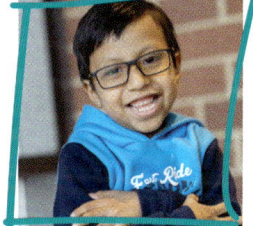
Aden S. age: 4
Kidney transplant

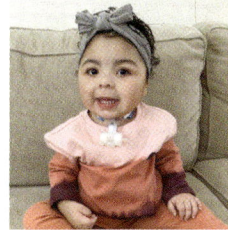
Ayla W. age: Newborn
Neonatal ECMO
Congenital diaphragmatic hernia

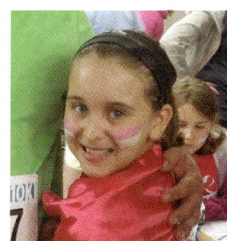
Cheyanne E. age: 13
Advanced hip dysplasia

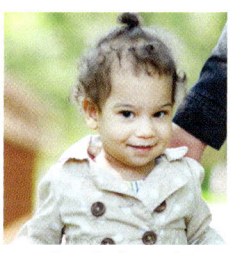
Emanta A. age: 1
Influenza & pediatric ECMO

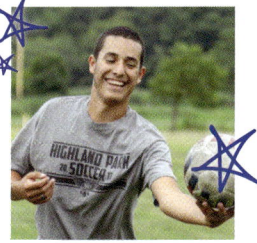
Joey C. age: 14
Pulmonary hemorrhage

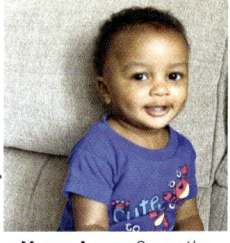
Mason A. age: 9 months
Brain bleed

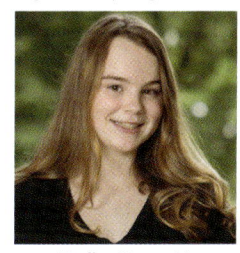
Hadley S. age: 14
Traumatic liver laceration

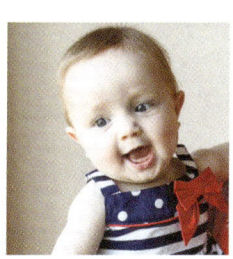
Carolyn R. age: Newborn
Brain surgery

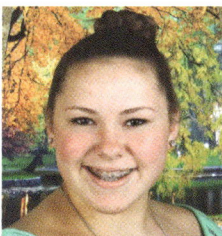
Selena D. age: 13
Rare kidney disorder

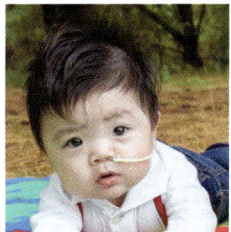
Kieran E. age: Preemie
Born at 25 weeks

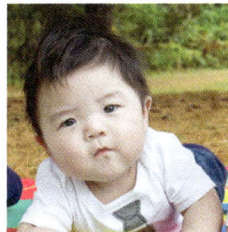
Grayson E. age: Preemie
Born at 25 weeks

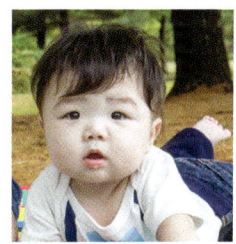
Colton E. age: Preemie
Born at 25 weeks

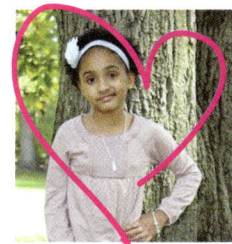
Ariana M. age: 8
Traumatic head injury

From newborns to teens, from broken bones to brain surgery, The Bristol-Myers Squibb Children's Hospital has cared for tens of thousands of children, each with their own unique story. In partnership with Rutgers Robert Wood Johnson Medical School, we offer advanced capabilities in urology, neurosurgery, orthopedics, pediatric emergency care and much more. Even though we've been in one place for two decades, it's been an incredible journey. Learn more at **rwjbh.org/BMSCH**

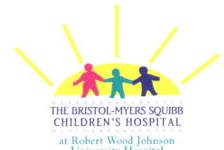

THE BRISTOL-MYERS SQUIBB CHILDREN'S HOSPITAL at Robert Wood Johnson University Hospital

Robert Wood Johnson University Hospital
RWJBarnabas HEALTH

Let's be healthy together.

kids can
show us the way

We're proud to be one of the nation's top 5 children's hospitals—and our numbers and rankings are only the beginning. From research to clinical care, we are passionate about bringing world-class healthcare to the next generation.

BEST CHILDREN'S HOSPITALS
U.S. News & World Report
HONOR ROLL 2021-22

See how we're changing the outcome at **cincinnatichildrens.org**

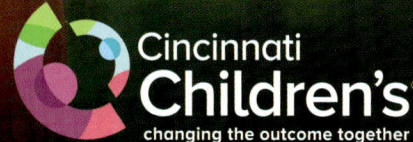

Cincinnati Children's®
changing the outcome together

CHAPTER 5

Best Children's Hospitals

BEST CHILDREN'S HOSPITALS
U.S. News & World Report
2021-22

168 The Honor Roll
173 A Key to the Rankings
178 Cancer
180 Cardiology & Heart Surgery
182 Diabetes & Endocrinology
184 Gastroenterology & GI Surgery
186 Neonatology
188 Nephrology
190 Neurology & Neurosurgery
191 Orthopedics
192 Pulmonology & Lung Surgery
194 Urology

U.S. NEWS & WORLD REPORT

Best Children's Hospitals
HONOR ROLL

BEST CHILDREN'S HOSPITALS
U.S.News & WORLD REPORT
HONOR ROLL 2021-22

This elite list showcases hospitals with unusual breadth of excellence in pediatric specialty care. For each specialty, each hospital that ranked among the top 50 earned points toward the Honor Roll: 25 points for ranking No. 1, 24 points for No. 2 and so on; hospitals ranked 21-50 received 5 points. The hospitals with the most points define the Honor Roll.

1 Boston Children's Hospital
237 points

2 Children's Hospital of Philadelphia
224 points

3 Texas Children's Hospital
Houston, 211 points

4 Cincinnati Children's Hospital Medical Center
205 points

5 Children's Hospital Los Angeles
178 points

6 Children's Hospital Colorado
Aurora
167 points

7 Children's National Hospital
Washington, D.C.
159 points

8 Nationwide Children's Hospital
Columbus, Ohio
146 points

9 UPMC Children's Hospital of Pittsburgh
145 points

10 Lucile Packard Children's Hospital Stanford
Palo Alto, California
137 points

DESERVE 166 YEARS OF EXCELLENCE.

Every child — every unique, wonderful kid — who seeks care at Children's Hospital of Philadelphia benefits from decade upon decade, layer upon layer of pioneering pediatric discovery and exceptional care. A storied history that has placed CHOP in the top tier of *U.S. News & World Report* rankings since their inception.

You can count the years.
But the impact is immeasurable.

CHOP.EDU

Oliver, 2.
Mischief maker, hot dog lover; CHOP cardiac, ENT and craniofacial surgery patient.

©2021 The Children's Hospital of Philadelphia

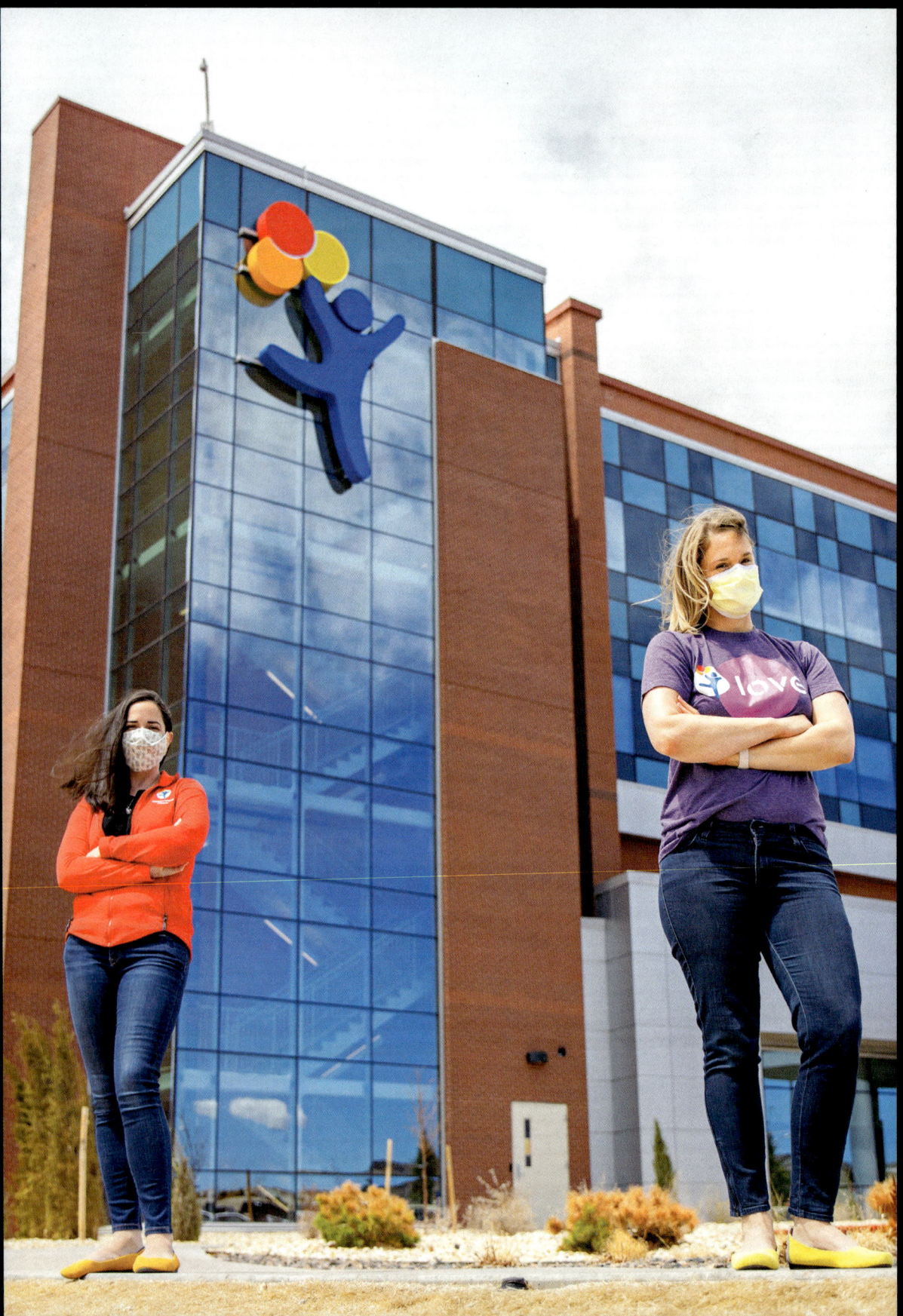

2 CHILDREN'S HOSPITAL OF PHILADELPHIA
THE COUNTRY'S FIRST HOSPITAL DEDICATED JUST TO PEDIATRIC CARE TYPICALLY COUNTS MORE THAN 1 MILLION ADMISSIONS AND OUTPATIENT VISITS ANNUALLY.

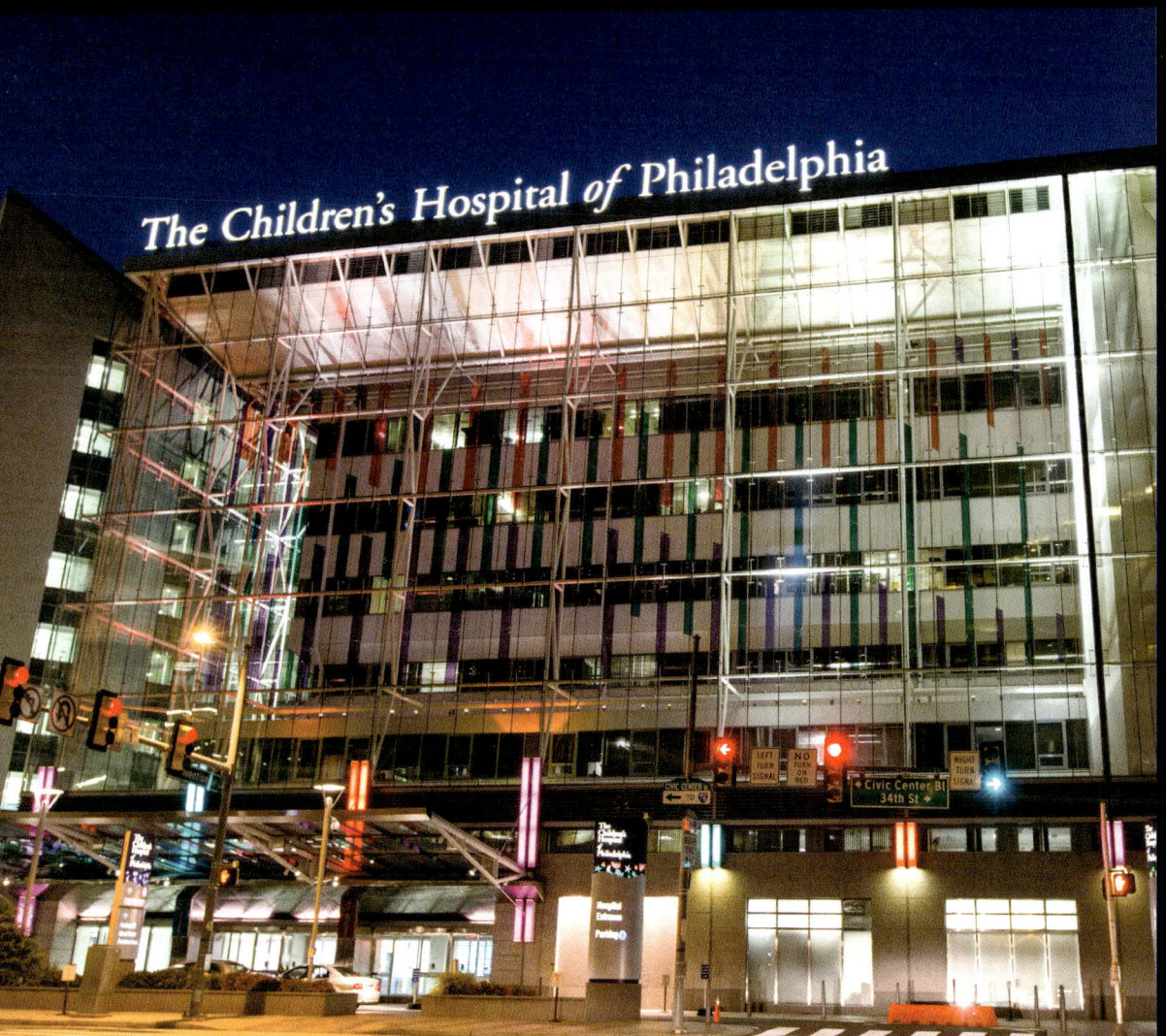

6 CHILDREN'S HOSPITAL COLORADO
INFECTIOUS DISEASE EXPERT DR. SARA SAPORTA-KEATING (LEFT) AND INFECTION PREVENTIONIST SHANNON ROWE AT THE COLORADO SPRINGS CAMPUS

TWO YEARS OF OLIVER ...

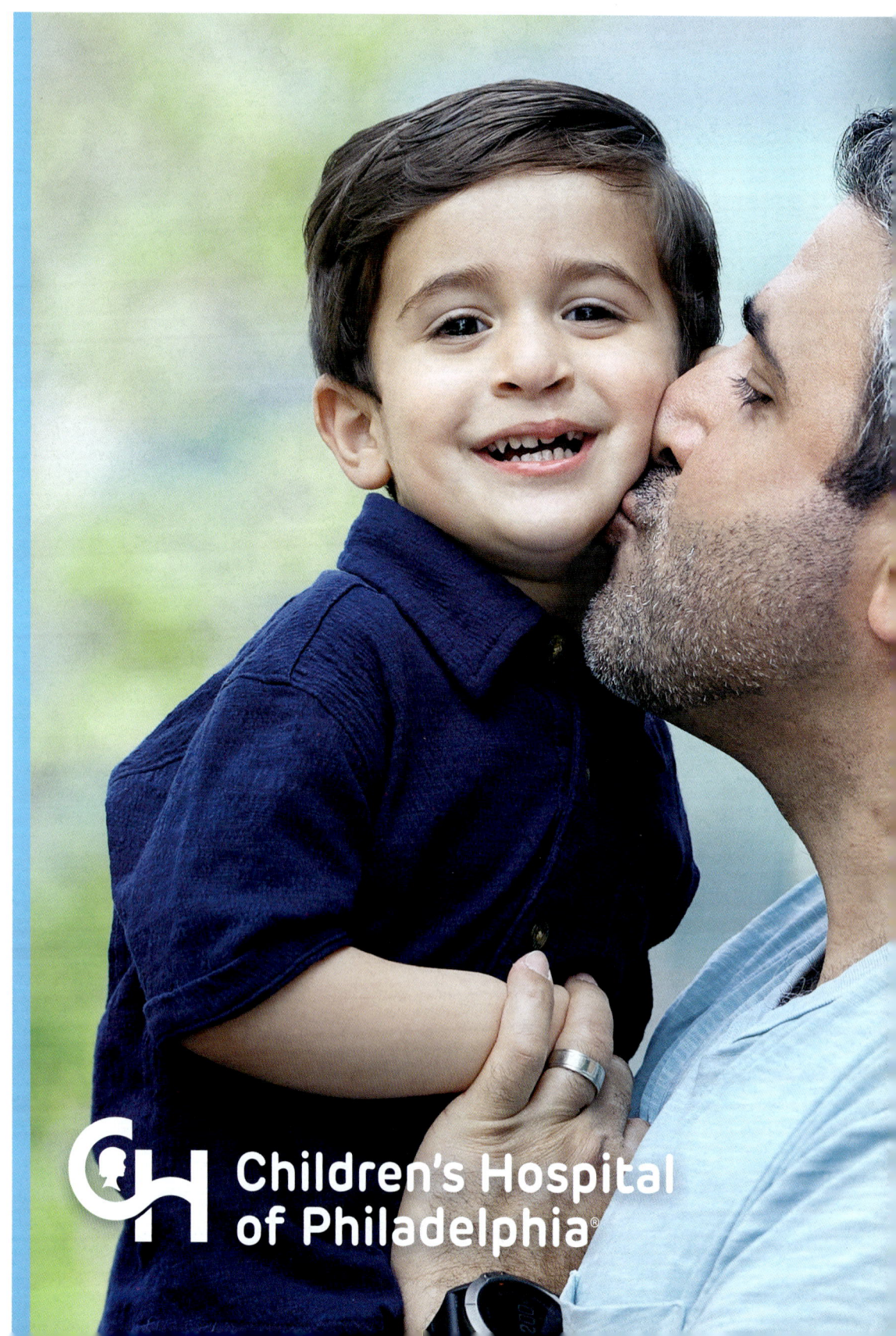

BEST CHILDREN'S HOSPITALS

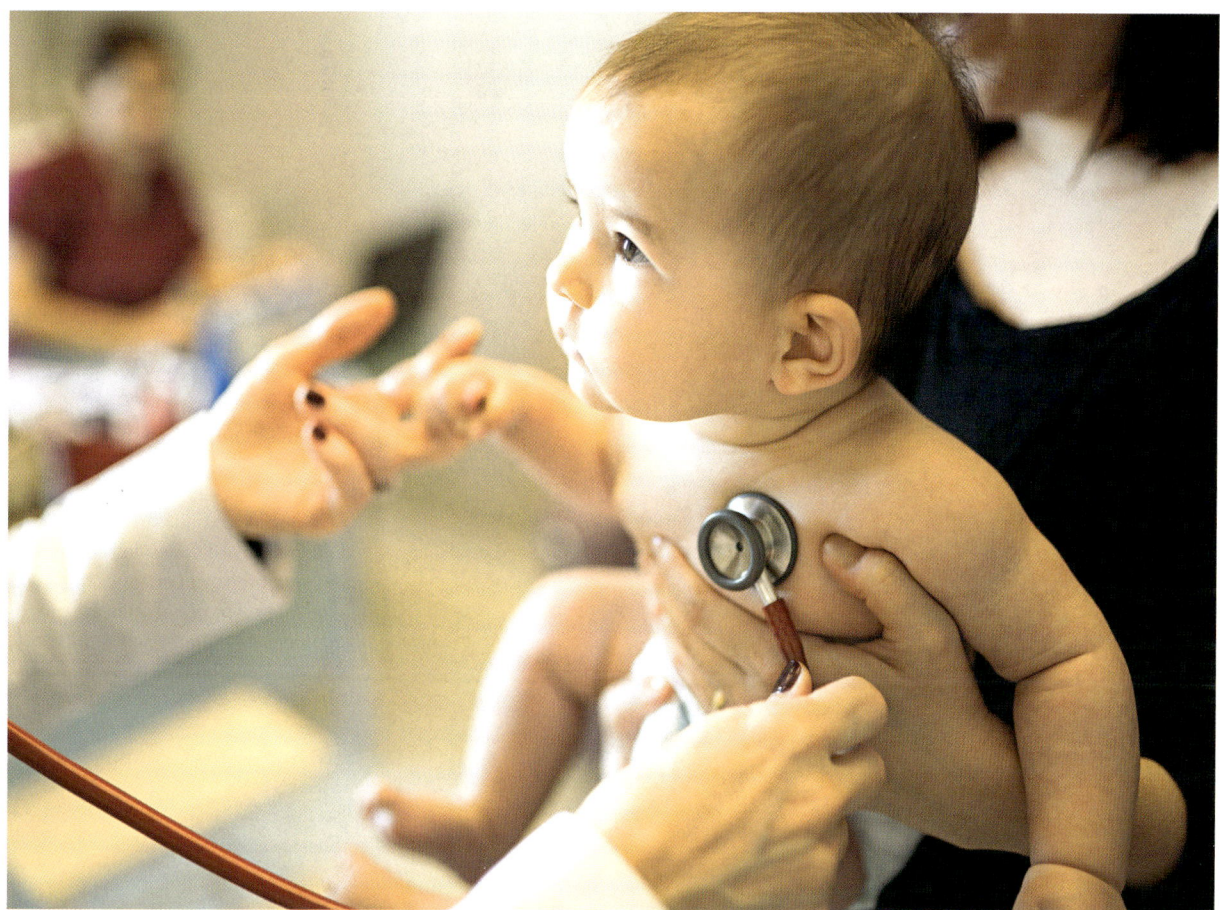

What Matters in Pediatrics

How we identified 89 outstanding children's hospitals

by **Ben Harder**

WHERE SHOULD anxious parents take a newborn with a life-threatening heart defect, or find ongoing care for a child with failing kidneys or lung-clogging cystic fibrosis? A local hospital's pediatric department might be perfectly capable of managing ear infections, allergies, flu and other common childhood ailments. But it may not have the expertise to treat severely ill kids. That's where children's hospitals come in. There are fewer than 200 hospitals in the country that either exclusively treat pediatric patients or possess a pediatric department that functions like a self-contained children's hospital. Even within that group, some centers are better than others. U.S. News created the Best Children's Hospitals rankings to help parents, in consultation with their doctors, find those best suited to their child.

The 2021-22 rankings highlight top children's centers in 10 specialties: cancer, cardiology and heart surgery, diabetes and endocrinology, gastroenterology and gastrointestinal surgery, neonatology, nephrology, neurology and neurosurgery, orthopedics, pulmonology and lung surgery, and urology. This year, 89 hospitals ranked in at least one specialty, and 10 were named to the Honor Roll for scoring near the top in most or all specialties. Newly introduced this year, regional rankings highlight hospi-

BEST CHILDREN'S HOSPITALS

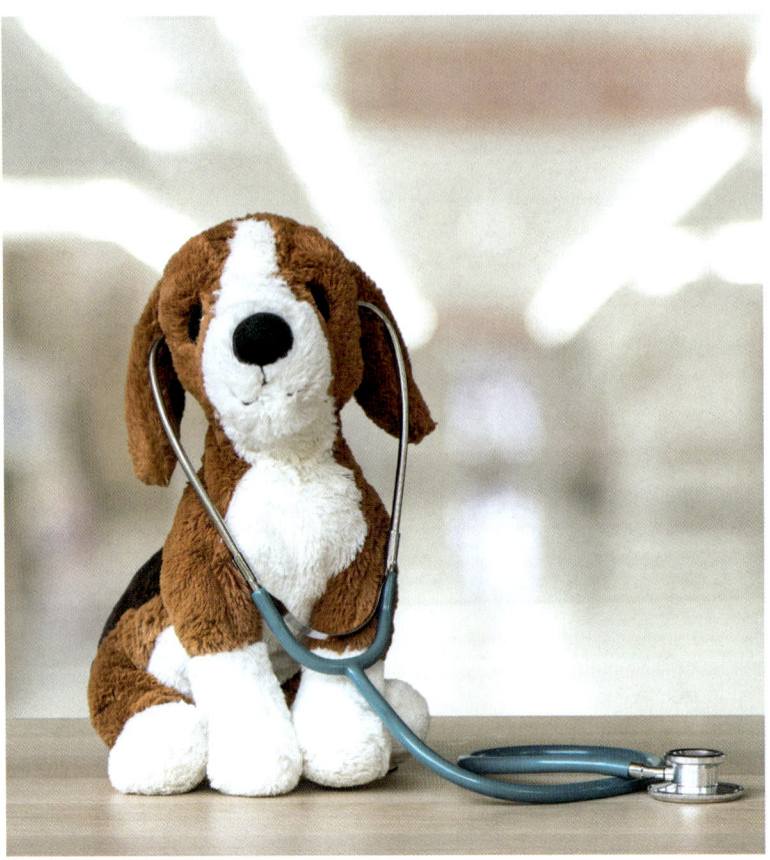

> **We gathered over 1,000 data points per hospital.**

tals that excel across a breadth of pediatric services; within each of seven multi-state regions, hospitals were ranked (Page 218) according to the number of specialties in which they were among the best.

Rich data. Judging the excellence of children's hospitals is challenging, and no single metric or ranking should be viewed as a definitive guide. U.S. News gathered more than 1,000 data points on each hospital to determine its strengths and weaknesses. Many summary measures appear in the ranking tables that follow; more can be found at usnews.com/childrenshospitals, which also features data on dozens of additional children's hospitals.

Almost all of the medical data used in these rankings were obtained by asking hospitals to complete a lengthy online data-collection process. This year, 110 hospitals surveyed by U.S. News provided enough data to be evaluated.

RTI International, a North Carolina-based research firm, oversaw data collection and produced the rankings. Working with RTI staff, pediatric experts serving in 12 working groups helped design the data-collection survey.

Whether and how high an institution was ranked depended on three elements: its clinical outcomes (such as survival and surgical complications), its delivery of care (such as adhering to safe and effective practices), and its resources (such as staffing and technology). Each element contributed one-third of a hospital's overall score in most specialties. A detailed FAQ about the rankings is available at usnews.com/aboutchildrens. Here are the basics:

Clinical outcomes. These reveal a hospital's success at keeping kids alive after their treatment or surgery, protecting them from infections and complications, and improving their quality of life. Though tough to measure, outcomes tend to matter most to families and doctors alike.

Delivery of care. How well a hospital handles day-to-day care was determined in part by compliance with accepted "best practices," such as having a full-time infection preventionist and holding regular conferences to discuss unexpected deaths and complications. U.S. News also surveyed pediatric specialists, asking them to identify up to 10 hospitals they consider best in their area of expertise for children with serious or difficult medical problems.

Resources. Surgical volume, nurse-patient ratio, clinics and programs for conditions such as asthma, and dozens of other measures were considered. ●

USNEWS.COM/BESTHOSPITALS

Visit usnews.com regularly while researching your health care choices, as U.S. News often adds content aimed at helping patients and families make decisions about their medical care. We also update the Best Hospitals, Best Children's Hospitals and Best Regional Hospitals content and data on the website when new content and data become available.

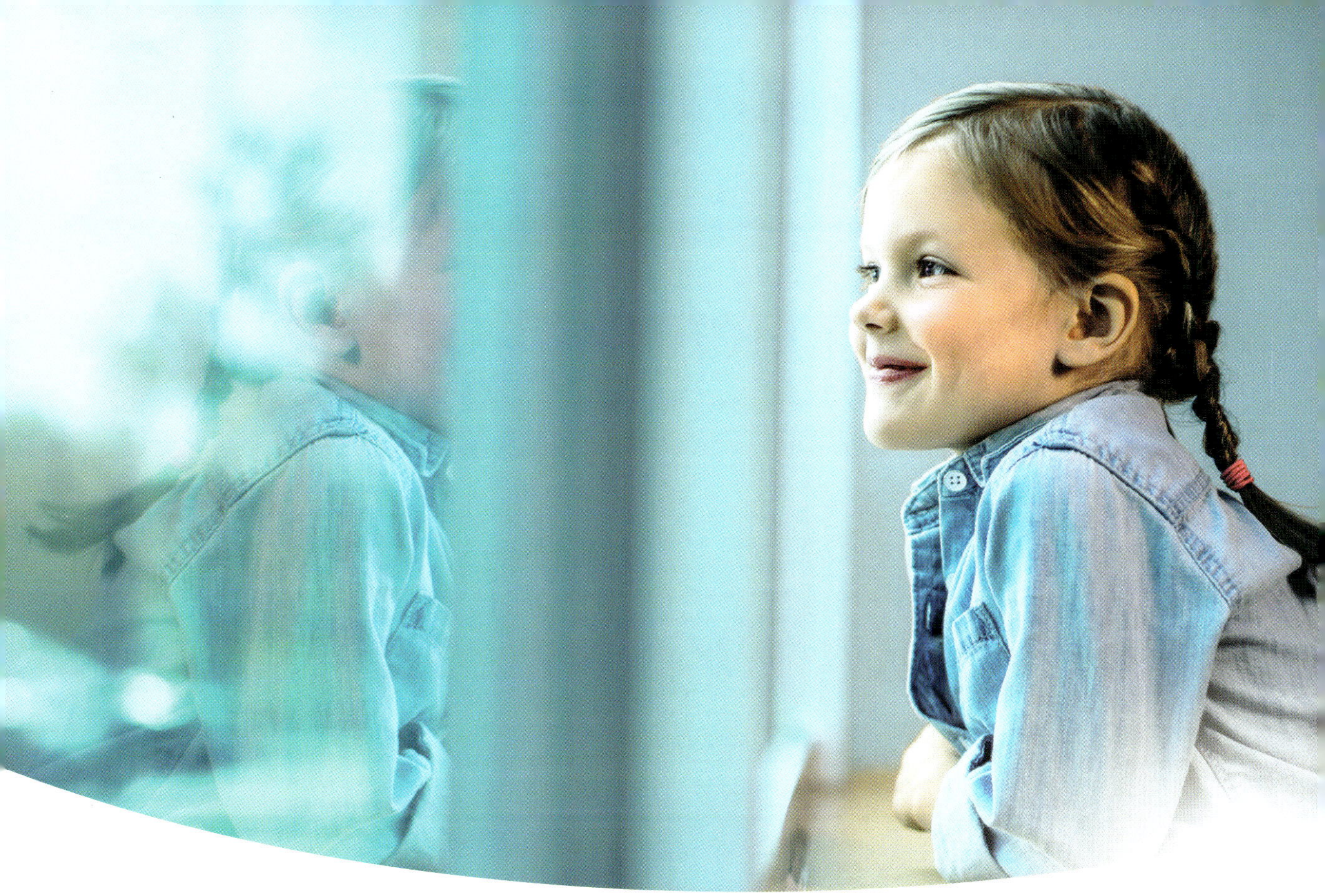

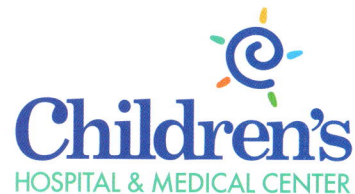

When children are your everything, **Anything can be.**

At Children's Hospital & Medical Center, science and heart lead us to even greater pediatric breakthroughs. We provide the very best in pediatric specialty care, advance pediatric research, educate tomorrow's experts and advocate for children, families and entire communities – to improve the future of medicine, and the life of every child.

To find a physician for your child, call **1.800.833.3100** or visit **ChildrensOmaha.org.**

Care · Advocacy · Research · Education

BEST CHILDREN'S HOSPITALS

A Word on the Terms

USED IN MORE THAN ONE SPECIALTY

A Nurse Magnet hospital: hospital recognized by American Nurses Credentialing Center as meeting standards for nursing excellence.
Infection prevention score, ICU: ability to prevent central-line bloodstream infections in intensive care units.
Infection prevention score, overall: ability to prevent infections through measures such as hand hygiene and vaccination.
No. of best practices: how well hospital adheres to recommended ways of diagnosing and treating patients, such as documenting blood sugar levels for a high percentage of outpatients (diabetes & endocrinology) and conducting hip exams with ultrasound specialists (orthopedics).
Nurse-patient ratio: balance of full-time registered nurses to inpatients.
Patient volume score: relative number of patients in past year with specified disorders.
% of specialists recommending hospital: percentage of physician specialists surveyed in 2019, 2020 and 2021 who named hospital among best for very challenging patients.
Procedure volume score: relative number of tests and nonsurgical procedures in past one, two or three years, such as implanting radioactive seeds in a cancerous thyroid (diabetes & endocrinology) and using an endoscope for diagnosis (gastroenterology). Surgical procedures are included in orthopedics.
Surgery volume score: relative number of patients who had specified surgical procedures in past year.
Surgical complications prevention score: ability to prevent surgery-related complications and readmissions within 30 days (neurology & neurosurgery, orthopedics, urology).
U.S. News score: 0 to 100 summary of overall performance in specialty.
NA: not applicable; service not provided by hospital.
NR: data not reported or unavailable.

USED IN ONE SPECIALTY

CANCER
Bone marrow transplant survival score: survival of stem cell recipients at 100 days.
Five-year survival score: survival five years after treatment for acute lymphoblastic leukemia, acute myeloid leukemia, and neuroblastoma.
Palliative care score: how well program meets specified training and staffing standards for children with terminal or life-limiting conditions, and number of cancer patients referred to program.

CARDIOLOGY & HEART SURGERY
Catheter procedure volume score: relative number of specified catheter-based procedures in past year, such as inserting stents and treating heart rhythm problems.
Length of stay after surgery score: success in minimizing how long certain congenital heart patients spend in the hospital for care related to their heart condition.
Norwood/hybrid surgery survival score: survival at one year after the first in a series of reconstructive surgeries, evaluated over past four years.
Risk-adjusted surgical survival score: survival in the hospital and 30 days from discharge after congenital heart surgery, adjusted for operative and patient risk, evaluated over past four years.

DIABETES & ENDOCRINOLOGY
Diabetes management score: ability to prevent serious problems in children with Type 1 diabetes and to keep blood sugar levels in check.
Hypothyroid management score: relative proportions of children treated for underactive thyroid who test normal and of infants who begin treatment by 3 weeks of age.

GASTROENTEROLOGY & GI SURGERY
Liver transplant survival score: one- and three-year survival after liver transplant.
Nonsurgical procedure volume score: relative number of tests and noninvasive procedures.
Selected treatments success score: shown, for example, by high remission rates for inflammatory bowel disease and few complications from endoscopic procedures.

NEONATOLOGY
Infection prevention score, NICU: ability to prevent central-line bloodstream infections in neonatal ICU.
Leaves NICU on breast milk score: relative percentage of infants discharged from NICU receiving some nutrition from breast milk.
Keeping breathing tube in place score: ability to minimize inappropriate breathing-tube removal in intubated infants.
NICU temperature management score: success in managing NICU patients' temperature at the time of admission and postoperatively.

NEPHROLOGY
Biopsy complications prevention score: ability to minimize complications after kidney biopsy.
Dialysis management score: relative proportion of dialysis patients in past two years who tested normal.
Infection prevention score, dialysis: ability to minimize dialysis-related infection.
Kidney transplant survival score: based on patient survival and functioning kidney at one and three years.

NEUROLOGY & NEUROSURGERY
Epilepsy management score: ability to treat children with epilepsy.
Surgical survival score: survival at 30 days after complex surgery and procedures, such as those involving brain tumors, epilepsy and head trauma.

ORTHOPEDICS
Fracture repair score: ability to treat complex leg and forearm fractures efficiently.

PULMONOLOGY & LUNG SURGERY
Asthma inpatient care score: ability to minimize asthmatic children's asthma-related deaths, length of stay and readmissions.
Cystic fibrosis management score: ability to improve lung function and nutritional status.
Lung transplant survival score: reflects number of transplants in past two years, one-year survival, and recognition by United Network for Organ Sharing.

UROLOGY
Minimally invasive volume score: relative number of patients in past year who had specified nonsurgical procedures.
Testicular torsion care score: promptness of emergency surgery to correct twisted spermatic cord.

Ranked #1 Children's Hospital in Florida

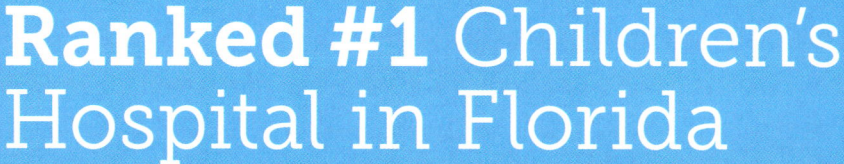

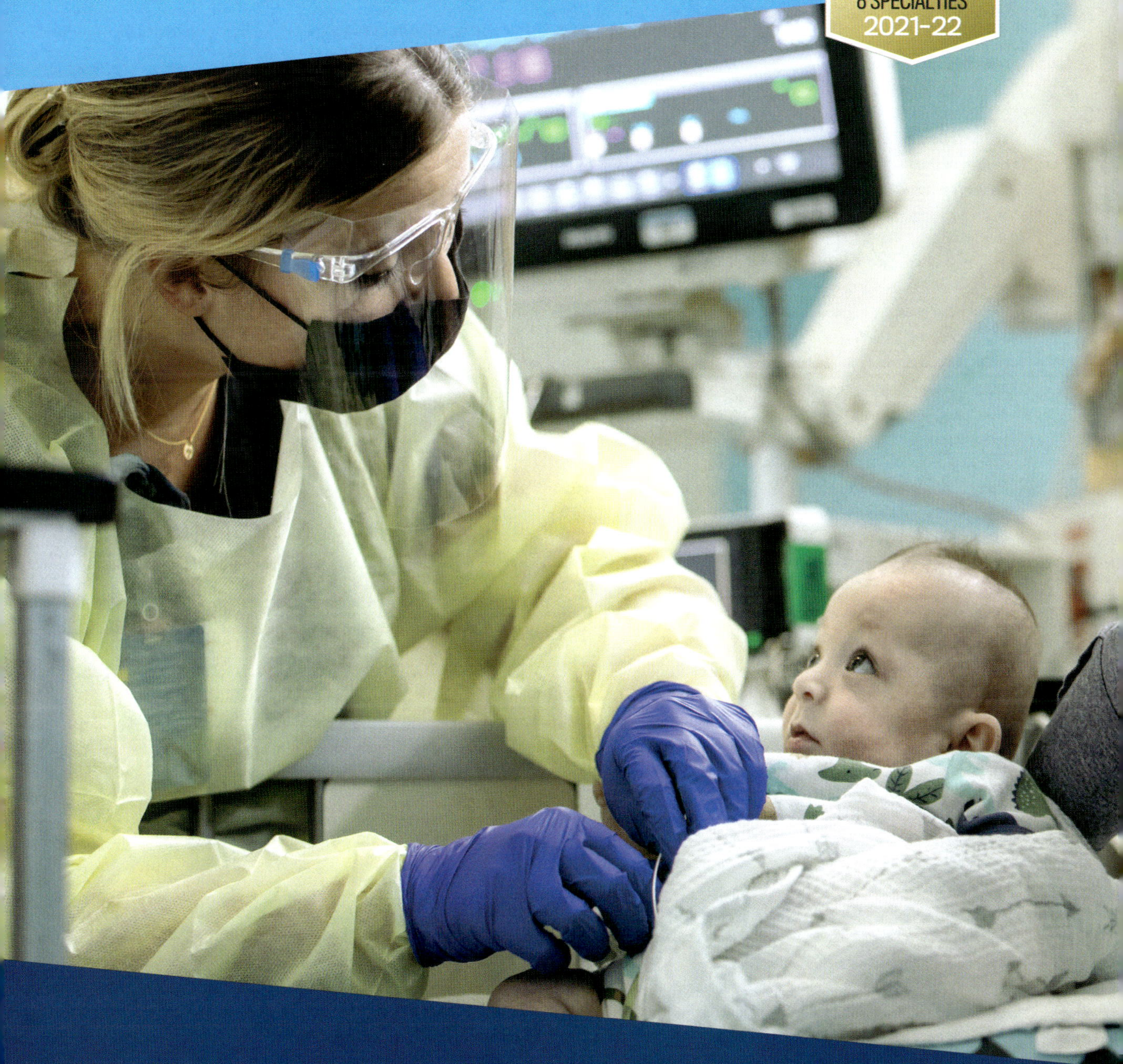

To heal a hurt, to elicit a smile, to save a life. We are inspired to excellence by the young patients we care for each and every day. Ranked nationally by *U.S. News & World Report* in eight specialties for the second consecutive year—we honor the commitment to do more, to heal more, to cure more.

Learn about our advanced specialty care at
HopkinsAllChildrens.org/ExpertPediatricCare

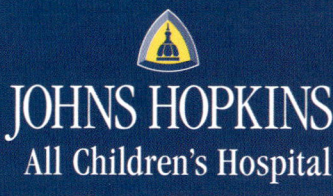

BEST CHILDREN'S HOSPITALS

Cancer

Rank	Hospital	U.S. News score	Five-year survival score (15=best)	Bone marrow transplant survival score (6=best)	Infection prevention score, overall (37=best)	Infection prevention score, ICU (15=best)	Patient volume score (30=best)	Nurse-patient ratio (higher is better)	A Nurse Magnet hospital	Palliative care score (8=best)	% of specialists recommending hospital
1	Children's Hospital of Philadelphia	100.0	14	6	36	9	30	4.3	Yes	8	47.0%
2	Dana-Farber/Boston Children's Cancer and Blood Disorders Center	99.6	14	5	35	15	30	3.9	Yes	8	48.9%
3	Cincinnati Children's Hospital Medical Center	99.0	15	5	36	13	30	4.1	Yes	8	37.3%
4	Texas Children's Hospital, Houston	97.1	13	6	37	9	30	4.6	Yes	8	36.0%
5	Children's National Hospital, Washington, D.C.	94.8	15	5	37	15	30	4.1	Yes	8	16.0%
6	Children's Healthcare of Atlanta	94.6	14	5	36	15	30	4.8	Yes	8	22.0%
7	Children's Hospital Los Angeles	94.2	15	5	34	15	29	3.8	Yes	8	22.5%
8	Nationwide Children's Hospital, Columbus, Ohio	93.4	13	6	35	15	30	3.3	Yes	8	14.2%
9	Children's Hospital Colorado, Aurora	92.9	14	5	36	14	30	4.3	Yes	8	17.8%
10	St. Jude Children's Research Hospital, Memphis, Tenn.	90.9	13	5	34	8	30	6.0	Yes	8	32.3%
11	Seattle Children's Hospital	88.8	13	5	35	11	20	3.4	Yes	8	28.0%
12	Johns Hopkins Children's Center, Baltimore	87.9	14	6	35	3	30	3.3	Yes	8	11.8%
13	Memorial Sloan Kettering Children's Cancer Center, New York	85.3	12	6	33	5	21	5.1	Yes	8	13.0%
14	UCSF Benioff Children's Hospitals, San Francisco and Oakland	84.6	12	5	35	13	25	4.1	Yes	7	10.9%
15	Ann and Robert H. Lurie Children's Hospital of Chicago	83.3	13	5	33	9	30	3.0	Yes	8	9.3%
16	Lucile Packard Children's Hospital Stanford, Palo Alto, Calif.	82.6	13	5	37	15	13	3.9	Yes	6	6.9%
17	Children's Hospital at Montefiore, New York	80.7	14	6	35	15	11	4.6	No	8	1.2%
18	Cleveland Clinic Children's Hospital	80.6	11	6	34	14	25	3.7	Yes	8	0.9%
19	UPMC Children's Hospital of Pittsburgh	80.3	12	5	32	15	27	3.5	Yes	8	4.2%
20	Riley Hospital for Children at IU Health, Indianapolis	80.1	13	5	32	11	27	4.3	Yes	8	2.0%
21	Monroe Carell Jr. Children's Hospital at Vanderbilt, Nashville, Tenn.	80.0	15	5	35	6	30	3.1	Yes	8	2.2%
22	Children's Medical Center Dallas	79.9	10	5	36	15	30	3.2	Yes	8	4.0%
23	Intermountain Primary Children's Hosp.-U. of Utah, Salt Lake City	78.8	14	6	35	10	27	3.4	No	8	1.7%
24	CHOC Children's Hospital, Orange, Calif.	78.5	11	6	35	9	20	3.6	Yes	8	3.8%
25	St. Louis Children's Hospital-Washington University	78.4	11	5	34	15	11	3.8	Yes	8	2.8%
26	C.S. Mott Children's Hospital-Michigan Medicine, Ann Arbor	78.1	12	4	36	15	30	3.7	Yes	8	3.8%
27	Children's Hospital of Alabama at UAB, Birmingham	77.9	12	6	35	12	24	3.4	No	8	2.4%
28	Children's Mercy Kansas City, Mo.	77.7	12	6	36	5	20	4.6	Yes	8	3.1%
28	Rainbow Babies and Children's Hospital, Cleveland	77.7	12	6	34	9	18	3.3	Yes	8	0.9%
30	Cohen Children's Medical Center, New Hyde Park, N.Y.	76.8	14	5	35	8	10	3.9	Yes	8	1.1%
30	UCLA Mattel Children's Hospital, Los Angeles	76.8	14	5	30	11	12	4.2	Yes	8	2.1%
32	Duke Children's Hospital and Health Center, Durham, N.C.	76.6	12	5	34	15	16	3.5	Yes	7	3.2%
32	Rady Children's Hospital, San Diego	76.6	11	5	35	9	22	3.2	Yes	8	2.8%
34	Levine Children's Hospital, Charlotte, N.C.	76.2	14	5	37	12	9	3.0	Yes	8	1.2%
35	Mayo Clinic Children's Center, Rochester, Minn.	75.6	12	5	32	8	13	4.1	Yes	8	0.9%
36	Phoenix Children's Hospital	75.3	14	4	36	15	30	3.0	No	8	1.8%
37	Children's Wisconsin, Milwaukee	74.5	12	4	31	15	15	4.3	Yes	8	1.7%
38	Penn State Children's Hospital, Hershey, Pa.	74.2	14	6	32	6	9	3.5	Yes	8	0.9%
39	Nemours Alfred I. duPont Hosp. for Children, Wilmington, Del.	74.0	13	6	30	2	10	3.5	Yes	8	1.9%
40	Doernbecher Children's Hospital, Portland, Ore.	73.9	15	4	29	9	24	3.9	Yes	8	1.2%
41	Children's Cancer Hosp.-U. of Tex. MD Anderson Cancer Ctr.	73.5	8	5	34	11	28	3.4	Yes	8	4.2%
42	Hackensack Meridian Hlth. Sanzari & Hovnanian Children's Hosps., N.J.	73.2	12	6	34	12	8	2.5	Yes	8	0.8%
43	Johns Hopkins All Children's Hospital, St. Petersburg, Fla.	73.1	10	5	35	13	11	3.8	Yes	8	1.0%
44	MUSC Shawn Jenkins Children's Hospital, Charleston, S.C.	73.0	13	5	32	15	12	2.5	Yes	8	0.7%
45	North Carolina Children's Hospital at UNC, Chapel Hill	72.8	9	5	36	9	26	4.7	Yes	8	1.0%
45	UF Health Shands Children's Hospital, Gainesville, Fla.	72.8	14	5	36	6	9	2.9	Yes	8	0.9%
47	New York-Presbyterian Hospital-Columbia and Cornell, New York	72.7	12	4	33	9	30	3.0	Yes	8	3.4%
48	Spectrum Hlth. Helen DeVos Children's Hosp., Grand Rapids, Mich.	72.0	11	6	29	13	12	2.7	Yes	7	0.8%
49	SSM Health Cardinal Glennon Children's Hosp.-St. Louis U., St. Louis	70.7	13	6	33	13	9	3.0	Yes	8	0.5%
50	Children's Hospital of Richmond at VCU, Va.	70.4	10	6	34	15	10	2.4	Yes	8	0.3%

Terms are explained on Page 176.

AWARD WINNING CARE FOR KIDS – YEAR AFTER YEAR.

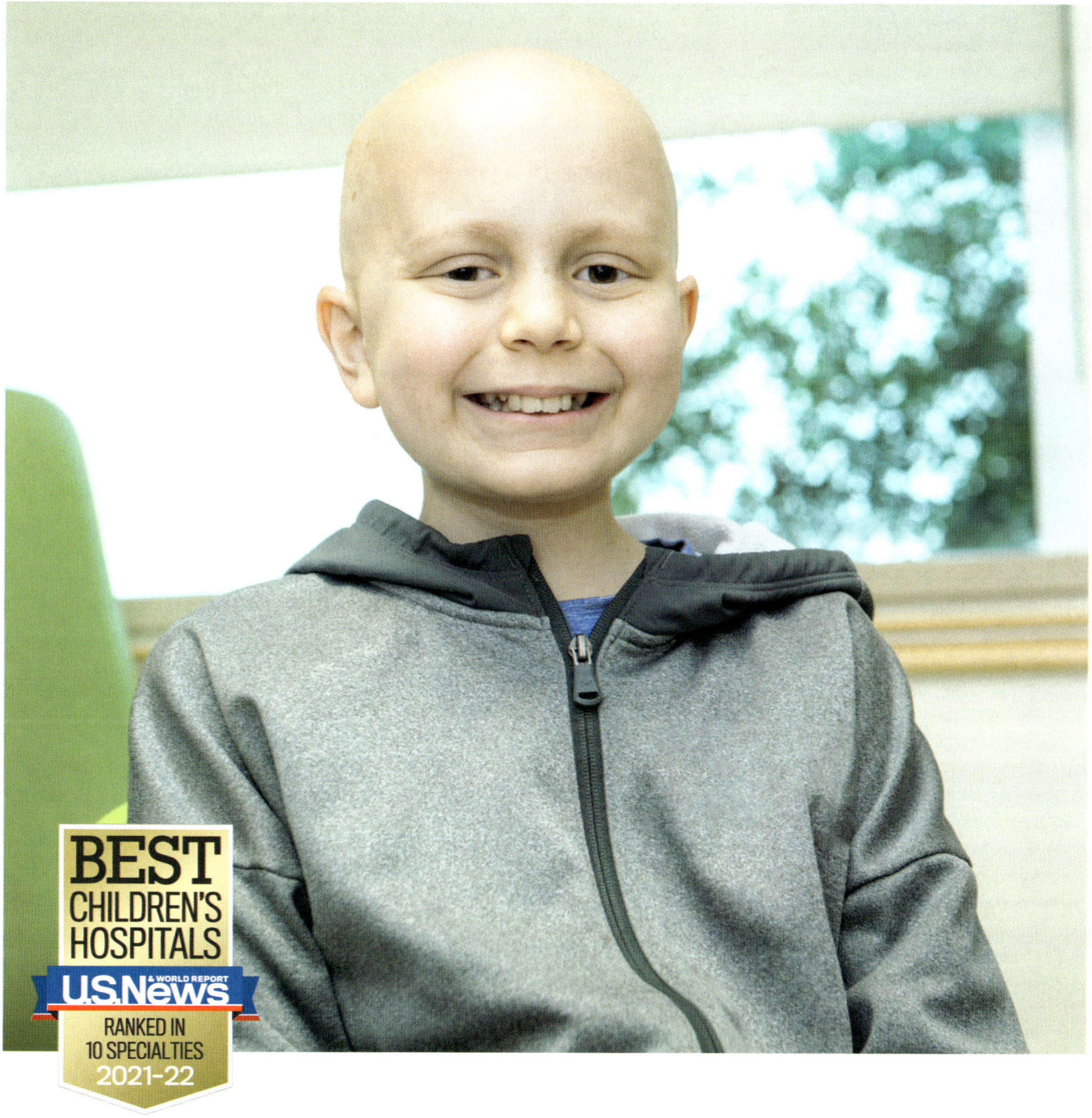

BEST CHILDREN'S HOSPITALS
U.S. News & WORLD REPORT
RANKED IN 10 SPECIALTIES 2021-22

Together with UT Southwestern Pediatric Group and private practices, we're advancing pediatrics.

At Children's Health℠ our team members provide care as strong as the kids we serve. In fact, Children's Medical Center Dallas was ranked in all 10 pediatric specialties by *U.S. News & World Report*.

Learn more at childrens.com/excellence

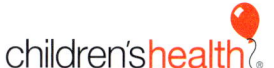 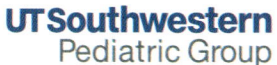

Specialty care provided by UT Southwestern physicians

BEST CHILDREN'S HOSPITALS
Cardiology & Heart Surgery

Rank	Hospital	U.S. News score	Risk-adjusted surgical survival score (5=best)	Norwood/hybrid surgery survival score (24=best)	Length of stay after surgery score (9=best)	Infection prevention score, overall (41=best)	Infection prevention score, ICU (5=best)	Surgery volume score (12=best)	Catheter procedure volume score (18=best)	Nurse-patient ratio (higher is better)	% of specialists recommending hospital
1	Texas Children's Hospital, Houston	100.0	5	22	6	41	3	10	18	4.6	46.4%
2	UPMC Children's Hospital of Pittsburgh	91.5	5	24	9	36	5	6	12	3.5	13.3%
3	Children's Hospital Los Angeles	90.7	4	22	8	38	5	11	12	3.8	17.3%
4	Boston Children's Hospital	89.9	3	19	7	39	5	12	18	3.9	60.8%
5	Riley Hospital for Children at IU Health, Indianapolis	89.7	5	22	7	36	5	9	13	4.3	3.1%
6	Children's Hospital Colorado, Aurora	88.0	3	22	8	40	4	9	16	4.3	13.6%
7	UF Health Shands Children's Hospital, Gainesville, Fla.	87.4	5	24	7	40	5	5	5	2.9	1.5%
8	Children's Hospital of Philadelphia	87.1	3	24	7	40	3	12	18	4.3	50.0%
9	Ann and Robert H. Lurie Children's Hospital of Chicago	86.9	4	21	7	37	3	6	11	3.0	17.7%
10	Children's Medical Center Dallas	85.6	4	24	7	40	5	7	13	3.2	4.5%
11	New York-Presbyterian Hospital-Columbia and Cornell, New York	84.9	4	24	7	37	3	10	12	3.0	16.6%
12	MUSC Children's Heart Network of South Carolina, Charleston	84.8	5	22	8	36	5	6	16	2.5	7.8%
13	Le Bonheur Children's Hospital, Memphis, Tenn.	84.1	5	23	8	38	2	5	12	3.0	3.7%
14	Seattle Children's Hospital	83.5	3	22	7	40	5	9	13	3.4	11.0%
15	Cincinnati Children's & Kentucky Children's Hosp. Joint Heart Program	82.6	2	24	8	40	3	9	18	4.1	27.6%
16	Cleveland Clinic Children's Hospital	81.7	4	18	8	38	4	6	13	3.7	1.6%
17	Penn State Children's Hospital, Hershey, Pa.	80.5	5	24	8	36	5	4	5	3.5	0.9%
17	St. Louis Children's Hospital-Washington University	80.5	3	17	7	39	5	6	16	3.8	3.3%
19	Children's Healthcare of Atlanta	80.4	2	18	9	40	5	12	16	4.8	16.5%
20	Children's Wisconsin, Milwaukee	79.9	4	21	8	35	5	7	13	4.3	6.4%
21	Lucile Packard Children's Hospital Stanford, Palo Alto, Calif.	79.5	1	17	7	41	5	11	17	3.9	34.1%
22	Rady Children's Hospital, San Diego	79.2	3	24	6	39	5	7	14	3.2	3.8%
23	Children's Memorial Hermann Hospital, Houston	79.0	5	22	7	35	5	5	8	3.4	1.8%
24	Children's Mercy Kansas City, Mo.	78.5	3	20	7	40	1	7	12	4.6	2.8%
25	Advocate Children's Heart Institute, Oak Lawn and Park Ridge, Ill.	78.4	4	22	9	36	4	8	12	4.3	2.1%
26	C.S. Mott Children's Hospital-Michigan Medicine, Ann Arbor	78.1	2	18	6	40	5	11	16	3.7	27.9%
27	UCSF Benioff Children's Hospitals, San Francisco and Oakland	77.1	3	18	6	40	3	8	14	4.1	6.9%
28	Phoenix Children's Hospital	76.9	4	16	8	40	5	9	15	3.0	3.4%
29	Children's Hospital of Alabama at UAB, Birmingham	76.5	4	22	7	39	2	6	12	3.4	2.0%
30	Johns Hopkins Children's Center, Baltimore	76.1	3	22	7	38	2	6	7	3.3	2.0%
31	Duke Children's Hospital and Health Center, Durham, N.C.	75.3	3	20	6	39	5	6	15	3.5	2.6%
32	Levine Children's Hospital, Charlotte, N.C.	74.2	3	23	8	41	4	6	12	3.0	2.2%
33	Spectrum Hlth. Helen DeVos Children's Hosp., Grand Rapids, Mich.	73.8	5	22	8	33	5	5	9	2.7	0.4%
34	Monroe Carell Jr. Children's Hospital at Vanderbilt, Nashville, Tenn.	73.7	3	19	7	39	2	9	17	3.1	4.7%
34	Nationwide Children's Hospital, Columbus, Ohio	73.7	1	18	7	39	5	7	14	3.3	10.2%
36	American Family Children's Hospital, Madison, Wis.	72.7	5	22	7	34	2	4	8	2.9	0.8%
37	University of Virginia Children's Hospital, Charlottesville	71.6	3	22	7	38	2	5	12	3.1	1.6%
38	Children's National Hospital, Washington, D.C.	70.7	1	14	6	41	5	6	14	4.1	10.6%
39	Children's Hospital and Medical Center, Omaha	70.6	3	18	8	39	2	6	11	4.5	1.5%
40	Arnold Palmer Hospital for Children, Orlando	70.5	4	22	6	39	4	4	7	3.0	1.0%
41	University of Maryland Children's Hospital, Baltimore	69.6	4	18	8	35	4	4	8	3.1	0.8%
42	Ochsner Hospital for Children, New Orleans	69.4	3	16	7	32	2	4	9	2.3	1.4%
43	Mayo Clinic Children's Minn. Cardiovascular Collaborative, Rochester	69.3	2	20	8	36	2	8	12	4.1	5.0%
44	Intermountain Primary Children's Hosp.-U. of Utah, Salt Lake City	69.1	2	24	8	39	2	9	12	3.4	5.1%
45	SSM Health Cardinal Glennon Children's Hosp.-St. Louis U., St. Louis	67.6	3	20	8	37	5	5	8	3.0	0.5%
46	Nicklaus Children's Hospital, Miami	67.0	3	18	6	31	5	6	12	2.7	1.9%
47	Loma Linda U. Children's Hospital, Loma Linda, Calif.	66.3	3	18	9	31	5	5	10	2.5	0.8%
48	Children's Hospital of Michigan, Detroit	66.0	3	16	6	36	5	5	13	3.1	1.4%
49	Joe DiMaggio Children's Hospital at Memorial, Hollywood, Fla.	65.7	3	17	7	37	5	4	11	3.5	1.2%
50	Arkansas Children's Hospital, Little Rock	65.1	3	19	6	30	5	5	14	3.2	1.1%

Terms are explained on Page 176.

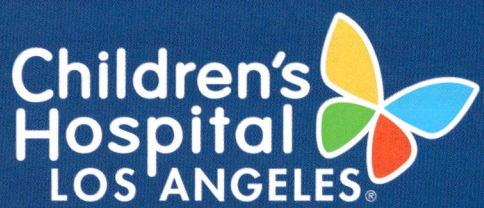

CHOOSE THE BEST CARE FOR KIDS IN CALIFORNIA.

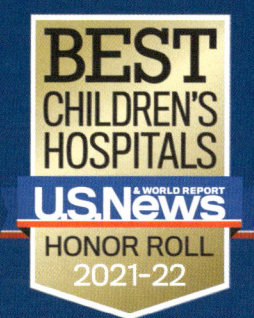

**#1 in California
#1 on the West Coast
#5 in the Nation**

RANKED IN ALL 10 SPECIALTIES

Cancer
Cardiology and Heart Surgery
Diabetes and Endocrinology
Gastroenterology and GI Surgery
Neonatology
Nephrology
Neurology and Neurosurgery
Orthopaedics
Pulmonology
Urology

No one in Southern California has more expertise treating children than us.

Find a doctor at CHLA.org

BEST CHILDREN'S HOSPITALS

Diabetes & Endocrinology

Rank	Hospital	U.S. News score	Diabetes management score (48=best)	Hypothyroid management score (6=best)	Infection prevention score, overall (37=best)	Patient volume score (36=best)	Procedure volume score (14=best)	Nurse-patient ratio (higher is better)	A Nurse Magnet hospital	No. of best practices (119=best)	% of specialists recommending hospital
1	Children's Hospital of Philadelphia	100.0	44	5	36	36	13	4.3	Yes	119	48.2%
2	Boston Children's Hospital	95.0	39	6	34	35	9	3.9	Yes	103	42.2%
3	Cincinnati Children's Hospital Medical Center	90.9	38	5	35	35	14	4.1	Yes	118	23.6%
4	Children's Hospital Colorado, Aurora	89.8	42	4	34	36	14	4.3	Yes	106	25.3%
5	Texas Children's Hospital, Houston	88.0	40	4	36	36	14	4.6	Yes	114	17.9%
6	Yale New Haven Children's Hospital, New Haven, Conn.	86.8	39	6	32	30	10	5.3	Yes	117	12.0%
7	UPMC Children's Hospital of Pittsburgh	85.2	38	5	30	36	12	3.5	Yes	114	15.9%
8	Children's Hospital Los Angeles	83.5	38	4	32	36	10	3.8	Yes	112	18.1%
9	Lucile Packard Children's Hospital Stanford, Palo Alto, Calif.	82.1	42	3	35	32	13	3.9	Yes	95	14.8%
10	Children's National Hospital, Washington, D.C.	78.5	34	3	37	35	14	4.1	Yes	112	10.3%
11	Nationwide Children's Hospital, Columbus, Ohio	77.1	31	5	34	36	9	3.3	Yes	108	7.3%
12	UF Health Shands Children's Hospital, Gainesville, Fla.	76.7	38	4	34	28	5	2.9	Yes	111	6.6%
13	Johns Hopkins Children's Center, Baltimore	76.2	36	4	34	26	11	3.3	Yes	108	8.0%
14	CHOC Children's Hospital, Orange, Calif.	75.7	43	4	34	34	12	3.6	Yes	108	2.1%
14	Rady Children's Hospital, San Diego	75.7	44	3	33	34	13	3.2	Yes	101	3.2%
16	North Carolina Children's Hospital at UNC, Chapel Hill	75.6	41	4	34	32	12	4.7	Yes	110	2.2%
17	UCSF Benioff Children's Hospitals, San Francisco and Oakland	75.5	30	4	34	34	12	4.1	Yes	98	12.9%
18	Norton Children's Hospital, Louisville, Ky.	75.3	45	4	35	34	14	3.1	No	106	1.6%
19	Seattle Children's Hospital	75.1	33	3	35	35	13	3.4	Yes	111	10.2%
20	Mount Sinai Kravis Children's Hospital, New York	75.0	35	6	30	29	14	3.7	Yes	112	3.3%
21	C.S. Mott Children's Hospital-Michigan Medicine, Ann Arbor	74.9	31	6	35	30	9	3.7	Yes	100	3.1%
22	Children's Medical Center Dallas	74.8	36	4	34	34	14	3.2	Yes	102	4.9%
23	Rainbow Babies and Children's Hospital, Cleveland	73.6	30	5	34	31	12	3.3	Yes	111	3.8%
23	St. Louis Children's Hospital-Washington University	73.6	31	4	33	34	14	3.8	Yes	101	5.0%
25	New York-Presbyterian Hospital-Columbia and Cornell, New York	73.2	35	4	30	29	13	3.0	Yes	97	9.0%
26	Riley Hospital for Children at IU Health, Indianapolis	72.2	33	3	31	35	11	4.3	Yes	95	8.5%
27	Cohen Children's Medical Center, New Hyde Park, N.Y.	71.6	35	4	34	33	13	3.9	Yes	108	2.4%
28	MassGeneral Hospital for Children, Boston	71.4	27	5	31	28	14	3.5	Yes	111	5.3%
29	Arnold Palmer Hospital for Children, Orlando	70.6	37	6	32	31	12	3.0	Yes	103	0.4%
30	Doernbecher Children's Hospital, Portland, Ore.	69.9	32	6	27	32	11	3.9	Yes	86	3.0%
30	Johns Hopkins All Children's Hospital, St. Petersburg, Fla.	69.9	32	6	34	32	8	3.8	Yes	99	0.8%
32	Monroe Carell Jr. Children's Hospital at Vanderbilt, Nashville, Tenn.	69.4	34	3	33	33	9	3.1	Yes	101	4.6%
33	Ann and Robert H. Lurie Children's Hospital of Chicago	69.0	32	4	31	33	10	3.0	Yes	96	7.3%
34	M Hlth. Fairview U. of Minn. Masonic Children's Hosp., Minneapolis	68.4	40	4	30	31	9	4.0	No	102	1.2%
35	Intermountain Primary Children's Hosp.-U. of Utah, Salt Lake City	68.2	39	5	33	32	9	3.4	No	96	1.6%
36	Connecticut Children's Medical Center, Hartford	67.3	34	4	33	32	11	3.1	Yes	104	1.7%
37	Phoenix Children's Hospital	67.1	26	6	34	36	14	3.0	No	104	0.9%
38	Children's Mercy Kansas City, Mo.	66.9	28	3	34	33	7	4.6	Yes	101	5.6%
38	Duke Children's Hospital and Health Center, Durham, N.C.	66.9	27	5	33	29	5	3.5	Yes	102	1.4%
38	Mayo Clinic Children's Center, Rochester, Minn.	66.9	32	3	30	30	14	4.1	Yes	110	2.5%
41	University of Iowa Stead Family Children's Hospital, Iowa City	66.6	39	3	30	29	7	3.4	Yes	94	1.4%
42	University of Virginia Children's Hospital, Charlottesville	66.4	30	4	32	26	10	3.1	Yes	106	1.8%
43	Cleveland Clinic Children's Hospital	66.3	29	4	33	34	12	3.7	Yes	110	1.1%
44	Wolfson Children's Hospital, Jacksonville, Fla.	66.2	32	4	32	32	11	2.6	Yes	98	2.1%
45	Children's Healthcare of Atlanta	66.1	24	4	34	36	8	4.8	Yes	103	2.5%
46	University of Chicago Comer Children's Hospital	65.8	32	4	30	23	12	2.8	Yes	98	1.7%
47	Holtz Children's Hospital at UM-Jackson Memorial Med. Ctr., Miami	65.7	42	5	26	27	10	2.2	No	114	1.6%
48	Valley Children's Healthcare and Hospital, Madera, Calif.	65.6	40	3	34	33	11	3.4	Yes	101	0.6%
49	Cook Children's Medical Center, Fort Worth	65.4	38	3	25	34	10	3.4	Yes	102	3.5%
49	Nicklaus Children's Hospital, Miami	65.3	32	6	25	34	8	2.7	Yes	105	1.7%
50	Children's Minnesota, Minneapolis	65.1	35	4	27	30	10	3.6	Yes	92	1.8%

Terms are explained on Page 176.

More @ usnews.com/childrenshospitals

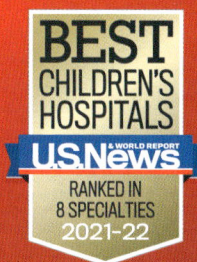

RANKED AMONG THE NATION'S **BEST CHILDREN'S HOSPITALS** FOR **15 YEARS** IN A ROW.

⌐ NewYork-Presbyterian

MORE TOP PEDIATRIC SPECIALISTS
IN NEW YORK CITY AND WESTCHESTER
THAN ANY OTHER HOSPITAL.

NewYork-Presbyterian Hospital as ranked by U.S. News & World Report 2021–22 and Castle Connolly's America's Top Doctors 2021

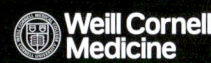 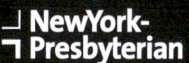 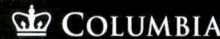

BEST CHILDREN'S HOSPITALS

Gastroenterology & GI Surgery

Rank	Hospital	U.S. News score	Selected treatments success score (9=best)	Liver transplant survival score (6=best)	Infection prevention score, overall (43=best)	Infection prevention score, ICU (5=best)	Patient volume score (27=best)	Surgery volume score (12=best)	Nonsurgical procedure volume score (18=best)	Nurse-patient ratio (higher is better)	A Nurse Magnet hospital	% of specialists recommending hospital
1	Children's Hospital Colorado, Aurora	100.0	9	5	42	4	27	11	18	4.3	Yes	30.5%
2	Boston Children's Hospital	99.0	7	5	41	5	27	12	18	3.9	Yes	51.8%
3	Children's Hospital of Philadelphia	98.6	8	5	42	3	27	12	18	4.3	Yes	47.0%
4	Texas Children's Hospital, Houston	97.8	9	5	43	3	27	11	18	4.6	Yes	27.6%
5	Cincinnati Children's Hospital Medical Center	96.2	8	4	42	3	27	12	18	4.1	Yes	45.9%
6	Children's Hospital Los Angeles	93.9	8	6	40	5	26	10	18	3.8	Yes	14.1%
7	Children's Medical Center Dallas	91.3	8	6	42	5	27	10	18	3.2	Yes	8.3%
8	Children's Healthcare of Atlanta	90.8	7	6	42	5	27	12	18	4.8	Yes	10.7%
9	UPMC Children's Hospital of Pittsburgh	88.7	7	6	37	5	27	10	13	3.5	Yes	16.2%
10	St. Louis Children's Hospital-Washington University	88.4	9	5	41	5	21	10	15	3.8	Yes	4.7%
11	Nationwide Children's Hospital, Columbus, Ohio	87.9	9	NR	41	5	26	12	16	3.3	Yes	29.9%
12	Seattle Children's Hospital	86.0	7	5	40	5	24	10	14	3.4	Yes	13.3%
13	Cleveland Clinic Children's Hospital	85.9	9	5	40	4	25	9	18	3.7	Yes	2.7%
14	Lucile Packard Children's Hospital Stanford, Palo Alto, Calif.	85.6	6	6	43	5	27	10	17	3.9	Yes	8.2%
15	Ann and Robert H. Lurie Children's Hospital of Chicago	84.7	7	5	39	3	26	10	18	3.0	Yes	15.5%
16	Children's Wisconsin, Milwaukee	83.5	7	6	38	5	23	11	15	4.3	Yes	4.8%
17	Children's Hospital at Montefiore, New York	83.4	9	5	41	5	19	9	14	4.6	No	2.6%
18	Monroe Carell Jr. Children's Hosp. at Vanderbilt, Nashville, Tenn.	82.8	8	6	41	2	26	11	18	3.1	Yes	3.3%
19	Johns Hopkins Children's Center, Baltimore	82.7	9	3	41	2	27	11	15	3.3	Yes	6.9%
20	Children's National Hospital, Washington, D.C.	81.5	6	5	43	5	25	11	15	4.1	Yes	4.9%
21	New York-Presbyterian Hosp.-Columbia and Cornell, New York	81.1	9	4	35	3	26	12	18	3.0	Yes	6.6%
21	Riley Hospital for Children at IU Health, Indianapolis	81.1	6	6	37	5	26	9	16	4.3	Yes	3.0%
23	Levine Children's Hospital, Charlotte, N.C.	80.7	8	6	43	4	23	9	15	3.0	Yes	1.3%
24	Mount Sinai Kravis Children's Hospital, New York	80.1	8	5	36	5	21	10	15	3.7	Yes	2.3%
25	UCLA Mattel Children's Hospital, Los Angeles	79.5	9	5	36	1	18	9	12	4.2	Yes	5.1%
26	MassGeneral Hospital for Children, Boston	79.2	6	6	39	5	20	10	14	3.5	Yes	3.6%
27	Children's Hospital of Michigan, Detroit	79.0	9	6	34	5	26	9	11	3.1	No	0.6%
28	C.S. Mott Children's Hospital-Michigan Medicine, Ann Arbor	78.6	8	4	40	5	27	9	15	3.7	Yes	2.6%
29	Duke Children's Hospital and Health Center, Durham, N.C.	78.5	7	6	40	5	20	9	16	3.5	Yes	1.6%
30	UCSF Benioff Children's Hospitals, San Francisco and Oakland	76.1	5	5	41	3	25	10	15	4.1	Yes	6.4%
31	Rady Children's Hospital, San Diego	76.0	7	3	40	5	27	7	17	3.2	Yes	2.7%
32	Children's Mercy Kansas City, Mo.	75.5	7	4	42	1	24	11	14	4.6	Yes	5.1%
33	Nemours Alfred I. duPont Hosp. for Children, Wilmington, Del.	74.0	9	4	35	1	20	9	7	3.5	Yes	2.6%
34	Le Bonheur Children's Hospital, Memphis, Tenn.	73.7	9	4	41	2	17	8	10	3.0	Yes	0.8%
34	University of Chicago Comer Children's Hospital	73.7	7	6	38	4	14	6	11	2.8	Yes	1.3%
36	Phoenix Children's Hospital	73.6	7	5	40	5	26	10	12	3.0	No	2.1%
37	Yale New Haven Children's Hospital, New Haven, Conn.	73.2	6	5	38	4	19	7	13	5.3	Yes	2.0%
38	Rainbow Babies and Children's Hospital, Cleveland	69.8	9	NA	40	5	16	6	12	3.3	Yes	1.9%
39	Cohen Children's Medical Center, New Hyde Park, N.Y.	69.3	8	NA	41	4	16	9	15	3.9	Yes	1.1%
40	SSM Health Cardinal Glennon Children's Hosp.-St. Louis U.	69.2	7	3	39	5	15	8	9	3.0	Yes	0.5%
41	Children's Hospital of Alabama at UAB, Birmingham	69.1	8	3	41	2	25	9	15	3.4	No	2.1%
42	MUSC Shawn Jenkins Children's Hospital, Charleston, S.C.	68.0	6	4	38	5	14	9	17	2.5	Yes	0.5%
43	Valley Children's Healthcare and Hospital, Madera, Calif.	67.8	9	NA	40	5	20	10	14	3.4	Yes	0.2%
44	Intermountain Primary Children's Hosp.-U. of Utah, Salt Lake City	67.4	6	5	39	2	26	9	17	3.4	No	2.6%
45	Mayo Clinic Children's Center, Rochester, Minn.	67.3	5	5	38	2	19	5	15	4.1	Yes	2.2%
45	North Carolina Children's Hospital at UNC, Chapel Hill	67.3	5	6	42	1	17	6	12	4.7	Yes	1.5%
47	Children's Hospital and Medical Center, Omaha	66.5	9	NA	37	2	13	7	14	4.5	Yes	1.6%
48	Connecticut Children's Medical Center, Hartford	66.2	9	NA	41	1	22	10	9	3.1	Yes	2.0%
49	M Hlth. Fairview U. of Minn. Masonic Children's Hosp., Minneapolis	65.8	6	6	37	1	25	9	13	4.0	No	1.4%
50	Akron Children's Hospital, Ohio	64.9	9	NA	36	4	19	7	9	3.5	Yes	1.0%

NA=not applicable. NR=not reported. Terms are explained on Page 176.

Among the Nation's Best

RANKED IN ALL 10 SPECIALTIES

CANCER | CARDIOLOGY & HEART SURGERY | DIABETES & ENDOCRINOLOGY
GASTROENTEROLOGY & GI SURGERY | NEONATOLOGY | NEPHROLOGY
NEUROLOGY & NEUROSURGERY | ORTHOPEDICS
PULMONOLOGY & LUNG SURGERY | UROLOGY

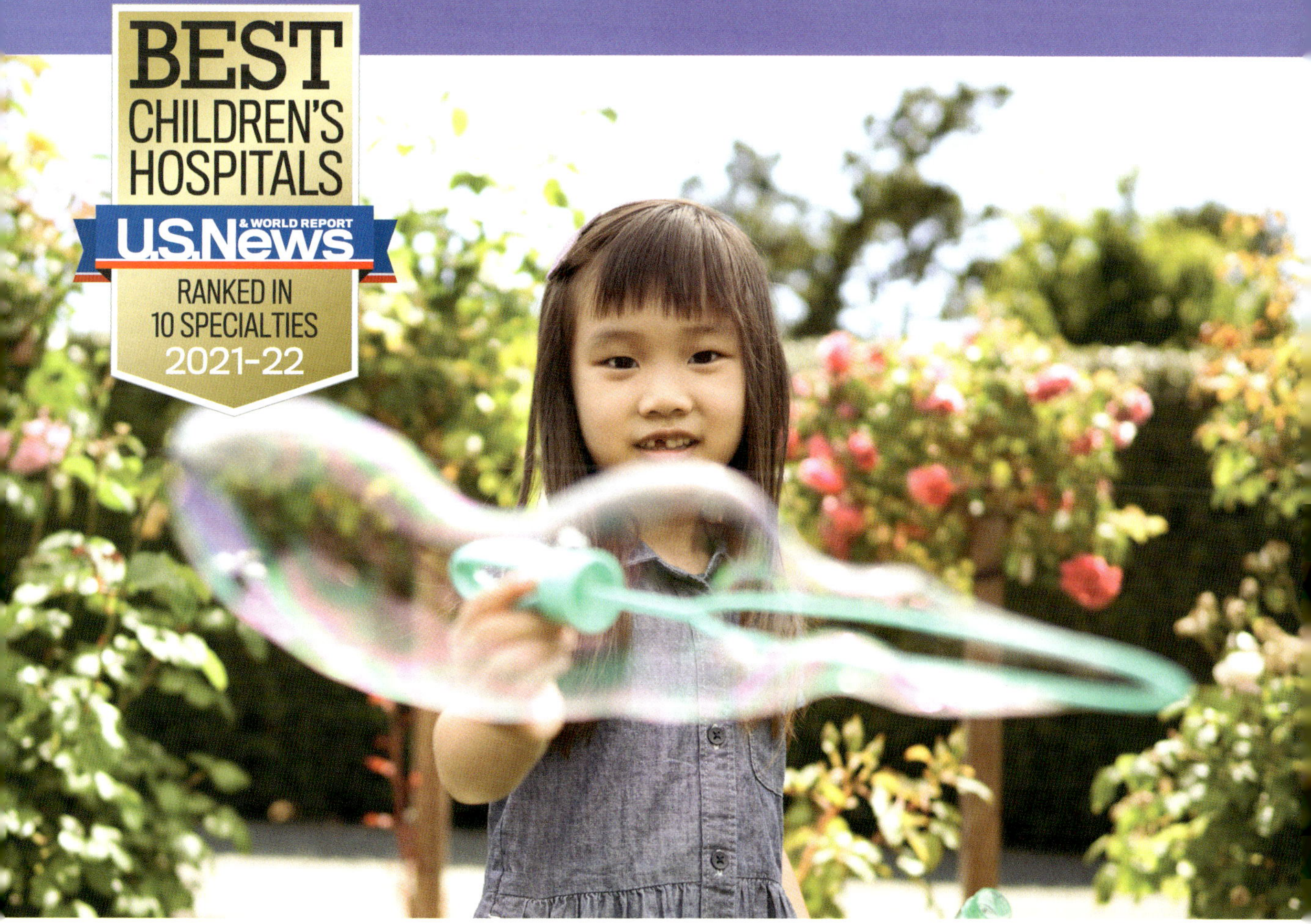

BEST CHILDREN'S HOSPITALS
U.S. News & World Report
RANKED IN 10 SPECIALTIES 2021-22

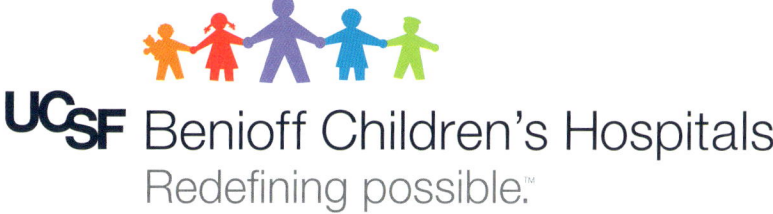

UCSF Benioff Children's Hospitals
Redefining possible.

BEST CHILDREN'S HOSPITALS

Neonatology

Rank	Hospital	U.S. News score	Leaves NICU on breast milk score (3=best)	Keeping breathing tube in place score (5=best)	NICU temperature management score (12=best)	Infection prevention score, overall (43=best)	Infection prevention score, NICU (5=best)	Patient volume score (33=best)	Nurse-patient ratio (higher is better)	No. of best practices (99=best)	% of specialists recommending hospital
1	Children's National Hospital, Washington, D.C.	100.0	3	5	12	43	5	32	4.0	98	20.0%
2	Children's Hospital Los Angeles	94.8	3	5	12	40	5	31	3.5	97	10.1%
3	Lucile Packard Children's Hospital Stanford, Palo Alto, Calif.	94.7	3	3	12	43	5	22	4.4	98	15.9%
4	UCSF Benioff Children's Hospitals, San Francisco and Oakland	93.3	3	3	12	42	5	28	3.4	96	13.7%
5	Rady Children's Hospital, San Diego	92.4	3	5	10	42	5	26	4.0	98	6.0%
6	Children's Hospital of Philadelphia	91.9	3	5	9	42	2	32	4.3	93	38.2%
7	Boston Children's Hospital	91.3	3	5	11	41	2	25	3.6	97	30.4%
8	Cincinnati Children's Hospital Medical Center	91.2	2	4	12	42	5	32	3.6	97	28.2%
9	Ann & Robert H. Lurie Children's Hosp.-Prentice Women's Hosp., Chicago	90.5	3	4	11	40	5	24	3.0	93	9.7%
10	New York-Presbyterian Hospital-Columbia and Cornell, New York	90.2	3	3	11	39	5	31	2.3	97	12.1%
11	Texas Children's Hospital, Houston	89.8	3	5	12	43	2	29	2.9	99	19.8%
12	Children's Healthcare of Atlanta	89.3	3	5	12	42	5	31	3.2	91	6.4%
13	Children's Hospital of Alabama at UAB, Birmingham	87.1	3	3	12	41	5	31	3.1	95	7.5%
14	Cleveland Clinic Children's Hospital	86.5	3	4	11	40	5	13	2.5	97	3.3%
15	UPMC Children's Hospital of Pittsburgh	86.4	2	4	10	38	5	25	3.1	97	5.9%
16	Riley Hospital for Children at IU Health, Indianapolis	85.9	2	5	10	38	5	30	3.1	94	3.2%
17	Monroe Carell Jr. Children's Hospital at Vanderbilt, Nashville, Tenn.	83.8	2	4	12	34	5	14	2.5	91	6.8%
18	Johns Hopkins Children's Center, Baltimore	83.7	2	4	7	41	5	22	3.0	86	6.6%
19	Children's Hospital at Montefiore, New York	83.2	3	5	12	41	4	11	4.2	98	1.9%
20	Phoenix Children's Hospital	83.0	3	5	11	41	5	25	2.8	96	0.6%
21	St. Louis Children's Hospital-Washington University	82.5	2	4	11	41	2	26	4.2	98	11.3%
21	UCLA Mattel Children's Hospital, Los Angeles	82.5	3	5	5	36	4	12	4.1	95	7.2%
21	University of Rochester-Golisano Children's Hospital, N.Y.	82.5	2	4	11	38	5	14	2.9	97	2.0%
24	Children's Hospital Colorado, Aurora	82.2	3	4	11	42	1	27	3.1	97	13.1%
25	Duke Children's Hospital and Health Center, Durham, N.C.	82.1	1	5	11	41	5	19	2.6	89	2.7%
25	University of Iowa Stead Family Children's Hospital, Iowa City	82.1	3	5	7	32	5	18	2.3	87	5.7%
27	Seattle Children's Hospital	81.9	3	5	12	36	2	29	3.8	92	13.3%
27	Yale New Haven Children's Hospital, New Haven, Conn.	81.9	2	5	10	37	5	15	2.3	94	2.2%
29	UC Davis Children's Hospital, Sacramento, Calif.	81.8	2	5	9	42	5	17	3.5	93	1.3%
30	SSM Health Cardinal Glennon Children's Hosp.-St. Louis U.	81.6	2	3	11	39	5	18	3.8	95	1.3%
31	Valley Children's Healthcare and Hospital, Madera, Calif.	81.5	2	4	12	40	5	21	3.3	91	1.2%
32	CHOC Children's Hospital, Orange, Calif.	81.0	3	5	12	41	2	30	3.4	96	3.1%
32	Cohen Children's Medical Center, New Hyde Park, N.Y.	81.0	3	3	6	41	5	20	2.5	95	1.3%
34	Doernbecher Children's Hospital, Portland, Ore.	80.8	3	5	9	35	5	18	2.6	94	1.1%
35	AdventHealth for Children, Orlando	80.6	2	5	12	36	5	14	2.3	95	1.5%
36	University of Virginia Children's Hospital, Charlottesville	80.4	2	5	10	36	5	14	2.7	93	1.4%
37	Connecticut Children's Medical Center, Hartford	79.8	2	4	11	40	5	11	2.2	95	1.8%
38	Levine Children's Hospital, Charlotte, N.C.	79.6	2	3	11	42	5	22	2.5	92	2.2%
38	Mayo Clinic Children's Center, Rochester, Minn.	79.6	2	5	12	38	4	12	3.9	87	0.6%
40	Children's Medical Center Dallas	79.4	2	4	9	42	5	24	2.3	92	3.6%
40	Inova Children's Hospital, Falls Church, Va.	79.4	3	4	5	40	5	17	2.9	96	0.9%
42	Penn State Children's Hospital, Hershey, Pa.	79.1	2	4	9	39	5	15	3.3	89	0.9%
43	Nationwide Children's Hospital, Columbus, Ohio	79.0	2	3	6	41	2	30	3.3	95	17.6%
44	MassGeneral Hospital for Children, Boston	78.9	3	3	8	37	5	15	3.2	91	1.4%
45	Johns Hopkins All Children's Hospital, St. Petersburg, Fla.	78.7	1	5	10	37	5	22	2.8	92	0.9%
46	C.S. Mott Children's Hospital-Michigan Medicine, Ann Arbor	78.6	2	3	10	42	5	27	2.6	87	3.4%
47	Children's Hosp. at St. Peter's University Hosp., New Brunswick, N.J.	78.5	3	5	9	41	4	10	3.6	98	0.0%
47	Rainbow Babies and Children's Hospital, Cleveland	78.5	2	4	9	40	2	11	4.5	96	12.0%
47	UF Health Shands Children's Hospital, Gainesville, Fla.	78.5	1	5	10	41	4	15	3.0	92	2.2%
50	Arnold Palmer Hospital for Children, Orlando	78.2	2	4	10	40	5	23	2.5	93	0.3%

Terms are explained on Page 176.

It's going to take all of us to help all of them.

Our kids' mental health is in a state of crisis.

And it's a crisis no one person, group or organization can fix alone.

That's why it's going to take all of us, whether you're a parent, a medical professional or a kind, concerned person, to help our kids through this. To make youth mental health a priority in the way we spend our time, money and resources. To use our collective skills and passions to give our kids the help they need, when they need it.

This is no small issue. To tackle it, we need everyone to work together: Talk to your community. Talk to your representatives and demand funding for pediatric mental health services.

And most importantly, talk to your kids.

Visit childrenscolorado.org/MentalHealthAdvice and start the conversation.

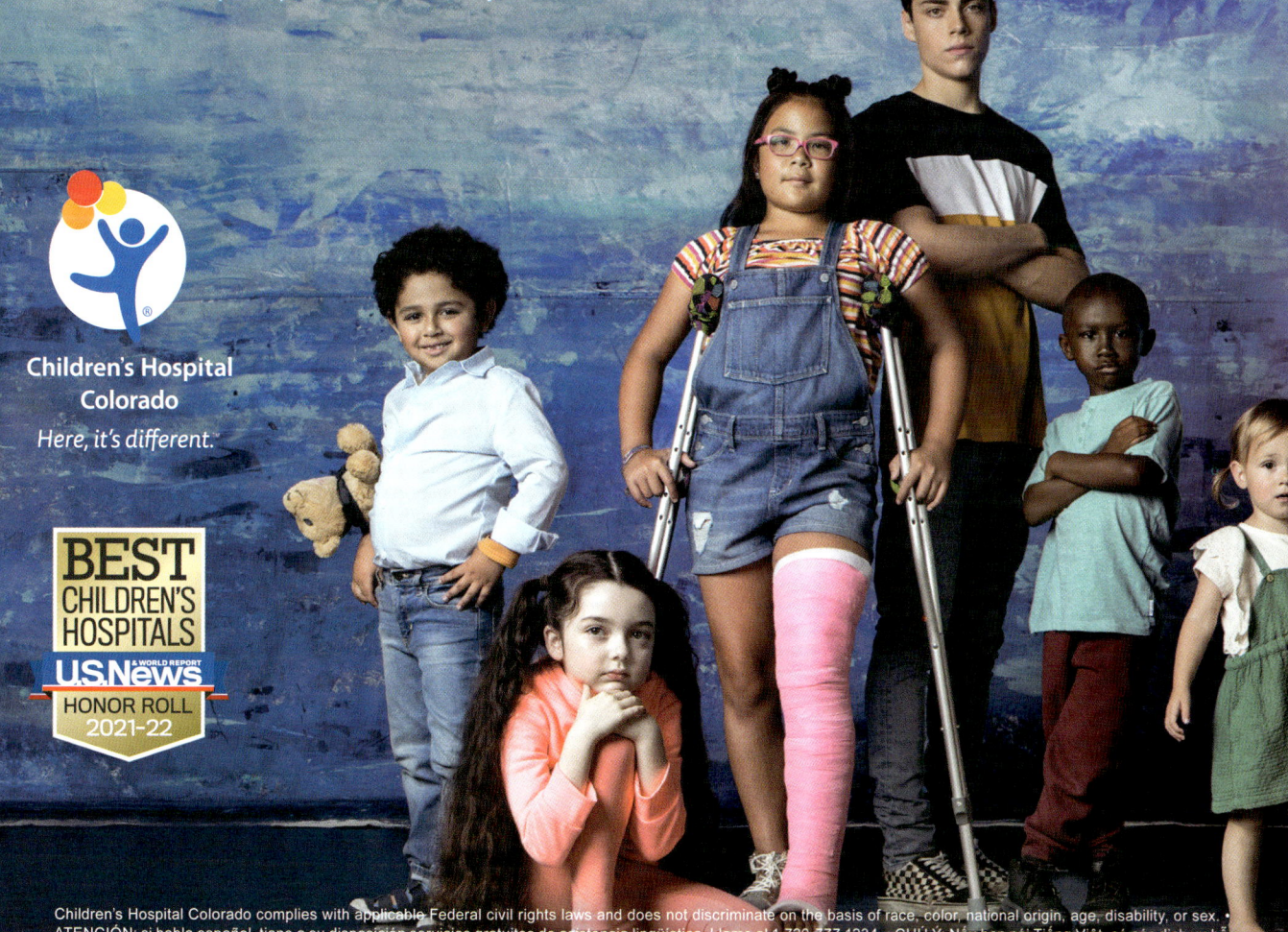

Children's Hospital Colorado
Here, it's different.

BEST CHILDREN'S HOSPITALS
U.S.News & World Report
HONOR ROLL 2021-22

Children's Hospital Colorado complies with applicable Federal civil rights laws and does not discriminate on the basis of race, color, national origin, age, disability, or sex. • ATENCIÓN: si habla español, tiene a su disposición servicios gratuitos de asistencia lingüística. Llame al 1-720-777-1234. • CHÚ Ý: Nếu bạn nói Tiếng Việt, có các dịch vụ hỗ trợ ngôn ngữ miễn phí dành cho bạn. Gọi số 1-720-777-1234.

BEST CHILDREN'S HOSPITALS

Nephrology

Rank	Hospital	U.S. News score	Kidney transplant survival score (24=best)	Biopsy complications prevention score (6=best)	Dialysis management score (12=best)	Infection prevention score, overall (60=best)	Infection prevention score, ICU (5=best)	Infection prevention score, dialysis (9=best)	Patient volume score (14=best)	Nurse-patient ratio (higher is better)	A Nurse Magnet hospital	% of specialists recommending hospital
1	Boston Children's Hospital	100.0	24	6	12	58	5	9	14	3.9	Yes	47.2%
2	Seattle Children's Hospital	93.7	23	6	12	57	5	6	14	3.4	Yes	42.5%
3	Texas Children's Hospital, Houston	92.6	23	6	12	60	3	9	14	4.6	Yes	28.3%
4	Lucile Packard Children's Hospital Stanford, Palo Alto, Calif.	92.5	24	6	11	60	5	9	14	3.9	Yes	24.5%
5	Cincinnati Children's Hospital Medical Center	92.3	22	6	12	59	3	8	12	4.1	Yes	43.4%
6	Children's Hospital of Philadelphia	90.7	24	6	9	59	3	8	13	4.3	Yes	39.7%
6	Children's National Hospital, Washington, D.C.	90.7	24	6	12	60	5	9	14	4.1	Yes	10.0%
8	Children's Healthcare of Atlanta	89.7	22	6	12	59	5	8	14	4.8	Yes	22.2%
9	Nationwide Children's Hospital, Columbus, Ohio	88.2	23	6	11	58	5	9	13	3.3	Yes	18.7%
10	Children's Mercy Kansas City, Mo.	87.0	24	6	12	59	1	9	14	4.6	Yes	20.6%
11	Ann and Robert H. Lurie Children's Hospital of Chicago	82.4	23	6	12	56	3	8	14	3.0	Yes	12.7%
12	UPMC Children's Hospital of Pittsburgh	82.2	24	6	12	55	5	9	10	3.5	Yes	8.8%
13	Johns Hopkins Children's Center, Baltimore	82.1	24	6	11	58	2	8	10	3.3	Yes	14.6%
14	Riley Hospital for Children at IU Health, Indianapolis	80.7	22	6	11	55	5	9	12	4.3	Yes	7.1%
15	Children's Hospital Los Angeles	79.7	23	6	12	57	5	9	13	3.8	Yes	5.5%
16	Children's Hospital Colorado, Aurora	79.3	24	6	10	59	4	7	13	4.3	Yes	6.3%
17	C.S. Mott Children's Hospital-Michigan Medicine, Ann Arbor	77.4	24	6	12	57	5	5	13	3.7	Yes	6.8%
18	Rady Children's Hospital, San Diego	77.1	24	5	12	58	5	9	12	3.2	Yes	2.7%
19	UCSF Benioff Children's Hospitals, San Francisco and Oakland	76.9	24	6	10	57	3	9	10	4.1	Yes	6.8%
20	St. Louis Children's Hospital-Washington University	76.3	22	5	12	57	5	7	11	3.8	Yes	4.1%
21	Children's Hospital at Montefiore, New York	75.2	23	6	12	58	5	6	12	4.6	No	4.7%
21	Duke Children's Hospital and Health Center, Durham, N.C.	75.2	24	6	11	58	5	8	12	3.5	Yes	5.2%
23	Children's Medical Center Dallas	74.9	24	5	10	55	5	7	12	3.2	Yes	6.0%
24	Levine Children's Hospital, Charlotte, N.C.	73.5	24	6	11	60	4	9	12	3.0	Yes	2.4%
25	UC Davis Children's Hospital, Sacramento, Calif.	72.6	21	6	12	59	4	8	9	6.9	Yes	1.6%
26	U. of Minn. Masonic Children's Hosp.-Children's Minn., Minneapolis	72.5	23	6	12	54	1	8	13	4.0	Yes	6.2%
27	UCLA Mattel Children's Hospital, Los Angeles	71.6	23	5	10	53	1	8	9	4.2	Yes	11.8%
27	Yale New Haven Children's Hospital, New Haven, Conn.	71.6	24	6	12	55	4	9	9	5.3	Yes	2.0%
29	New York-Presbyterian Hosp.-Columbia and Cornell, New York	71.2	23	6	11	56	3	8	11	3.0	Yes	4.4%
30	MUSC Shawn Jenkins Children's Hospital, Charleston, S.C.	70.1	24	6	10	55	5	8	14	2.5	Yes	0.9%
31	Doernbecher Children's Hospital, Portland, Ore.	68.8	24	6	12	51	1	9	10	3.9	Yes	2.5%
32	Cohen Children's Medical Center, New Hyde Park, N.Y.	68.7	12	5	12	58	4	8	12	3.9	Yes	0.9%
33	Cleveland Clinic Children's Hospital	68.2	17	6	12	56	4	8	10	3.7	Yes	2.1%
33	Rainbow Babies and Children's Hospital, Cleveland	68.2	22	6	12	57	5	8	7	3.3	Yes	1.6%
35	North Carolina Children's Hospital at UNC, Chapel Hill	68.1	24	6	10	59	1	8	11	4.7	Yes	1.8%
35	Phoenix Children's Hospital	68.1	22	6	12	59	5	8	14	3.0	No	1.8%
37	Spectrum Hlth. Helen DeVos Children's Hosp., Grand Rapids, Mich.	67.9	22	6	12	52	5	7	11	2.7	Yes	1.2%
38	Children's Hospital of Alabama at UAB, Birmingham	67.8	24	6	8	56	2	7	14	3.4	No	6.7%
39	Johns Hopkins All Children's Hospital, St. Petersburg, Fla.	67.0	23	6	10	59	5	9	8	3.8	Yes	0.7%
40	Mount Sinai Kravis Children's Hospital, New York	66.4	24	6	10	53	5	7	8	3.7	Yes	3.2%
41	Intermountain Primary Children's Hosp.-U. of Utah, Salt Lake City	65.4	24	6	12	58	2	7	12	3.4	No	2.2%
42	Children's Hospital of Richmond at VCU, Va.	65.2	18	6	11	56	5	6	13	2.4	Yes	1.7%
42	Monroe Carell Jr. Children's Hosp. at Vanderbilt, Nashville, Tenn.	65.2	23	6	9	58	2	9	10	3.1	Yes	1.4%
42	University of Iowa Stead Family Children's Hospital, Iowa City	65.2	24	5	9	54	4	8	10	3.4	Yes	4.2%
45	Children's Hospital of Michigan, Detroit	64.1	22	6	10	53	5	7	12	3.1	No	1.4%
45	Le Bonheur Children's Hospital, Memphis, Tenn.	64.1	23	6	8	57	2	8	12	3.0	Yes	2.9%
47	OSF HealthCare Children's Hospital of Illinois, Peoria	63.4	18	6	12	59	5	8	9	3.8	Yes	0.1%
48	UF Health Shands Children's Hospital, Gainesville, Fla.	63.2	19	6	11	58	5	8	10	2.9	Yes	1.1%
49	Penn State Children's Hospital, Hershey, Pa.	63.1	24	6	8	55	5	6	6	3.5	Yes	0.8%
50	Arkansas Children's Hospital, Little Rock	63.0	22	6	10	49	5	8	11	3.2	Yes	0.1%

Terms are explained on Page 176.

LIVE AND LET LIVE

Become a living organ donor with
a national leader in transplant.
See Adriana and Nicole's story at
liveandletlive.com/adriana

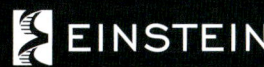

BEST CHILDREN'S HOSPITALS

Neurology & Neurosurgery

Rank	Hospital	U.S. News score	Surgical survival score (12=best)	Surgical complications prevention score (22=best)	Epilepsy management score (6=best)	Infection prevention score, overall (41=best)	Surgery volume score (42=best)	Nurse-patient ratio (higher is better)	A Nurse Magnet hospital	% of specialists recommending hospital
1	Boston Children's Hospital	100.0	12	22	6	39	39	3.9	Yes	46.4%
2	Texas Children's Hospital, Houston	97.0	12	22	6	41	41	4.6	Yes	26.6%
3	Children's National Hospital, Washington, D.C.	95.7	12	22	6	41	39	4.1	Yes	20.5%
4	Children's Hospital of Philadelphia	94.1	12	19	5	40	35	4.3	Yes	38.3%
5	Cincinnati Children's Hospital Medical Center	92.1	12	21	5	40	40	4.1	Yes	21.9%
6	Nationwide Children's Hospital, Columbus, Ohio	91.3	12	21	6	39	34	3.3	Yes	14.6%
7	St. Louis Children's Hospital-Washington University	89.1	12	16	6	39	38	3.8	Yes	18.9%
8	Lucile Packard Children's Hospital Stanford, Palo Alto, Calif.	88.7	12	21	6	41	34	3.9	Yes	8.7%
9	Children's Hospital Los Angeles	88.6	12	22	6	38	42	3.8	Yes	7.5%
10	Children's Hospital Colorado, Aurora	87.6	12	16	6	40	38	4.3	Yes	15.4%
11	Ann and Robert H. Lurie Children's Hospital of Chicago	86.7	12	20	6	36	38	3.0	Yes	14.0%
12	UCSF Benioff Children's Hospitals, San Francisco and Oakland	85.8	11	16	6	39	33	4.1	Yes	12.5%
13	Children's Healthcare of Atlanta	85.7	12	21	6	40	34	4.8	Yes	3.6%
14	UPMC Children's Hospital of Pittsburgh	85.2	11	20	6	35	27	3.5	Yes	9.5%
15	Seattle Children's Hospital	85.0	11	17	6	40	32	3.4	Yes	18.7%
16	Johns Hopkins Children's Center, Baltimore	84.5	12	21	4	39	32	3.3	Yes	15.2%
17	Rady Children's Hospital, San Diego	84.2	12	21	6	39	42	3.2	Yes	3.1%
18	Children's Medical Center Dallas	83.4	12	22	5	40	41	3.2	Yes	3.5%
19	New York-Presbyterian Hospital-Columbia and Cornell, New York	83.3	12	21	6	36	31	3.0	Yes	6.9%
20	C.S. Mott Children's Hospital-Michigan Medicine, Ann Arbor	82.9	12	20	6	40	31	3.7	Yes	5.1%
21	Cohen Children's Medical Center, New Hyde Park, N.Y.	82.8	12	22	6	39	34	3.9	Yes	2.3%
22	Intermountain Primary Children's Hosp.-U. of Utah, Salt Lake City	82.7	12	22	6	38	39	3.4	No	7.7%
23	Riley Hospital for Children at IU Health, Indianapolis	81.7	11	22	6	36	40	4.3	Yes	1.8%
24	Nicklaus Children's Hospital, Miami	80.8	12	22	6	31	28	2.7	Yes	6.7%
25	Children's Mercy Kansas City, Mo.	79.2	12	18	6	40	32	4.6	Yes	1.9%
25	Johns Hopkins All Children's Hospital, St. Petersburg, Fla.	79.2	12	21	6	40	30	3.8	Yes	1.2%
27	Cleveland Clinic Children's Hospital	79.0	12	20	4	38	26	3.7	Yes	6.1%
28	Monroe Carell Jr. Children's Hospital at Vanderbilt, Nashville, Tenn.	78.9	12	16	6	39	37	3.1	Yes	4.4%
29	Cook Children's Medical Center, Fort Worth	77.6	12	21	6	31	29	3.4	Yes	3.9%
30	Phoenix Children's Hospital	77.1	11	16	6	40	36	3.0	No	4.4%
31	CHOC Children's Hospital, Orange, Calif.	77.0	12	15	6	39	25	3.6	Yes	2.9%
32	Children's Memorial Hermann Hospital, Houston	76.7	12	20	6	36	26	3.4	Yes	1.4%
33	Children's Hospital of Alabama at UAB, Birmingham	76.3	12	21	4	39	40	3.4	No	5.5%
34	Duke Children's Hospital and Health Center, Durham, N.C.	75.7	12	15	6	38	31	3.5	Yes	2.9%
35	Le Bonheur Children's Hospital, Memphis, Tenn.	74.9	11	14	6	39	25	3.0	Yes	4.8%
36	Doernbecher Children's Hospital, Portland, Ore.	74.5	12	18	5	33	26	3.9	Yes	2.0%
37	Valley Children's Healthcare and Hospital, Madera, Calif.	73.8	12	22	6	38	20	3.4	Yes	0.8%
38	Mount Sinai Kravis Children's Hospital, New York	73.2	12	20	6	33	19	3.7	Yes	0.7%
39	Mayo Clinic Children's Center, Rochester, Minn.	73.1	12	12	5	36	22	4.1	Yes	5.2%
40	Spectrum Hlth. Helen DeVos Children's Hosp., Grand Rapids, Mich.	72.9	12	18	6	32	23	2.7	Yes	0.6%
40	UCLA Mattel Children's Hospital, Los Angeles	72.9	12	17	4	33	17	4.2	Yes	6.2%
42	Children's Wisconsin, Milwaukee	72.7	12	13	6	36	25	4.3	Yes	1.9%
43	Children's Hospital of Michigan, Detroit	72.4	11	19	6	35	26	3.1	No	0.6%
43	Levine Children's Hospital, Charlotte, N.C.	72.4	12	19	5	41	26	3.0	Yes	0.7%
45	UF Health Shands Children's Hospital, Gainesville, Fla.	71.7	12	19	4	39	17	2.9	Yes	1.4%
46	Nemours Alfred I. duPont Hosp. for Children, Wilmington, Del.	71.5	11	19	6	33	15	3.5	Yes	1.0%
47	Yale New Haven Children's Hospital, New Haven, Conn.	71.4	12	19	4	35	19	5.3	Yes	1.0%
48	Children's Hospital at Montefiore, New York	70.4	12	22	2	38	17	4.6	No	3.2%
49	Akron Children's Hospital, Ohio	70.1	12	15	6	34	23	3.5	Yes	1.0%
50	University of Iowa Stead Family Children's Hospital, Iowa City	69.9	12	16	5	35	25	3.4	Yes	1.3%

Terms are explained on Page 176.

Orthopedics

Rank	Hospital	U.S. News score	Fracture repair score (8=best)	Surgical complications prevention score (13=best)	Infection prevention score, overall (38=best)	Patient volume score (24=best)	Procedure volume score (26=best)	Nurse-patient ratio (higher is better)	A Nurse Magnet hospital	No. of best practices (82=best)	% of specialists recommending hospital
1	Children's Hospital of Philadelphia	100.0	8	12	37	24	23	4.3	Yes	82	41.2%
2	Boston Children's Hospital	97.5	8	11	36	22	26	3.9	Yes	77	47.0%
3	Children's Medical Ctr. Dallas-Texas Scottish Rite Hosp. for Children	91.7	8	9	37	21	26	3.2	Yes	82	38.4%
4	Children's Hospital Los Angeles	90.3	8	12	35	20	23	3.8	Yes	77	17.7%
5	Cincinnati Children's Hospital Medical Center	87.7	8	10	37	19	24	4.1	Yes	77	18.2%
6	Children's National Hospital, Washington, D.C.	86.2	8	13	38	21	15	4.1	Yes	71	6.5%
7	St. Louis Children's Hospital-Washington University/Shriners Hospital	85.9	8	11	36	21	25	3.8	Yes	79	9.3%
8	Rady Children's Hospital, San Diego	85.8	8	8	36	22	20	3.2	Yes	79	33.5%
9	Nationwide Children's Hospital, Columbus, Ohio	83.7	8	11	36	19	23	3.3	Yes	77	8.9%
10	Children's Healthcare of Atlanta	80.9	7	10	37	23	22	4.8	Yes	76	11.2%
11	Texas Children's Hospital, Houston	79.6	7	9	38	20	25	4.6	Yes	77	11.2%
12	Mayo Clinic Children's Center, Rochester, Minn.	78.5	8	13	33	8	13	4.1	Yes	74	3.3%
13	UPMC Children's Hosp. of Pittsburgh-Shriners Hosps. for Children Erie	77.3	8	12	33	20	16	3.5	Yes	69	2.2%
14	Nemours Alfred I. duPont Hosp. for Children, Wilmington, Del.	77.0	7	9	31	21	22	3.5	Yes	80	16.1%
15	Children's Hospital Colorado, Aurora	76.0	6	9	37	20	24	4.3	Yes	74	14.0%
16	Lerner Children's Pavilion-Hospital for Special Surgery, New York	75.4	8	9	38	14	23	4.1	Yes	78	4.4%
17	UCLA Mattel Children's Hospital, Los Angeles	75.2	8	10	31	19	16	4.2	Yes	81	3.8%
18	Seattle Children's Hospital	74.8	8	9	37	21	18	3.4	Yes	66	8.5%
19	Rainbow Babies and Children's Hospital, Cleveland	74.5	8	9	35	19	19	3.3	Yes	78	6.4%
20	CHOC Children's Hospital, Orange, Calif.	74.3	8	13	36	14	15	3.6	Yes	70	1.3%
21	Johns Hopkins Children's Center, Baltimore	73.3	8	9	36	12	12	3.3	Yes	77	5.1%
22	UC Davis Children's Hospital/Shriners Hosps. N. Calif., Sacramento	72.9	8	7	37	19	24	6.9	Yes	76	6.5%
23	C.S. Mott Children's Hospital-Michigan Medicine, Ann Arbor	72.2	7	10	37	18	15	3.7	Yes	73	2.7%
24	Le Bonheur Children's Hospital, Memphis, Tenn.	71.4	8	9	36	15	16	3.0	Yes	74	3.7%
24	Valley Children's Healthcare and Hospital, Madera, Calif.	71.4	8	12	35	18	18	3.4	Yes	74	0.3%
26	Cohen Children's Medical Center, New Hyde Park, N.Y.	71.0	7	11	36	17	18	3.9	Yes	77	0.7%
27	Levine Children's Hospital, Charlotte, N.C.	70.5	8	11	38	14	12	3.0	Yes	67	1.2%
28	Intermountain Primary Children's Hosp.-Shriners Hosps. for Children-U. of Utah	70.4	7	10	36	21	24	3.4	No	70	7.5%
29	Cleveland Clinic Children's Hospital	69.4	8	11	35	12	10	3.7	Yes	70	1.6%
30	Lucile Packard Children's Hospital Stanford, Palo Alto, Calif.	69.2	6	11	38	11	17	3.9	Yes	66	3.1%
31	Children's Mercy Kansas City, Mo.	68.1	8	6	37	22	21	4.6	Yes	77	3.4%
32	Joe DiMaggio Children's Hospital at Memorial, Hollywood, Fla.	67.6	8	11	34	19	22	3.5	No	76	1.4%
33	Phoenix Children's Hospital	67.4	8	9	37	15	23	3.0	No	77	0.8%
34	Ann and Robert H. Lurie Children's Hospital of Chicago	67.3	7	10	34	16	23	3.0	Yes	67	4.8%
35	University of Iowa Stead Family Children's Hospital, Iowa City	67.0	6	13	32	19	13	3.4	Yes	65	1.3%
36	North Carolina Children's Hospital at UNC, Chapel Hill	66.9	7	11	37	11	12	4.7	Yes	68	1.0%
37	Dayton Children's Hospital, Ohio	66.6	8	8	37	18	17	4.1	Yes	73	1.3%
38	Children's Wisconsin, Milwaukee	66.4	7	10	33	15	17	4.3	Yes	71	1.0%
39	Monroe Carell Jr. Children's Hospital at Vanderbilt, Nashville, Tenn.	66.0	7	7	36	16	18	3.1	Yes	75	5.3%
40	Nicklaus Children's Hospital, Miami	64.3	8	8	28	22	17	2.7	Yes	79	2.4%
41	Kentucky Children's Hosp.-Shriners Hosps. for Children, Lexington, Ky.	63.7	6	12	33	10	14	3.1	Yes	71	4.7%
42	University of Virginia Children's Hospital, Charlottesville	62.6	8	8	35	8	9	3.1	Yes	80	0.7%
43	Spectrum Hlth. Helen DeVos Children's Hosp., Grand Rapids, Mich.	62.0	8	10	30	10	6	2.7	Yes	70	0.5%
44	Children's Hospital of Michigan, Detroit	61.4	7	10	33	20	12	3.1	No	75	0.2%
45	Connecticut Children's Medical Center, Hartford	60.8	7	8	36	12	13	3.1	Yes	75	0.7%
45	Johns Hopkins All Children's Hospital, St. Petersburg, Fla.	60.8	8	6	37	11	11	3.8	Yes	75	1.7%
45	Wolfson Children's Hospital, Jacksonville, Fla.	60.8	6	12	33	11	11	2.6	Yes	73	2.1%
48	Arnold Palmer Hospital for Children, Orlando	60.3	7	10	36	14	10	3.0	Yes	57	1.6%
49	Children's Hospital of Alabama at UAB, Birmingham	60.1	7	9	36	19	16	3.4	No	72	0.9%
50	UCSF Benioff Children's Hospitals, San Francisco and Oakland	60.0	5	8	37	16	15	4.1	Yes	73	3.2%

Terms are explained on Page 176.

More @ usnews.com/childrenshospitals

BEST CHILDREN'S HOSPITALS
Pulmonology & Lung Surgery

Rank	Hospital	U.S. News score	Asthma inpatient care score (8=best)	Lung transplant survival score (5=best)	Cystic fibrosis management score (19=best)	Infection prevention score, overall (50=best)	Infection prevention score, ICU (5=best)	Patient volume score (17=best)	Nurse-patient ratio (higher is better)	A Nurse Magnet hospital	% of specialists recommending hospital
1	Boston Children's Hospital	100.0	8	2	15	48	5	17	3.9	Yes	45.2%
2	Children's Hospital of Philadelphia	99.5	7	5	17	49	3	17	4.3	Yes	49.2%
3	Texas Children's Hospital, Houston	97.8	8	5	14	49	3	17	4.6	Yes	36.9%
4	Cincinnati Children's Hospital Medical Center	95.3	7	2	16	48	3	17	4.1	Yes	43.2%
5	Children's Hospital Colorado, Aurora	93.2	6	NA	15	48	4	15	4.3	Yes	42.1%
6	Lucile Packard Children's Hospital Stanford, Palo Alto, Calif.	92.1	8	4	13	49	5	16	3.9	Yes	14.2%
7	Nationwide Children's Hospital, Columbus, Ohio	91.8	7	3	15	48	5	17	3.3	Yes	18.7%
8	Children's National Hospital, Washington, D.C.	91.0	8	NA	17	50	5	14	4.1	Yes	10.2%
9	St. Louis Children's Hospital-Washington University	89.9	7	3	17	43	5	12	3.8	Yes	13.5%
10	Seattle Children's Hospital	88.1	8	NA	14	48	5	13	3.4	Yes	23.8%
11	UPMC Children's Hospital of Pittsburgh	86.9	6	5	15	44	5	15	3.5	Yes	15.9%
12	Children's Hospital Los Angeles	85.4	8	NA	13	47	5	14	3.8	Yes	13.0%
13	Rainbow Babies and Children's Hospital, Cleveland	83.6	8	NA	16	47	5	12	3.3	Yes	7.3%
14	Riley Hospital for Children at IU Health, Indianapolis	83.1	6	2	14	42	5	15	4.3	Yes	13.8%
15	Children's Wisconsin, Milwaukee	81.1	7	NA	18	44	5	14	4.3	Yes	1.4%
16	Children's Healthcare of Atlanta	80.6	7	NR	14	45	5	15	4.8	Yes	2.8%
17	C.S. Mott Children's Hospital-Michigan Medicine, Ann Arbor	79.7	7	NA	15	47	5	13	3.7	Yes	2.9%
17	Monroe Carell Jr. Children's Hosp. at Vanderbilt, Nashville, Tenn.	79.7	7	NR	17	46	2	13	3.1	Yes	8.4%
19	Rady Children's Hospital, San Diego	79.5	7	NA	15	46	5	12	3.2	Yes	3.3%
20	Ann and Robert H. Lurie Children's Hospital of Chicago	79.0	6	NA	15	43	3	11	3.0	Yes	10.2%
21	UF Health Shands Children's Hospital, Gainesville, Fla.	78.3	8	4	11	48	5	12	2.9	Yes	1.2%
22	MassGeneral Hospital for Children, Boston	78.2	7	NA	15	46	5	8	3.5	Yes	3.4%
23	Johns Hopkins Children's Center, Baltimore	77.8	5	NR	14	48	2	15	3.3	Yes	12.0%
24	Cohen Children's Medical Center, New Hyde Park, N.Y.	76.9	8	NA	15	48	4	8	3.9	Yes	0.8%
24	North Carolina Children's Hospital at UNC, Chapel Hill	76.9	7	3	14	49	1	11	4.7	Yes	13.1%
26	Children's Medical Center Dallas	76.6	7	NA	15	47	5	14	3.2	Yes	2.6%
27	CHOC Children's Hospital, Orange, Calif.	76.0	7	NA	14	48	5	12	3.6	Yes	1.7%
28	New York-Presbyterian Hospital-Columbia and Cornell, New York	75.3	7	5	11	40	3	14	3.0	Yes	6.1%
29	UCSF Benioff Children's Hospitals, San Francisco and Oakland	74.7	6	NA	14	48	3	8	4.1	Yes	3.3%
30	Children's Hospital of Richmond at VCU, Va.	74.5	8	NA	17	47	5	10	2.4	Yes	1.3%
31	Valley Children's Healthcare and Hospital, Madera, Calif.	74.4	8	NA	15	47	5	9	3.4	Yes	0.1%
32	Children's Hospital of Alabama at UAB, Birmingham	74.0	8	NA	16	44	2	14	3.4	No	3.6%
33	Duke Children's Hospital and Health Center, Durham, N.C.	73.8	7	NR	14	46	5	10	3.5	Yes	1.7%
34	Arkansas Children's Hospital, Little Rock	73.6	8	NA	15	34	5	9	3.2	Yes	1.3%
35	Cleveland Clinic Children's Hospital	73.4	4	NA	18	43	4	11	3.7	Yes	1.5%
36	Nicklaus Children's Hospital, Miami	73.2	8	NA	17	40	5	11	2.7	Yes	0.4%
37	Children's Mercy Kansas City, Mo.	73.1	7	NA	15	46	1	10	4.6	Yes	3.1%
37	Levine Children's Hospital, Charlotte, N.C.	73.1	7	NA	14	49	4	11	3.0	Yes	1.3%
39	Penn State Children's Hospital, Hershey, Pa.	72.8	7	NA	15	40	5	10	3.5	Yes	0.5%
40	Phoenix Children's Hospital	72.4	8	NA	14	44	5	14	3.0	No	0.9%
41	Dayton Children's Hospital, Ohio	71.3	8	NA	12	48	4	10	4.1	Yes	0.9%
42	Children's Minnesota, Minneapolis	70.6	7	NA	16	38	3	13	3.6	Yes	1.4%
43	Spectrum Hlth. Helen DeVos Children's Hosp., Grand Rapids, Mich.	70.5	6	NA	17	35	5	11	2.7	Yes	1.2%
43	Yale New Haven Children's Hospital, New Haven, Conn.	70.5	6	NA	15	45	4	8	5.3	Yes	1.2%
45	Le Bonheur Children's Hospital, Memphis, Tenn.	70.3	8	NA	13	46	2	10	3.0	Yes	2.5%
46	Johns Hopkins All Children's Hospital, St. Petersburg, Fla.	70.1	3	NA	16	48	5	8	3.8	Yes	0.7%
46	MemorialCare Miller Children's & Women's Hosp. Long Beach, Calif.	70.1	6	NA	17	38	4	12	4.2	Yes	0.9%
48	SSM Hlth. Cardinal Glennon Children's Hosp.-St. Louis U., St. Louis	70.0	8	NA	14	42	5	11	3.0	Yes	1.4%
49	Children's Hospital and Medical Center, Omaha	69.6	5	NA	14	48	2	11	4.5	Yes	0.9%
50	Akron Children's Hospital, Ohio	68.2	6	NA	15	39	4	6	3.5	Yes	0.9%

NA=not applicable. NR=not reported. Terms are explained on Page 176.

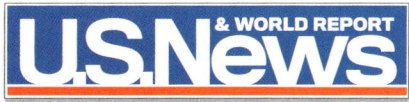

Shop the U.S. News Store

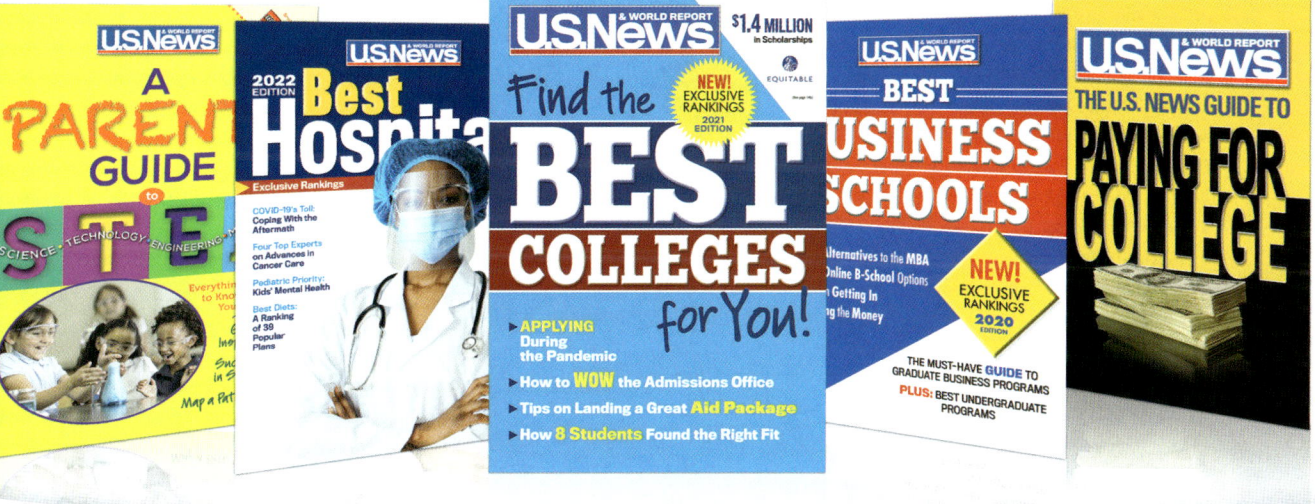

Find Your Perfect School
U.S. News College Compass

- See complete U.S. News rankings
- Premium data on more than 1,800 schools
- Compare schools side by side
- Detailed financial aid and alumni salary information
- See entering student SAT scores and GPAs
- Match schools to your preferences with the MyFit Engine
- See how you stack up with the Admissions Calculator

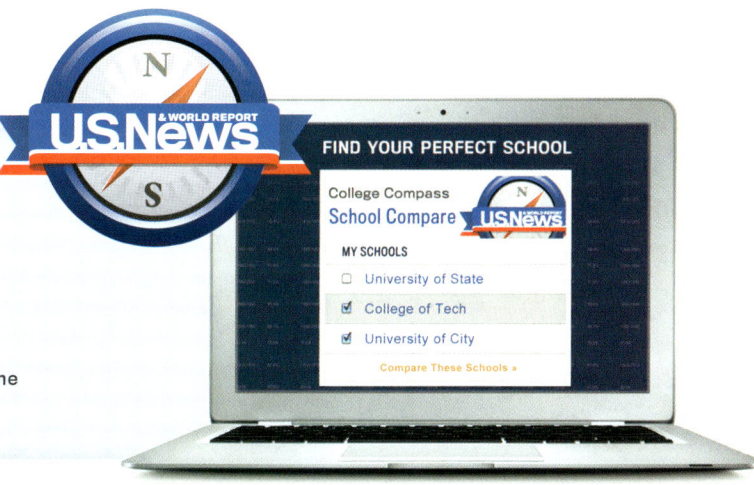

visit usnews.com/store

For discounted bulk orders, or to order by phone, call 1-800-836-6397.

BEST CHILDREN'S HOSPITALS

Urology

Rank	Hospital	U.S. News score	Surgical complications prevention score (15=best)	Testicular torsion care score (2=best)	Infection prevention score, overall (32=best)	Patient volume score (27=best)	Surgery volume score (20=best)	Minimally invasive volume score (9=best)	Nurse-patient ratio (higher is better)	A Nurse Magnet hospital	% of specialists recommending hospital
1	Boston Children's Hospital	100.0	14	2	30	26	18	9	3.9	Yes	60.6%
2	Cincinnati Children's Hospital Medical Center	94.8	14	2	31	23	14	9	4.1	Yes	38.7%
3	Riley Hospital for Children at IU Health, Indianapolis	93.2	14	2	27	26	18	9	4.3	Yes	40.8%
4	Children's Hospital of Philadelphia	92.0	11	2	31	26	19	9	4.3	Yes	61.3%
5	Texas Children's Hospital, Houston	88.3	12	2	32	27	19	9	4.6	Yes	31.4%
6	Children's Hospital Colorado, Aurora	87.1	15	2	31	26	17	9	4.3	Yes	11.0%
7	Ann and Robert H. Lurie Children's Hospital of Chicago	85.9	12	2	28	25	16	9	3.0	Yes	42.9%
8	Monroe Carell Jr. Children's Hospital at Vanderbilt, Nashville, Tenn.	85.5	13	2	30	21	17	8	3.1	Yes	31.4%
9	Seattle Children's Hospital	81.7	12	2	31	20	15	8	3.4	Yes	27.2%
10	Rady Children's Hospital, San Diego	79.1	15	2	30	20	14	8	3.2	Yes	9.5%
11	Nationwide Children's Hospital, Columbus, Ohio	78.4	11	2	30	23	18	9	3.3	Yes	25.2%
12	St. Louis Children's Hospital-Washington University	75.0	15	2	30	19	14	8	3.8	Yes	2.2%
13	UPMC Children's Hospital of Pittsburgh	74.4	13	2	27	21	15	9	3.5	Yes	8.6%
14	Children's Medical Center Dallas	72.0	11	2	31	19	15	9	3.2	Yes	15.3%
15	UCSF Benioff Children's Hospitals, San Francisco and Oakland	71.9	12	2	31	24	14	9	4.1	Yes	8.5%
16	Children's Hospital Los Angeles	71.6	11	2	29	25	18	9	3.8	Yes	13.3%
17	Children's Healthcare of Atlanta	71.5	11	2	31	23	18	9	4.8	Yes	9.4%
18	Cohen Children's Medical Center, New Hyde Park, N.Y.	70.7	14	2	30	18	13	8	3.9	Yes	2.1%
19	Children's Mercy Kansas City, Mo.	70.0	13	2	31	18	16	8	4.6	Yes	2.6%
20	C.S. Mott Children's Hospital-Michigan Medicine, Ann Arbor	69.7	13	2	31	19	10	7	3.7	Yes	5.1%
21	Mayo Clinic Children's Center, Rochester, Minn.	69.5	13	2	27	23	11	5	4.1	Yes	10.0%
22	Cleveland Clinic Children's Hospital	68.6	14	2	29	13	10	7	3.7	Yes	0.9%
22	Le Bonheur Children's Hospital, Memphis, Tenn.	68.6	15	2	30	11	12	8	3.0	Yes	3.5%
24	Lucile Packard Children's Hospital Stanford, Palo Alto, Calif.	68.4	12	2	32	20	9	6	3.9	Yes	3.9%
25	Children's National Hospital, Washington, D.C.	65.0	8	2	32	23	13	9	4.1	Yes	12.2%
26	Johns Hopkins Children's Center, Baltimore	62.7	9	2	30	18	13	6	3.3	Yes	12.7%
27	Duke Children's Hospital and Health Center, Durham, N.C.	62.2	11	2	30	21	13	6	3.5	Yes	6.8%
28	Children's Hospital of Richmond at VCU, Va.	62.1	15	2	30	14	14	8	2.4	Yes	1.7%
29	Children's Hospital and Medical Center, Omaha	61.6	14	2	30	11	11	8	4.5	Yes	0.6%
30	CHOC Children's Hospital, Orange, Calif.	60.6	11	2	30	20	15	7	3.6	Yes	3.7%
31	Rainbow Babies and Children's Hospital, Cleveland	59.6	14	2	29	11	5	4	3.3	Yes	1.5%
32	Children's Hospital of Michigan, Detroit	58.1	14	2	27	12	11	7	3.1	No	2.4%
33	Intermountain Primary Children's Hosp.-U. of Utah, Salt Lake City	56.0	11	2	30	26	16	8	3.4	No	3.5%
34	North Carolina Children's Hospital at UNC, Chapel Hill	55.3	11	2	31	9	12	6	4.7	Yes	1.5%
35	West Virginia U. Children's Hospital, Morgantown	55.2	13	2	30	10	9	6	4.6	Yes	0.6%
36	SSM Hlth. Cardinal Glennon Children's Hosp.-St. Louis U., St. Louis	54.9	13	2	28	11	8	5	3.0	Yes	0.9%
37	UC Davis Children's Hospital/Shriners Hosps. N. Calif., Sacramento	54.4	10	2	31	17	10	8	6.9	Yes	1.4%
38	Spectrum Hlth. Helen DeVos Children's Hosp., Grand Rapids, Mich.	54.0	14	2	24	13	12	8	2.7	Yes	0.1%
39	Connecticut Children's Medical Center, Hartford	53.8	13	2	30	10	8	4	3.1	Yes	0.2%
40	Norton Children's Hospital, Louisville, Ky.	53.7	13	2	31	18	12	4	3.1	No	0.4%
41	Akron Children's Hospital, Ohio	53.4	13	2	25	13	10	5	3.5	Yes	1.9%
42	Valley Children's Healthcare and Hospital, Madera, Calif.	53.1	13	2	29	15	14	8	3.4	Yes	1.3%
43	Children's Hospital of Alabama at UAB, Birmingham	52.6	11	2	30	17	15	8	3.4	No	2.8%
43	University of Virginia Children's Hospital, Charlottesville	52.6	12	2	29	8	12	7	3.1	Yes	2.8%
45	Johns Hopkins All Children's Hospital, St. Petersburg, Fla.	52.3	15	2	31	8	11	5	3.8	Yes	1.3%
46	UF Health Shands Children's Hospital, Gainesville, Fla.	52.0	13	2	31	12	8	6	2.9	Yes	0.4%
47	Arkansas Children's Hospital, Little Rock	51.3	11	2	21	15	13	7	3.2	Yes	1.7%
48	Phoenix Children's Hospital	51.2	10	2	31	22	12	8	3.0	No	2.4%
49	Arnold Palmer Hospital for Children, Orlando	50.8	12	2	30	12	8	4	3.0	Yes	0.4%
50	MassGeneral Hospital for Children, Boston	50.3	10	2	28	14	6	4	3.5	Yes	2.0%

Terms are explained on Page 176.

Translating real patient needs into real-world treatments.

At CHOC, we know that research can lead to lifesaving decisions. A key part of our vision is to address a critical need in rare disease research, so every child can live the healthiest life possible.

BEST CHILDREN'S HOSPITALS — U.S. News & World Report — RANKED IN 7 SPECIALTIES 2021-22

Finding the answers that each child needs to thrive

Start With One Child. This is one of our guiding principles as we seek the answers for each child to thrive. Our "bedside-to-bedside" approach to research means we learn from every child and when we know the answer for one, we can extrapolate to find the answer for many. With more than 530 active studies in over 30 specialties, CHOC is committed to personalized, precision-medicine research for the neonatal, pediatric, adolescent, and young adult populations.

A destination for kids with rare conditions

Kids from around the world come to CHOC for treatment of their rare conditions. We are the largest center in the United States, and second largest in the world, for Brineura treatment for kids with CLN2-associated Batten disease, a neurological disorder that leads to blindness, loss of ability to speak or move, dementia, and death.

CHOC is on track to become an active site for a gene therapy clinical trial to give brain cells the ability to produce the missing enzyme that causes Batten disease.

Success in rapidly diagnosing genetic diseases

In the last four years, CHOC has ordered the comprehensive and cutting-edge test of rapid whole genome sequencing (rWGS) on 150 patients, with more than half of them getting a precise diagnosis that, in many cases, has resulted in life-changing care.

- rWGS can identify the cause of rare diseases in a manner of days, leading to faster, more customized treatments.
- This level of early intervention can eliminate the need for further tests, reduce costs and save lives in the short and long term.

READ STORIES OF INNOVATIVE RESEARCH
CHOC.org/research-usnwr

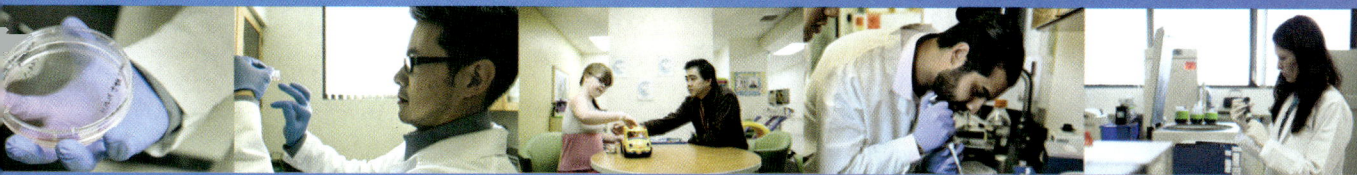

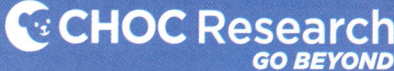

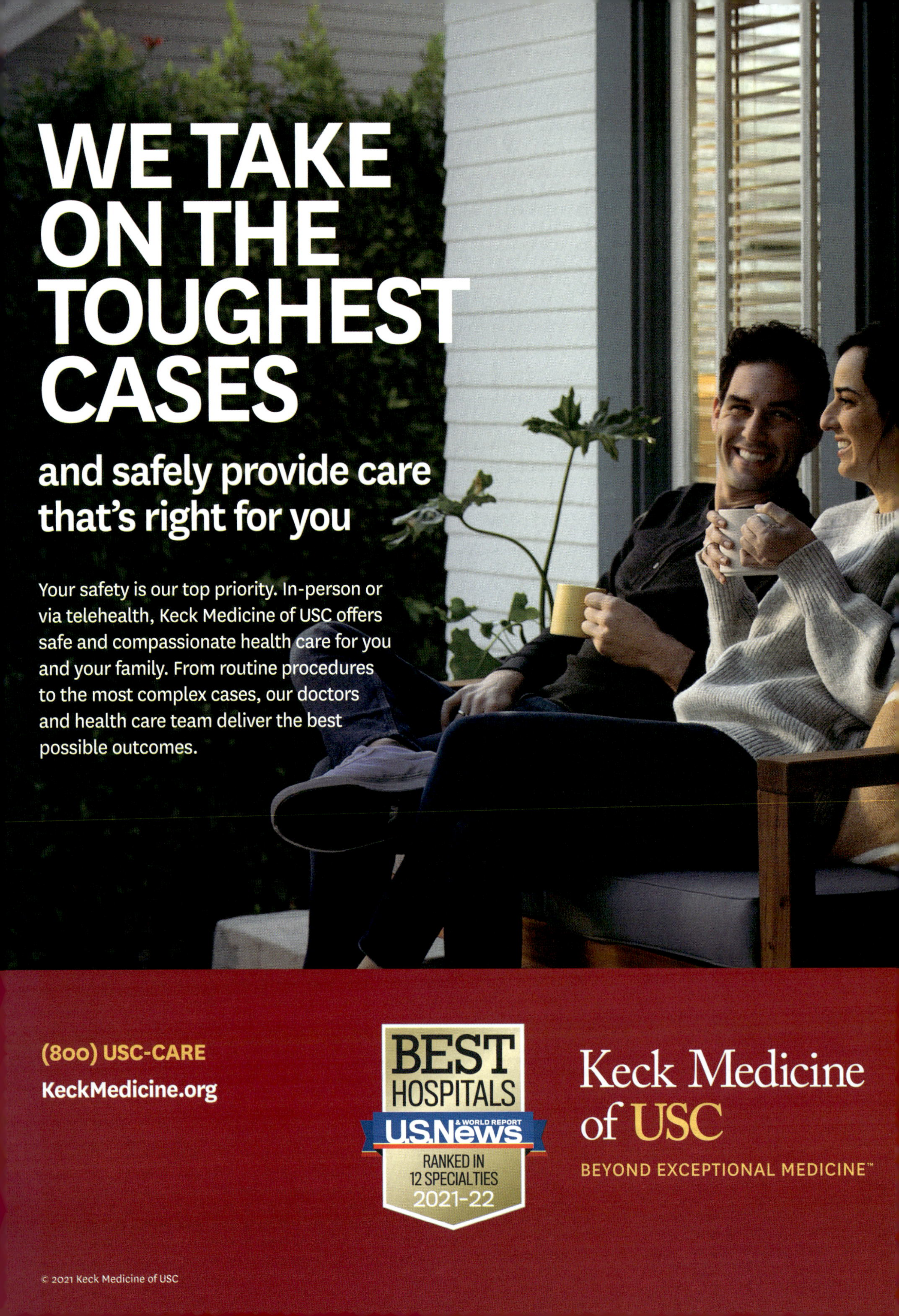

WE TAKE ON THE TOUGHEST CASES

and safely provide care that's right for you

Your safety is our top priority. In-person or via telehealth, Keck Medicine of USC offers safe and compassionate health care for you and your family. From routine procedures to the most complex cases, our doctors and health care team deliver the best possible outcomes.

(800) USC-CARE
KeckMedicine.org

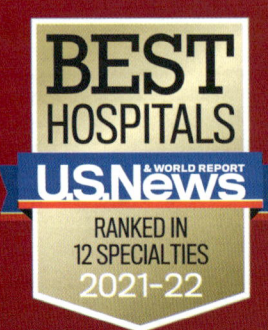

Keck Medicine of USC

BEYOND EXCEPTIONAL MEDICINE™

© 2021 Keck Medicine of USC

CHAPTER 6

Best Regional Hospitals

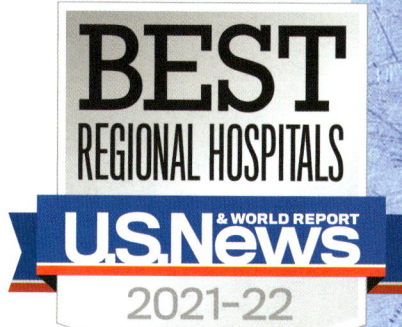

198 **Great Care Near Home:** Read about how U.S. News identified and ranked top hospitals in each state.

200 **The Rankings:** See how nearby hospitals performed in areas of specialty care and in common procedures and conditions.

218 **Best Regional Children's Hospitals:** A region-by-region ranking based on performance in 10 specialties

BEST REGIONAL HOSPITALS

Great Care Near Home

How we identified and ranked the top hospitals state by state

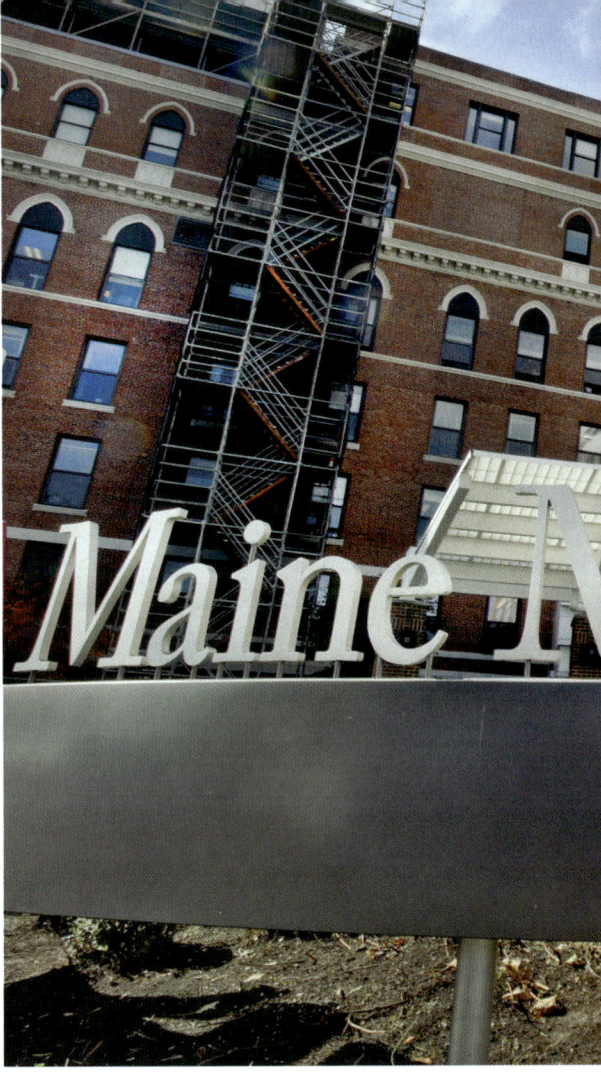

by **Ben Harder**

IF YOU'RE LIKE MOST people facing hospitalization, you'd prefer to stay close to home. It's more convenient. It might avoid a battle with your health insurer over out-of-network coverage. Friends and family may be able to visit you. And getting follow-up care from the same medical team will be more practical.

Our Best Regional Hospitals listings showcase hundreds of hospitals around the U.S. that offer high-quality care across a range of clinical services. These services include both complex, highly specialized care for the sickest patients – the focus of the Best Hospitals specialty rankings (Page 110) – and safe, effective treatment for those whose medical needs are more commonplace, such as patients seeking hip or knee replacement surgery for age-related arthritis. Found in their entirety at usnews.com/bestregionalhospitals, the Best Regional Hospitals rankings offer readers in most parts of the country a number of high-quality choices near home.

These evaluations include ratings of how well hospitals handle 17 relatively common procedures and conditions in addition to their assessments in 11 specialties.* The 17 areas of care are colon cancer surgery, lung cancer surgery, heart attack, heart failure, heart bypass surgery, heart valve surgery, transcatheter aortic valve replacement, abdominal aortic aneurysm repair, stroke, back surgery, hip replacement, knee replacement, hip fracture, diabetes, kidney failure, pneumonia and chronic obstructive pulmonary disease. Hospitals are assigned a rating of "high performing," "average" or "below average" in each area in which they treated enough patients to be evaluated.

Recognition as a Best Regional Hospital means a hospital was nationally ranked in at least one of 11 specialties that use objective data, or that it earned at least six "high performing" ratings across the procedures and conditions. Each such hospital also had to meet certain other criteria; an FAQ at usnews.com/best-hospitals offers more details.

This year, 531 hospitals merited Best Regional Hospitals status. They appear ranked by state on the following pages. Hospitals are numerically ordered according to the following rules:

1. The higher rank went to the hospital with the better status in the Best Hospitals Honor Roll ranking (Page 109), if applicable.

*Cancer; cardiology & heart surgery; diabetes & endocrinology; ear, nose & throat; gastroenterology & GI surgery; geriatrics; gynecology; neurology & neurosurgery; orthopedics; pulmonology & lung surgery; and urology.

USNEWS.COM/BESTHOSPITALS

Visit usnews.com regularly while researching your health care choices, as U.S. News often adds content aimed at helping patients make decisions about their care. We also update the Best Hospitals, Best Children's Hospitals and Best Regional Hospitals content and data on the website when new content and data become available.

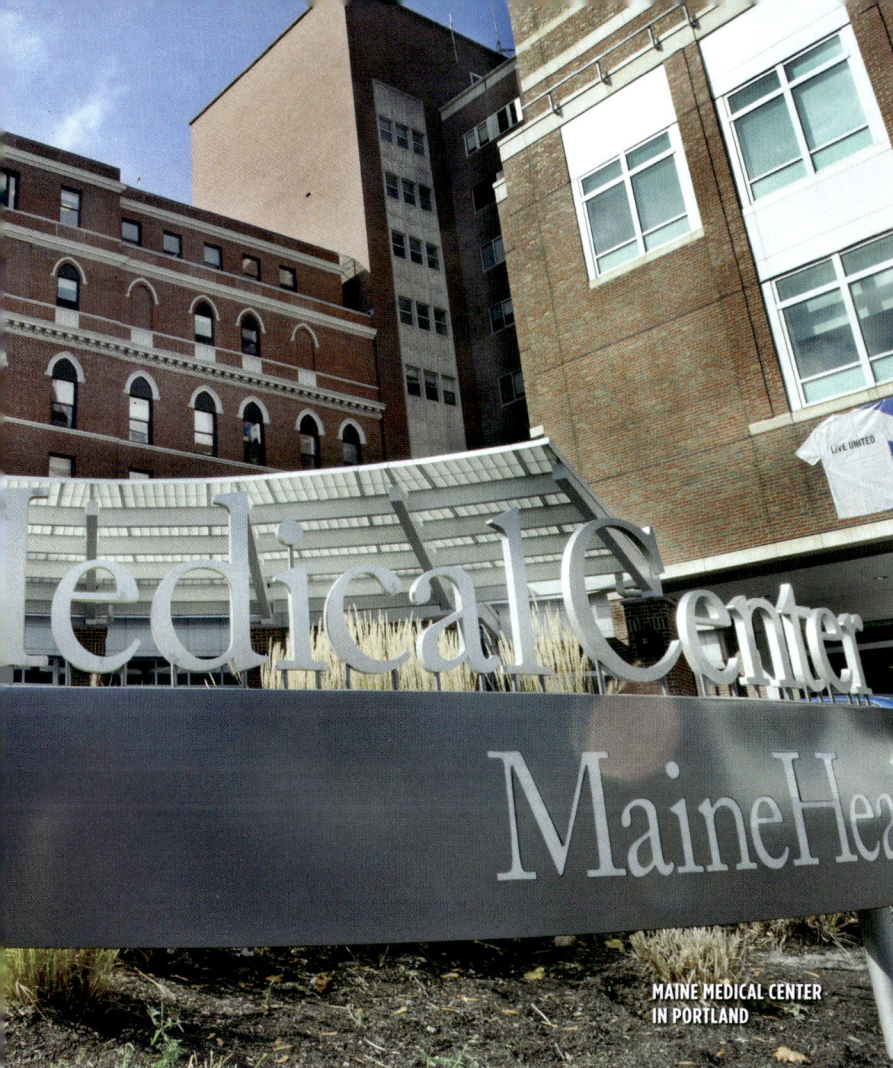

MAINE MEDICAL CENTER IN PORTLAND

Tops at Routine Care

U.S. NEWS EVALUATED nearly 4,500 hospitals on their handling of up to seven medical conditions – heart attack, heart failure, stroke, pneumonia, chronic obstructive pulmonary disease, diabetes and kidney failure – and 10 procedures: colon cancer surgery, lung cancer surgery, heart bypass surgery, heart valve surgery, transcatheter aortic valve replacement, abdominal aortic aneurysm repair, knee replacement, hip replacement, hip fracture repair, and the back surgery known as spinal fusion. Nearly half of those hospitals earned a top rating of "high performing" in at least one of those procedures and conditions. But only these 11 standout hospitals, barely 0.2% of those evaluated, got the top rating in all 17 areas of care.

- **Cedars-Sinai Medical Center,** Los Angeles
- **Cleveland Clinic**
- **Hoag Memorial Hospital Presbyterian,** Newport Beach, California
- **Houston Methodist Hospital**
- **Massachusetts General Hospital,** Boston
- **Mayo Clinic-Phoenix**
- **Scripps La Jolla Hospitals,** La Jolla, California
- **UCLA Medical Center,** Los Angeles
- **UNC Rex Hospital,** Raleigh, North Carolina
- **University of Michigan Hospitals-Michigan Medicine,** Ann Arbor
- **University of Wisconsin Hospitals,** Madison

2. Next, the higher rank went to the hospital that earned more points according to the following three rules: (a) A hospital received two points for each of the 11 specialties in which it was ranked among the top 50. (b) A hospital received one point for each specialty, procedure or condition in which it was rated high performing. (c) A hospital lost one point for each procedure or condition in which it was rated below average. Certain rare exceptions apply.

Based on the same rules, hospitals in major metropolitan areas also were ranked against other top hospitals in the metropolis. Our website displays these rankings for 92 metro areas with approximately 500,000 or more residents. The website also lists top hospitals in more than 100 U.S. News-defined regions, such as Kentucky's Bluegrass Region, the Ozarks in Arkansas and the Florida Panhandle, to help consumers outside the biggest urban centers searching for high-quality care.

Our goal with the state and metro area rankings is to identify general medical-surgical hospitals that provide both breadth and quality, so only hospitals that deliver a wide range of clinical services for adults were considered for the Best Regional Hospitals rankings.

Pediatric care did not factor into these rankings; instead, children's hospitals are separately ranked by region (Page 218) based on their performance across the 10 children's specialties (Page 173).

How a hospital performed in ophthalmology, psychiatry, rehabilitation and rheumatology did not factor into the Best Regional Hospitals rankings, either. While these four specialties are undeniably important, many hospitals treat few, if any, inpatients in these specialty areas. Additionally, specialty hospitals such as dedicated cancer centers, surgical hospitals and rehabilitation facilities were not considered for the regional rankings.

When choosing a hospital, you'll want to consult with your physician or other health professional and combine your own research with ours to find the best possible care. ●

Best Regional Hospitals

To help patients identify top hospitals near home, the state rankings below compare hospitals across 11 areas of complex specialty care (for all specialties, see Page 110) and 17 procedures and conditions.

Legend:
- COMPLEX SPECIALTY CARE: ● Nationally ranked, ● High performing
- COMMON PROCEDURES & CONDITIONS: ● High performing, ● Average, ● Below average

State Rank Hospital	Cancer	Cardiology & Heart Surgery	Orthopedics	Other Specialties (Nationally Ranked)	Other Specialties (High Performing)	Colon Cancer Surgery	Lung Cancer Surgery	Heart Attack	Heart Failure	Heart Bypass Surgery	Heart Valve Surgery	TAVR*	Abdominal Aortic Aneurysm	Stroke	Back Surgery	Hip Replacement	Knee Replacement	Hip Fracture	Diabetes	Kidney Failure	Pneumonia	COPD*
ALABAMA																						
1 University of Alabama at Birmingham Hospital, Birmingham	●	●	–	6	2	●	●	●	●	●	●	●	●	●	●	●	●	●	●	●	●	●
2 Huntsville Hospital, Huntsville	–	–	–	–	–	●	●	●	●	●	●	●	●	●	●	●	●	●	●	●	●	●
3 Ascension St. Vincent's Birmingham, Birmingham	–	–	–	–	–	●	●	●	●	●	●	●	●	●	●	●	●	●	●	●	●	●
ALASKA																						
1 Providence Alaska Medical Center, Anchorage	–	–	●	1	3	●	●	●	●	●	●	●	●	●	●	●	●	●	●	●	●	●
ARIZONA																						
1 Mayo Clinic-Phoenix	●	●	●	7	1	●	●	●	●	●	●	●	●	●	●	●	●	●	●	●	●	●
2 Banner Boswell Medical Center, Sun City	–	–	–	1	1	●	●	●	●	●	●	●	●	●	●	●	●	●	●	●	●	●
2 Banner-University Medical Center Phoenix	–	–	–	–	3	●	●	●	●	●	●	●	●	●	●	●	●	●	●	●	●	●
2 St. Joseph's Hospital and Medical Center, Phoenix[1]	–	–	–	1	2	●	●	●	●	●	●	●	●	●	●	●	●	●	●	●	●	●
5 Chandler Regional Medical Center, Chandler	–	–	–	–	–	●	●	●	●	●	●	●	●	●	●	●	●	●	●	●	●	●
5 TMC Healthcare-Tucson	–	–	–	–	–	●	●	●	●	●	●	●	●	●	●	●	●	●	●	●	●	●
7 Abrazo Arrowhead Campus, Glendale	–	–	–	–	–	●	–	●	●	●	●	●	●	●	●	●	●	●	●	●	●	●
7 Banner-University Medical Center Tucson	–	–	–	–	–	●	●	●	●	●	●	●	●	●	●	●	●	●	●	●	●	●
9 Banner Baywood Medical Center, Mesa	–	–	–	–	–	●	–	●	–	–	–	–	●	●	●	●	●	●	●	●	●	●
ARKANSAS																						
1 Washington Regional Medical Center, Fayetteville	–	–	–	–	–	●	●	●	●	●	●	●	●	●	●	●	●	●	●	●	●	●
2 Baptist Health Medical Center-Little Rock	–	–	–	–	–	●	●	●	●	●	●	●	●	●	●	●	●	●	●	●	●	●
2 UAMS Medical Center, Little Rock	–	–	–	–	1	●	●	●	●	●	●	●	●	–	●	●	●	●	●	●	●	●
CALIFORNIA																						
1 UCLA Medical Center, Los Angeles	●	●	●	11	–	●	●	●	●	●	●	●	●	●	●	●	●	●	●	●	●	●
2 Cedars-Sinai Medical Center, Los Angeles	●	●	●	8	1	●	●	●	●	●	●	●	●	●	●	●	●	●	●	●	●	●
3 UCSF Medical Center, San Francisco	●	●	●	11	–	●	●	●	●	●	●	●	●	●	●	●	●	●	●	●	●	●
4 Stanford Health Care-Stanford Hospital, Stanford	●	●	●	8	1	●	●	●	●	●	●	●	●	●	●	●	●	●	●	●	●	●
5 Keck Medical Center of USC, Los Angeles[2]	●	●	●	9	–	●	●	●	●	●	●	●	●	●	●	●	●	●	●	●	●	●
5 UC San Diego Health-Jacobs Medical Center, La Jolla[3]	●	●	●	7	–	●	●	●	●	●	●	●	●	●	●	●	●	●	●	●	●	●
7 Scripps La Jolla Hospitals, La Jolla	●	●	●	4	3	●	●	●	●	●	●	●	●	●	●	●	●	●	●	●	●	●

In complex care specialties, (-) indicates hospital is not nationally ranked or high performing. In procedures and conditions, (-) indicates care not offered or hospital has too few Medicare patients to be rated. *TAVR: Transcatheter aortic valve replacement. *COPD: Chronic obstructive pulmonary disease

A footnote indicates that another hospital's results are included, that the hospital has a different name in one or more areas of care, or both. [1]Barrow Neurological Institute. [2]USC Norris Cancer Hospital-Keck Medical Center of USC. [3]UC San Diego Health-Moores Cancer Center; UC San Diego Health-Cardiovascular Institute

UCLA Health

#1

IN CALIFORNIA
AND *TOP 3* IN THE NATION

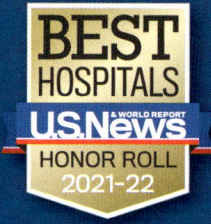

U.S. News & World Report Best Hospitals

BEST REGIONAL HOSPITALS

COMPLEX SPECIALTY CARE
- 🔴 Nationally ranked
- 🔵 High performing

COMMON PROCEDURES & CONDITIONS
- 🔵 High performing
- 🟠 Average
- ⚫ Below average

Legend for cells below: R = 🔴 nationally ranked, B = 🔵 high performing, O = 🟠 average, K = ⚫ below average, − = dash

State Rank	Hospital	Cancer	Cardiology & Heart Surgery	Orthopedics	Other Specialties (Nat. Ranked)	Other Specialties (High Perf.)	Colon Cancer Surgery	Lung Cancer Surgery	Heart Attack	Heart Failure	Heart Bypass Surgery	Heart Valve Surgery	TAVR*	Abdominal Aortic Aneurysm	Stroke	Back Surgery	Hip Replacement	Knee Replacement	Hip Fracture	Diabetes	Kidney Failure	Pneumonia	COPD*
CALIFORNIA continued																							
7	UC Davis Medical Center, Sacramento	R	R	R	6	2	B	B	B	B	B	B	B	B	B	B	B	B	B	B	B	B	B
9	Hoag Memorial Hospital Presbyterian, Newport Beach[4]	B	−	R	4	1	B	B	B	B	B	B	−	−	B	B	B	B	B	B	B	B	B
10	John Muir Health-Walnut Creek Medical Center, Walnut Creek	−	−	R	3	4	B	B	O	B	B	B	−	−	B	B	B	B	B	B	B	B	B
11	Torrance Memorial Medical Center, Torrance	−	−	B	−	6	B	B	B	B	B	O	B	B	B	B	B	B	B	B	B	B	B
12	Providence Mission Hospital-Mission Viejo & Laguna Beach	−	−	R	1	5	B	B	B	B	B	B	B	−	B	B	B	B	B	B	B	B	B
13	Loma Linda University Medical Center, Loma Linda	B	−	B	1	5	B	B	B	B	B	B	B	B	B	B	B	B	B	B	B	B	B
13	MemorialCare Long Beach Medical Center, Long Beach	B	−	B	1	6	B	B	B	B	B	B	B	B	B	B	B	B	B	B	B	B	B
15	UCI Medical Center, Orange	B	−	B	2	4	B	B	B	B	B	B	−	B	B	B	B	B	B	B	B	B	B
16	John Muir Health-Concord Medical Center, Concord	−	−	B	−	5	B	B	B	B	B	B	−	−	B	B	B	B	B	B	B	B	B
17	Sharp Memorial Hospital, San Diego[5]	−	−	B	1	1	B	B	B	B	B	B	B	B	B	B	B	B	B	B	B	B	B
18	Kaiser Permanente Anaheim and Irvine Med. Centers, Anaheim	−	−	B	−	3	B	B	B	B	−	−	−	−	B	B	B	B	B	B	B	B	B
18	Providence St. John's Health Center, Santa Monica	−	−	B	1	4	B	B	O	B	B	B	−	−	B	B	B	B	B	B	B	B	B
20	PIH Health Hospital-Whittier	−	−	−	−	−	B	B	B	B	B	B	B	B	B	B	B	B	B	B	B	B	B
21	Adventist Health-Glendale	−	−	B	−	4	B	B	B	B	B	B	B	B	B	B	B	B	B	B	B	B	B
21	Eisenhower Medical Center, Rancho Mirage	−	−	−	−	−	B	B	B	B	B	B	B	B	B	B	B	B	B	B	B	B	B
21	Providence St. Joseph Hospital-Orange	−	−	B	−	3	B	B	B	B	B	B	B	−	B	B	B	B	B	B	B	B	B
24	Community Hospital of the Monterey Peninsula, Monterey	−	−	−	−	−	B	B	B	B	B	B	−	−	B	B	B	B	B	B	B	B	B
24	Kaiser Permanente Fontana and Ontario Med. Centers, Fontana	−	−	−	−	−	O	B	B	B	B	B	−	−	B	B	B	B	B	B	B	B	B
24	Kaiser Permanente San Diego Zion and San Diego Med. Ctr.	−	−	−	−	1	B	B	B	B	−	−	−	−	B	B	B	B	B	B	B	B	B
24	MemorialCare Orange Coast Medical Center, Fountain Valley	B	−	−	−	2	B	B	B	B	B	B	−	−	B	B	B	B	B	B	B	B	B
24	Providence Holy Cross Medical Center, Mission Hills	−	−	B	−	4	B	B	B	B	B	B	−	B	B	B	B	B	B	B	B	B	B
24	Providence St. Joseph Medical Center-Burbank	−	−	−	−	4	B	B	B	B	B	B	B	−	B	B	B	B	B	B	B	B	B
30	Kaiser Permanente Los Angeles Medical Center	−	−	−	−	2	B	B	B	B	B	B	−	−	B	B	B	B	B	B	B	B	B
30	Mercy General Hospital, Sacramento	−	−	−	−	−	B	−	B	B	B	B	B	B	B	B	B	B	B	B	B	B	B
32	Huntington Hospital, Pasadena	−	−	B	−	4	B	B	B	B	B	B	B	K	O	B	B	B	B	B	B	B	B
32	Providence Little Company of Mary Medical Center Torrance	−	−	−	−	−	B	B	B	B	B	B	B	−	B	B	B	B	B	B	B	B	B
32	Santa Barbara Cottage Hospital, Santa Barbara	−	−	−	−	−	B	B	B	B	B	B	B	B	B	B	B	B	B	B	B	B	B
32	Sequoia Hospital, Redwood City	−	−	−	−	−	B	B	B	B	B	B	B	−	B	B	B	B	B	B	B	B	B
32	Sharp Chula Vista Medical Center, Chula Vista	−	−	−	−	2	B	B	B	B	B	B	B	−	B	O	B	B	B	B	B	B	B
37	Kaiser Permanente Roseville Medical Center, Roseville	−	−	−	−	−	B	B	B	B	B	B	−	−	B	B	B	B	B	B	B	B	B
37	Kaiser Permanente San Francisco Medical Center	−	−	−	−	1	B	B	B	B	B	B	−	−	B	B	B	B	B	B	B	B	B
37	Kaiser Permanente Santa Clara Medical Center, Santa Clara	−	−	−	−	−	−	B	B	B	B	B	−	−	B	B	B	B	B	B	B	B	B
37	MemorialCare Saddleback Medical Center, Laguna Hills	−	−	−	−	−	B	B	B	B	B	B	−	−	B	B	B	B	B	B	B	B	B
37	Providence Tarzana Medical Center, Tarzana	−	−	−	−	4	B	K	B	B	B	B	−	−	B	B	B	B	B	B	B	B	B
42	Community Memorial Hospital-Ventura	−	−	−	−	−	B	B	B	B	B	B	B	−	B	B	B	B	B	B	B	B	B
42	Enloe Medical Center, Chico	−	−	−	−	−	B	K	B	B	B	B	−	−	B	B	B	B	B	B	B	B	B
42	Kaiser Permanente Downey Medical Center, Downey	−	−	−	−	−	B	B	B	B	B	B	−	−	B	B	B	B	B	B	B	B	B
42	Pomona Valley Hospital Medical Center, Pomona	−	−	−	−	−	B	B	B	O	B	B	−	−	B	B	B	B	B	B	B	B	B
42	Providence St. Jude Medical Center, Fullerton	−	−	−	1	1	B	B	B	B	B	B	−	−	B	B	B	B	B	B	B	B	B
42	Scripps Mercy Hospital, San Diego	−	−	−	−	−	O	B	B	B	B	B	−	−	B	B	O	B	B	B	B	B	B
42	Sharp Grossmont Women's Hospital, La Mesa	−	−	−	−	−	B	B	B	B	K	B	−	−	B	B	B	B	B	B	B	B	B
42	Sutter Medical Center, Sacramento	−	−	−	−	−	O	B	O	B	B	B	B	B	B	B	B	B	O	B	B	B	B

In complex care specialties, (-) indicates hospital is not nationally ranked or high performing. In procedures and conditions, (-) indicates care not offered or hospital has too few Medicare patients to be rated. *TAVR: Transcatheter aortic valve replacement. *COPD: Chronic obstructive pulmonary disease

A footnote indicates that another hospital's results are included, that the hospital has a different name in one or more areas of care, or both.
[4]Hoag Orthopedic Institute. [5]Sharp Mary Birch Hospital for Women and Newborns-Sharp Memorial Hospital.

COMPLEX SPECIALTY CARE
- 🔴 Nationally ranked
- 🔵 High performing

COMMON PROCEDURES & CONDITIONS
- 🔵 High performing
- 🟠 Average
- ⚫ Below average

Legend for table cells below: R = nationally ranked (red), B = high performing (blue), O = average (orange), K = below average (black), – = not ranked / not offered / too few patients. Number in "Other Specialties – Nationally Ranked" column indicates count of nationally ranked specialties.

Columns (left to right):
- Complex Specialty Care: Cancer | Cardiology & Heart Surgery | Orthopedics | Other Specialties (Nationally Ranked) | Other Specialties (High Performing)
- Common Procedures & Conditions: Colon Cancer Surgery | Lung Cancer Surgery | Heart Attack | Heart Failure | Heart Bypass Surgery | Heart Valve Surgery | TAVR* | Abdominal Aortic Aneurysm | Stroke | Back Surgery | Hip Replacement | Knee Replacement | Hip Fracture | Diabetes | Kidney Failure | Pneumonia | COPD*

State Rank	Hospital	Can	CHS	Ort	OS-NR	OS-HP	CC	LC	HA	HF	HB	HV	TAVR	AAA	Str	BS	HipR	KneeR	HipF	Diab	KF	Pne	COPD
CALIFORNIA continued																							
50	Kaiser Permanente Baldwin Park Medical Center, Baldwin Park	–	–	–	–	–	B	–	O	B	–	–	–	B	B	–	O	B	B	O	B	O	O
50	Kaiser Permanente Oakland & Richmond Med. Centers, Oakland	–	–	–	–	–	B	B	O	B	–	–	–	O	B	O	–	B	O	O	B	O	B
50	Kaiser Permanente South Bay Medical Center, Harbor City	–	–	–	–	–	B	–	O	B	–	–	–	B	B	O	B	B	O	O	B	O	O
50	Methodist Hospital of Southern California, Arcadia	–	–	–	–	–	B	–	B	B	O	–	–	O	B	O	B	B	O	O	B	O	O
50	NorthBay Medical Center, Fairfield	–	–	–	–	1	B	–	B	B	–	–	–	–	B	–	B	B	O	O	B	O	B
50	Scripps Memorial Hospital-Encinitas	–	–	–	–	–	B	O	B	B	–	–	–	–	B	O	B	B	O	O	B	O	O
56	California Pacific Medical Center, San Francisco	–	–	–	–	–	B	O	B	B	–	–	–	B	B	O	B	B	O	O	B	O	O
56	El Camino Hospital, Mountain View	–	–	–	–	–	B	–	O	B	–	–	–	–	B	O	O	B	O	O	B	O	O
56	Henry Mayo Newhall Hospital, Valencia	–	–	–	–	–	B	–	B	B	–	–	–	–	B	–	B	B	O	O	O	O	B
56	Kaiser Permanente Sacramento Medical Center, Sacramento	–	–	–	–	–	B	–	B	B	–	–	–	–	B	–	B	B	O	O	B	O	B
56	Kaiser Permanente San Leandro Medical Center, San Leandro	–	–	–	–	–	B	–	B	B	–	–	–	–	B	O	B	B	O	B	B	O	B
56	Kaiser Permanente South Sacramento Medical Ctr., Sacramento	–	–	–	–	–	B	–	O	B	–	–	–	–	B	–	B	B	O	O	B	O	B
56	Kaiser Permanente Woodland Hills Med. Ctr., Woodland Hills	–	–	–	–	–	B	–	B	B	–	–	–	–	B	–	–	B	–	B	B	O	B
56	Salinas Valley Memorial Healthcare System, Salinas	–	–	–	–	–	B	–	O	B	O	–	–	–	B	O	B	B	O	O	B	O	O
56	San Joaquin Community Hospital, Bakersfield	–	–	–	–	–	B	–	B	O	O	O	K	–	B	O	B	B	O	O	B	O	O
65	Good Samaritan Hospital-Los Angeles	–	–	–	–	–	B	K	B	O	O	–	–	O	B	B	B	B	O	O	B	O	O
65	Kaweah Delta Medical Center, Visalia	–	–	–	–	–	B	K	B	B	–	–	–	O	B	O	B	B	O	O	B	O	B
65	Palomar Medical Center Escondido	–	–	–	–	–	B	K	B	B	O	–	–	O	B	O	B	B	O	O	B	O	O
68	Fountain Valley Reg. Hosp. and Med. Ctr., Fountain Valley	–	–	–	–	–	B	O	O	B	–	–	–	K	B	K	K	B	K	O	B	O	B
COLORADO																							
1	UCHealth University of Colorado Hospital, Aurora[6]	R	–	B	7	2	B	B	B	B	B	B	B	B	B	B	B	B	O	B	B	B	B
2	UCHealth Medical Center of the Rockies, Loveland	–	–	–	–	2	O	B	B	B	B	B	O	B	B	B	B	B	O	B	B	B	B
3	SCL Health Saint Joseph Hospital, Denver	–	–	–	–	1	B	B	B	B	O	B	O	B	B	B	B	B	O	B	B	B	B
4	UCHealth Poudre Valley Hospital, Fort Collins	–	–	B	–	1	B	–	B	B	–	–	–	B	B	O	B	B	O	B	B	B	B
5	Sky Ridge Medical Center, Lone Tree	–	–	B	–	–	B	O	B	B	O	B	O	B	B	B	B	B	O	B	B	B	B
6	SCL Health Good Samaritan Medical Center, Lafayette	–	–	–	–	–	B	–	B	B	–	–	–	B	B	O	B	B	O	B	B	B	B
7	Parkview Medical Center, Pueblo	–	–	–	–	–	O	K	B	B	O	O	–	B	B	B	B	B	O	B	B	B	B
7	Porter Adventist Hospital, Denver	–	–	–	–	–	O	–	B	B	O	O	–	O	B	B	B	B	O	O	B	B	B
7	St. Mary's Medical Center, Grand Junction	–	–	–	–	–	B	–	B	B	O	O	–	B	B	O	B	B	O	B	B	B	B
CONNECTICUT																							
1	Yale-New Haven Hospital, New Haven[7]	B	–	B	8	1	B	B	B	B	B	B	B	B	B	B	B	B	O	B	B	B	B
2	Hartford Hospital, Hartford	–	B	–	–	1	B	B	B	B	B	B	B	B	B	B	B	B	O	O	B	B	B
3	St. Francis Hospital and Medical Center, Hartford	–	B	–	–	–	B	O	B	B	B	B	B	B	B	O	B	B	O	O	B	B	B
DELAWARE																							
1	Christiana Care Hospitals, Newark	–	–	B	–	–	B	B	B	B	O	O	O	B	B	O	B	B	O	O	B	B	B
DISTRICT OF COLUMBIA**																							
	MedStar Washington Hospital Center[8]	–	R	–	–	1	B	O	B	B	B	B	B	B	B	K	B	K	O	B	B	B	B
	Sibley Memorial Hospital, Washington	–	–	–	–	–	B	O	O	B	–	–	–	–	B	O	B	B	O	O	B	O	O
FLORIDA																							
1	Mayo Clinic-Jacksonville	R	–	R	5	1	B	B	B	B	B	B	B	B	B	B	B	B	O	B	B	B	B
2	UF Health Shands Hospital, Gainesville	B	R	B	5	3	B	B	B	B	B	B	B	B	B	B	B	B	O	B	B	B	B
3	AdventHealth Orlando	B	B	B	3	3	B	B	B	B	B	B	O	B	B	B	B	O	O	B	B	B	B

In complex care specialties, (–) indicates hospital is not nationally ranked or high performing. In procedures and conditions, (–) indicates care not offered or hospital has too few Medicare patients to be rated. *TAVR: Transcatheter aortic valve replacement. *COPD: Chronic obstructive pulmonary disease

**MedStar Washington Hospital Center is ranked No. 2 and Sibley Memorial Hospital is ranked No. 4 in the Washington, D.C., metro area rankings, which include hospitals in and around the District of Columbia. These two hospitals in D.C. are presented here alphabetically.

A footnote indicates that another hospital's results are included, that the hospital has a different name in one or more areas of care, or both.
[6]National Jewish Health, Denver-University of Colorado Hospital. [7]Smilow Cancer Hospital at Yale New Haven.
[8]MedStar Heart & Vascular Institute at MedStar Washington Hospital Center.

More @ usnews.com/bestregionalhospitals

BEST REGIONAL HOSPITALS

COMPLEX SPECIALTY CARE
- ● Nationally ranked (red)
- ● High performing (blue)

COMMON PROCEDURES & CONDITIONS
- ● High performing (blue)
- ● Average (orange)
- ● Below average (black)

In complex care specialties, (-) indicates hospital is not nationally ranked or high performing. In procedures and conditions, (-) indicates care not offered or hospital has too few Medicare patients to be rated. *TAVR: Transcatheter aortic valve replacement. *COPD: Chronic obstructive pulmonary disease

Legend for table cells below: ℝ = nationally ranked (red), 🅗 = high performing (blue), 🅐 = average (orange), 🅑 = below average (black), – = dash

Complex Specialty Care columns: Cancer | Cardiology & Heart Surgery | Orthopedics | Other Specialties (Nationally Ranked count) | Other Specialties (High Performing count)

Common Procedures & Conditions columns: Colon Cancer Surgery | Lung Cancer Surgery | Heart Attack | Heart Failure | Heart Bypass Surgery | Heart Valve Surgery | TAVR* | Abdominal Aortic Aneurysm | Stroke | Back Surgery | Hip Replacement | Knee Replacement | Hip Fracture | Diabetes | Kidney Failure | Pneumonia | COPD*

State Rank	Hospital	Can	Card	Ortho	OS-NR	OS-HP	Colon	Lung	HAtk	HFail	HByp	HValv	TAVR	AAA	Strk	Back	HipR	KneeR	HipFx	Diab	KidF	Pneu	COPD
FLORIDA continued																							
4	Tampa General Hospital	🅗	–	🅐	4	3	🅗	🅗	🅗	🅗	🅗	🅗	🅗	🅗	🅗	🅗	🅗	🅗	🅗	🅗	🅗	🅗	🅗
5	Cleveland Clinic Weston	–	–	–	1	4	🅗	🅐	🅗	🅗	🅗	🅗	🅗	🅗	🅗	🅗	🅗	🅗	🅗	🅐	🅗	🅐	🅗
6	Morton Plant Hospital, Clearwater	–	–	–	–	–	🅗	🅗	🅗	🅗	🅗	🅗	🅗	🅗	🅗	🅗	🅗	🅗	🅗	🅗	🅗	🅗	🅗
6	Sarasota Memorial Hospital, Sarasota	–	–	–	1	–	🅗	🅗	🅗	🅗	🅗	🅗	🅗	🅗	🅗	🅗	🅗	🅗	🅗	🅗	🅗	🅗	🅗
8	Orlando Regional Medical Center	–	–	–	–	–	🅗	🅗	🅗	🅗	🅗	🅗	🅗	🅗	🅗	🅗	🅗	🅗	🅗	🅗	🅗	🅗	🅗
9	Baptist Health Baptist Hospital, Miami[9]	🅗	–	–	–	2	🅗	🅗	🅗	🅗	🅗	🅗	🅗	🅗	🅗	🅗	🅗	🅗	🅗	🅗	🅗	🅗	🅗
9	Lee Memorial Hospital, Fort Myers	–	–	–	–	–	🅗	🅗	🅗	🅗	🅗	🅗	🅗	🅗	🅗	🅗	🅗	🅗	🅗	🅗	🅗	🅗	🅗
9	University of Miami Hospital and Clinics-UHealth Tower[10]	🅗	–	–	3	–	🅗	🅗	🅗	🅗	🅗	🅗	🅗	🅗	🅗	🅗	🅗	🅗	🅗	🅗	🅗	🅗	🅗
12	Baptist Medical Center Jacksonville	–	–	–	–	1	🅗	🅗	🅗	🅗	🅗	🅗	🅗	🅗	🅗	🅗	🅗	🅗	🅗	🅗	🅗	🅗	🅗
12	Mount Sinai Medical Center, Miami Beach	–	–	–	1	1	🅗	🅗	🅗	🅗	🅗	🅗	🅑	🅗	🅗	🅗	🅗	🅗	🅗	🅗	🅗	🅐	🅗
12	NCH Downtown Naples Hospital, Naples	–	–	–	–	–	🅗	🅗	🅗	🅗	🅗	🅗	🅗	🅗	🅗	🅑	🅗	🅗	🅗	🅗	🅗	🅗	🅗
12	St. Joseph's Hospital-Tampa	–	–	–	–	–	🅗	🅗	🅗	🅗	🅗	🅗	🅗	🅗	🅗	🅗	🅗	🅗	🅗	🅗	🅗	🅗	🅗
16	AdventHealth Daytona Beach	–	–	–	–	–	🅗	🅗	🅗	🅗	🅗	🅗	🅗	🅗	🅗	🅗	🅗	🅗	🅗	🅗	🅗	🅗	🅗
16	Baptist Health Doctors Hospital, Coral Gables[11]	–	–	🅗	–	1	🅗	–	🅗	🅗	–	–	–	🅗	🅗	🅗	🅗	🅗	🅗	🅗	🅗	🅗	🅗
16	Gulf Coast Medical Center, Fort Myers	–	–	–	–	–	🅗	🅗	🅗	🅗	🅗	🅗	🅗	🅗	🅗	🅗	🅗	🅗	🅗	🅗	🅗	🅗	🅗
16	Memorial Hospital West, Pembroke Pines	–	–	–	–	1	🅗	–	🅗	🅗	–	–	–	🅗	🅗	🅗	🅗	🅗	🅗	🅗	🅗	🅗	🅗
16	Memorial Regional Hospital, Hollywood	–	–	–	–	–	🅗	🅗	🅗	🅗	🅗	🅗	🅗	🅗	🅗	🅗	🅗	🅗	🅗	🅗	🅗	🅗	🅗
16	UF Health Jacksonville	–	–	–	1	1	🅗	🅗	🅑	🅑	🅑	🅗	🅗	🅗	🅗	🅗	🅗	🅗	🅗	🅗	🅗	🅗	🅗
22	Ascension Sacred Heart Hospital Pensacola	–	–	–	–	–	🅗	🅗	🅗	🅗	🅗	🅗	🅗	🅗	🅗	🅗	🅗	🅗	🅗	🅗	🅗	🅗	🅗
22	Baptist Health South Miami Hospital, South Miami[12]	–	–	🅗	–	1	🅗	–	🅗	🅗	–	🅑	–	🅗	🅗	🅗	🅗	🅗	🅗	🅗	🅗	🅗	🅗
22	Health First Holmes Regional Medical Center, Melbourne	–	–	–	–	–	🅗	🅗	🅗	🅗	🅗	🅗	🅗	🅗	🅗	🅗	🅗	🅗	🅗	🅗	🅗	🅗	🅗
25	AdventHealth Tampa	–	–	–	–	–	🅗	🅑	🅗	🅗	🅗	🅗	🅗	🅗	🅗	🅗	🅗	🅗	🅗	🅗	🅗	🅗	🅗
25	Ascension St. Vincent's Hospital Riverside, Jacksonville	–	–	–	–	–	🅗	🅗	🅗	🅗	🅗	🅗	🅗	🅗	🅗	🅑	🅗	🅗	🅗	🅗	🅗	🅗	🅗
25	Baptist Health Boca Raton Regional Hospital, Boca Raton[13]	–	–	–	–	–	🅗	🅗	🅗	🅗	🅑	🅗	🅗	🅗	🅗	🅗	🅗	🅗	🅗	🅗	🅗	🅗	🅗
25	Cleveland Clinic Martin Heath, Stuart	–	–	–	–	–	🅗	🅗	🅗	🅗	🅑	🅑	🅗	🅗	🅗	🅗	🅗	🅗	🅗	🅗	🅗	🅗	🅗
25	Holy Cross Health-Fort Lauderdale	–	–	–	–	–	🅗	🅗	🅗	🅑	🅗	🅗	🅗	🅑	🅗	🅗	🅗	🅗	🅗	🅗	🅗	🅗	🅗
25	St. Anthony's Hospital, Saint Petersburg	–	–	–	–	–	🅗	🅗	🅗	🅗	–	–	–	🅗	🅗	🅗	🅗	🅗	🅗	🅗	🅗	🅗	🅗
31	AdventHealth Waterman, Tavares	–	–	–	–	–	🅗	🅗	🅗	🅗	–	🅑	–	🅗	🅗	🅑	🅗	🅗	🅗	🅗	🅗	🅗	🅗
31	Cleveland Clinic Indian River Hospital, Vero Beach	–	–	–	–	–	🅗	🅗	🅗	🅗	–	–	–	🅗	🅗	🅗	🅑	🅗	🅗	🅗	🅗	🅗	🅗
31	Tallahassee Memorial Healthcare, Tallahassee	–	–	–	–	–	🅗	🅗	🅗	🅗	🅗	🅗	🅗	🅗	🅗	🅗	🅑	🅗	🅗	🅗	🅗	🅗	🅗
34	Broward Health Medical Center, Fort Lauderdale	–	–	–	–	–	🅗	🅑	🅗	🅗	🅗	🅗	🅗	🅗	🅗	🅗	🅗	🅗	🅑	🅗	🅗	🅗	🅗
34	Jackson Health System-Miami	–	–	–	–	–	🅗	🅗	🅗	–	🅑	🅗	🅗	🅑	🅗	🅗	🅗	🅗	🅑	🅗	🅑	🅗	🅗
GEORGIA																							
1	Emory University Hospital, Atlanta[14]	🔴	–	🅗	4	2	🅗	🅗	🅗	🅗	🅗	🅗	🅗	🅗	🅗	🅗	🅗	🅗	🅗	🅗	🅗	🅗	🅗
2	Emory St. Joseph's Hospital, Atlanta	🅗	🅗	🅗	–	5	🅗	🅗	🅗	🅗	🅗	🅗	🅗	🅗	🅗	🅗	🅗	🅗	🅗	🅗	🅗	🅗	🅗
3	Piedmont Atlanta Hospital[15]	🅗	–	🅗	–	2	🅗	🅗	🅗	🅗	🅗	🅗	🅗	🅗	🅗	🅗	🅗	🅗	🅗	🅗	🅗	🅗	🅗
4	Northside Hospital Atlanta	–	–	–	1	–	🅗	🅗	🅗	–	–	–	–	🅗	🅗	🅗	🅗	🅗	🅗	🅗	🅗	🅗	🅗
5	Emory University Hospital Midtown, Atlanta	🅗	–	🅗	1	1	🅗	🅗	🅗	🅗	🅗	🅗	🅗	🅗	🅗	🅗	🅗	🅗	🅗	🅗	🅗	🅗	🅗
6	Northeast Georgia Medical Center, Gainesville	–	–	–	–	–	🅗	🅗	🅗	🅗	🅗	🅗	🅗	🅗	🅗	🅗	🅗	🅗	🅗	🅗	🅗	🅗	🅗
7	WellStar Kennestone Hospital, Marietta	–	–	–	1	–	🅗	🅗	🅗	🅗	🅗	🅗	🅗	🅗	🅗	🅗	🅗	🅗	🅗	🅗	🅗	🅗	🅗

A footnote indicates that another hospital's results are included, that the hospital has a different name in one or more areas of care, or both.
[9]Miami Cancer Institute at Baptist Hospital of Miami; Miami Cardiac & Vascular Institute at Baptist Hospital of Miami; Baptist Hospital of Miami; Miami Orthopedics & Sports Medicine Institute at Baptist Hospital of Miami. [10]Sylvester Comprehensive Cancer Center-University of Miami Hospital and Clinics. [11]Baptist Health Doctors Hospital; Miami Cardiac & Vascular Institute at Baptist Health Doctors Hospital; Baptist Health Neuroscience Center at Baptist Health Doctors Hospital; Miami Orthopedics & Sports Medicine Institute at Baptist Health Doctors Hospital. [12]South Miami Hospital; Miami Cardiac & Vascular Institute at South Miami Hospital; Miami Orthopedics & Sports Medicine Institute at South Miami Hospital. [13]Lynn Cancer Institute at Baptist Health Boca Raton Regional Hospital; Lynn Heart & Vascular Institute at Baptist Health Boca Raton Regional Hospital; Marcus Neuroscience Institute at Baptist Health Boca Raton Regional Hospital; Baptist Health Orthopedics & Sports Medicine at Baptist Health Boca Raton Regional Hospital. [14]Emory University Hospital at Wesley Woods. [15]Piedmont Heart Institute at Piedmont Atlanta Hospital.

NCH NAMED AMONG THE
TOP FIVE PERCENT OF U.S. HOSPITALS
BY HEALTHGRADES FOR THE FOURTH YEAR IN A ROW

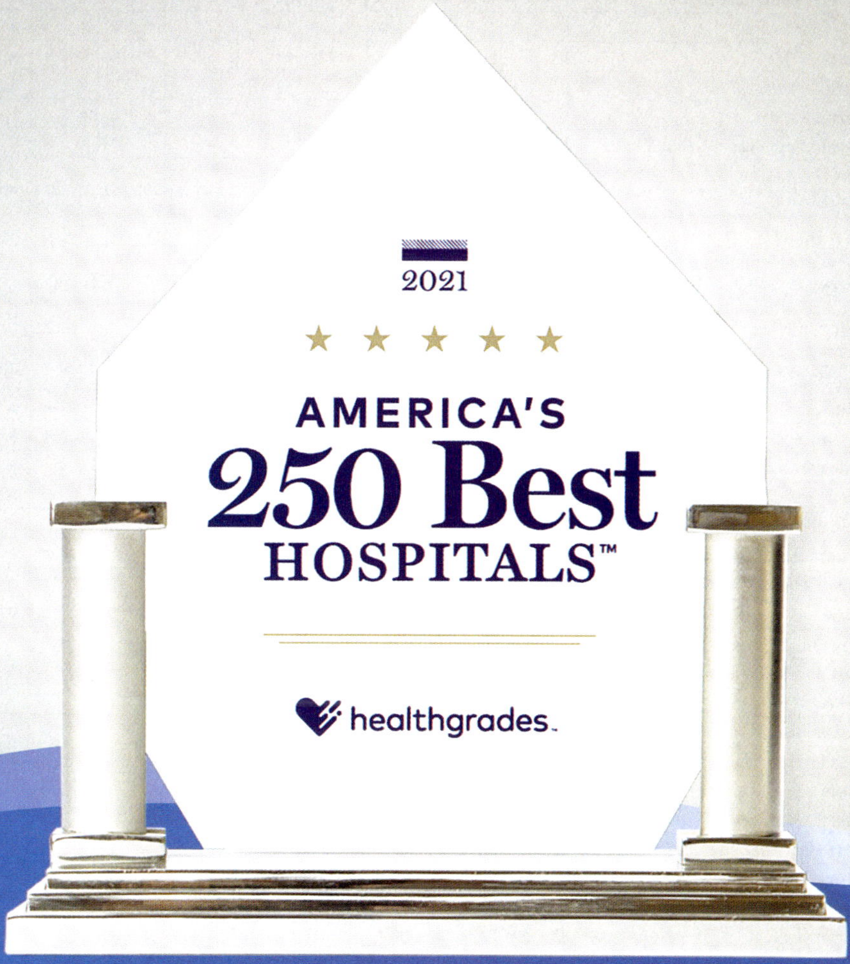

2021

★★★★★

AMERICA'S 250 Best HOSPITALS™

♥ healthgrades.

The NCH Healthcare System has received the Healthgrades 2021 America's 250 Best Hospitals Award™ for the fourth year in a row. The distinction places NCH in the top five percent of nearly 4,500 hospitals assessed nationwide for its superior clinical performance as measured by Healthgrades, the leading resource that connects consumers, physicians and health systems.

For more information on the award-winning services of the NCH Healthcare System, please visit **NCHmd.org**.

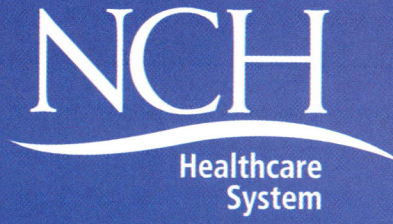

BEST REGIONAL HOSPITALS

COMPLEX SPECIALTY CARE
- ● Nationally ranked
- ● High performing

COMMON PROCEDURES & CONDITIONS
- ● High performing
- ● Average
- ● Below average

Legend note: *TAVR: Transcatheter aortic valve replacement. *COPD: Chronic obstructive pulmonary disease

State / Rank / Hospital	Cancer	Cardiology & Heart Surgery	Orthopedics	Other Specialties	Other Specialties (Nationally Ranked / High Performing)	Colon Cancer Surgery	Lung Cancer Surgery	Heart Attack	Heart Failure	Heart Bypass Surgery	Heart Valve Surgery	TAVR*	Abdominal Aortic Aneurysm	Stroke	Back Surgery	Hip Replacement	Knee Replacement	Hip Fracture	Diabetes	Kidney Failure	Pneumonia	COPD*
GEORGIA continued																						
8 Northside Hospital Gwinnett, Lawrenceville	–	–	–	–	–	●	●	●	●	●	●	●	●	●	●	●	●	●	●	●	●	●
9 Navicent Health Medical Center, Macon	–	–	–	–	–	●	●	●	●	●	●	●	●	●	●	●	●	●	●	●	●	●
9 University Hospital-Augusta	–	–	–	–	–	●	●	●	●	●	●	●	●	●	●	●	●	●	●	●	●	●
11 Northside Hospital Forsyth, Cumming	–	–	–	–	–	●	●	●	●	–	–	–	●	●	●	●	●	●	●	●	●	●
12 Northside Hospital Cherokee, Canton	–	–	–	–	–	●	–	●	●	–	–	–	●	●	●	●	●	●	●	●	●	●
12 Piedmont Athens Regional Medical Center, Athens	–	–	–	–	–	●	●	●	●	●	●	●	●	●	●	●	●	●	●	●	●	●
12 Piedmont Fayette Hospital, Fayetteville	–	–	–	–	–	●	–	●	●	●	●	●	●	●	●	●	●	●	●	●	●	●
HAWAII																						
1 Queen's Medical Center, Honolulu	●	–	●	–	5	●	●	●	●	●	●	●	●	●	●	●	●	●	●	●	●	●
2 Kaiser Permanente Moanalua Medical Center, Honolulu	–	–	–	–	1	●	●	●	●	●	●	●	●	●	●	●	●	●	●	●	●	●
IDAHO																						
1 St. Luke's Regional Medical Center, Boise	–	–	–	–	2	●	●	●	●	●	●	●	●	●	●	●	●	●	●	●	●	●
2 St. Alphonsus Regional Medical Center, Boise	–	–	–	–	–	●	●	●	●	●	●	●	●	●	●	●	●	●	●	●	●	●
ILLINOIS																						
1 Northwestern Memorial Hospital, Chicago	●	●	●	7	1	●	●	●	●	●	●	●	●	●	●	●	●	●	●	●	●	●
2 Rush University Medical Center, Chicago	●	●	●	6	1	●	●	●	●	●	●	●	●	●	●	●	●	●	●	●	●	●
3 University of Chicago Medical Center	●	●	●	5	2	●	●	●	●	●	●	●	●	●	●	●	●	●	●	●	●	●
4 Advocate Christ Medical Center, Oak Lawn	●	●	●	1	6	●	●	●	●	●	●	●	●	●	●	●	●	●	●	●	●	●
5 Loyola University Medical Center, Maywood	●	●	●	3	3	●	●	●	●	●	●	●	●	●	●	●	●	●	●	●	●	●
6 NorthShore University HealthSystem-Metro Chicago, Evanston	–	–	●	–	6	●	●	●	●	●	●	●	●	●	●	●	●	●	●	●	●	●
7 Advocate Lutheran General Hospital, Park Ridge	–	–	●	3	1	●	●	●	●	●	●	●	●	●	●	●	●	●	●	●	●	●
8 Edward Hospital, Naperville[16]	–	–	–	–	4	●	●	●	●	●	●	●	●	●	●	●	●	●	●	●	●	●
9 Advocate Good Samaritan Hospital, Downers Grove	–	–	●	–	5	●	●	●	●	●	●	●	●	●	●	●	●	●	●	●	●	●
10 Carle Foundation Hospital, Urbana	–	–	–	1	3	●	●	●	●	●	●	●	●	●	–	●	●	●	●	●	●	●
10 Northwestern Medicine Central DuPage Hospital, Winfield	–	–	–	–	–	●	●	●	●	●	●	●	●	●	●	●	●	●	●	●	●	●
12 Advocate Good Shepherd Hospital, Barrington	–	–	–	–	5	●	●	●	●	●	●	●	●	●	●	●	●	●	●	●	●	●
13 Advocate Illinois Masonic Medical Center, Chicago	–	–	●	1	2	●	●	●	●	●	●	●	●	●	●	●	●	●	●	●	●	●
13 OSF HealthCare St. Francis Medical Center, Peoria	–	–	–	–	1	●	●	●	●	●	●	●	●	●	●	●	●	●	●	●	●	●
15 Northwestern Lake Forest Hospital, Lake Forest	–	–	●	1	2	●	–	●	●	–	–	–	●	●	●	●	●	●	●	●	●	●
16 Northwestern Medicine-McHenry, Huntley & Woodstock, McHenry	–	●	●	–	–	●	●	●	●	–	–	–	●	●	●	●	●	●	●	●	●	●
17 Elmhurst Hospital, Elmhurst	–	–	–	–	1	●	●	●	●	●	●	●	●	●	●	●	●	●	●	●	●	●
17 Silver Cross Hospital, New Lenox[17]	–	–	–	–	–	●	●	●	●	–	–	–	●	●	●	●	●	●	●	●	●	●
19 Advocate Trinity Hospital, Chicago	–	–	–	–	1	●	–	●	●	–	–	–	●	●	–	●	●	–	●	●	●	●
19 Memorial Medical Center-Springfield	–	–	–	–	–	●	●	●	●	●	●	●	●	●	●	●	●	●	●	●	●	●
19 Northwestern Medicine Delnor Hospital, Geneva	–	–	●	–	–	●	–	●	●	–	–	–	●	●	●	●	●	●	●	●	●	●
22 Advocate Condell Medical Center, Libertyville	–	–	–	–	1	●	●	●	●	–	–	–	●	●	●	●	●	●	●	●	●	●
22 St. John's Hospital, Springfield	–	–	–	–	–	●	●	●	●	●	●	●	●	●	●	●	●	●	●	●	●	●
24 Advocate South Suburban Hospital, Hazel Crest	–	–	–	–	–	●	–	●	●	–	–	–	●	●	●	●	●	●	●	●	●	●
24 Rush Copley Medical Center, Aurora	–	–	–	–	–	●	●	●	●	–	–	–	●	●	●	●	●	●	●	●	●	●
26 Blessing Hospital, Quincy	–	–	–	–	–	●	●	●	●	–	–	–	●	●	–	●	●	●	●	●	●	●
INDIANA																						
1 Indiana University Health Medical Center, Indianapolis	–	–	–	2	3	●	●	●	●	●	●	●	●	●	●	●	●	●	●	●	●	●
2 Deaconess Hospital, Evansville	–	–	–	–	–	●	●	●	●	●	●	●	●	●	●	●	●	●	●	●	●	●
3 Ascension St. Vincent Hospital, Indianapolis	–	–	–	–	–	●	●	●	●	●	–	●	●	●	●	●	●	●	●	●	●	●

In complex care specialties, (–) indicates hospital is not nationally ranked or high performing. In procedures and conditions, (–) indicates care not offered or hospital has too few Medicare patients to be rated. *TAVR: Transcatheter aortic valve replacement. *COPD: Chronic obstructive pulmonary disease

A footnote indicates that another hospital's results are included, that the hospital has a different name in one or more areas of care, or both.
[16] Edward Cancer Center; Edward Heart Hospital. [17] Shirley Ryan AbilityLab at Silver Cross Hospital.

Best Hospitals

Legend:
- **COMPLEX SPECIALTY CARE:** ● Nationally ranked (red) | ● High performing (blue)
- **COMMON PROCEDURES & CONDITIONS:** ● High performing (blue) | ● Average (orange) | ● Below average (black)

Symbols used in table below: **N** = nationally ranked (red), **H** = high performing (blue), **A** = average (orange), **B** = below average (black), **–** = dash (not ranked / not rated)

State / Rank / Hospital	Cancer	Cardiology & Heart Surgery	Orthopedics	Other Specialties (Nat'l Ranked)	Other Specialties (High Perf.)	Colon Cancer Surgery	Lung Cancer Surgery	Heart Attack	Heart Failure	Heart Bypass Surgery	Heart Valve Surgery	TAVR*	Abdominal Aortic Aneurysm	Stroke	Back Surgery	Hip Replacement	Knee Replacement	Hip Fracture	Diabetes	Kidney Failure	Pneumonia	COPD*
INDIANA continued																						
4 Community Hospital of Anderson and Madison County, Anderson	–	–	–	–	–	H	–	A	H	–	–	–	H	H	H	H	H	H	A	H	H	H
4 Franciscan St. Francis Health-Indianapolis	–	–	–	–	–	H	H	H	H	H	B	A	H	H	H	H	H	H	H	H	H	H
4 Indiana University Health Ball Memorial Hospital, Muncie	–	–	–	–	–	H	H	H	H	A	–	–	H	H	H	H	H	H	A	H	H	H
4 Memorial Hospital of South Bend	–	–	–	–	–	H	H	H	H	A	A	A	A	H	H	H	H	H	A	H	H	H
4 Parkview Regional Medical Center, Fort Wayne	–	–	–	–	–	H	H	H	H	H	A	A	H	H	H	H	H	H	H	H	H	H
9 St. Joseph Regional Medical Center, Mishawaka	–	–	–	–	–	H	H	H	H	B	–	A	H	H	H	H	H	H	A	H	H	H
IOWA																						
1 University of Iowa Hospitals and Clinics, Iowa City	N	–	H	3	5	H	H	H	H	H	H	H	H	H	H	H	H	H	H	H	H	H
2 MercyOne Des Moines Medical Center	–	–	–	–	–	H	H	H	H	H	H	A	H	H	H	H	H	H	H	H	H	H
3 UnityPoint Health-St. Luke's Hospital, Cedar Rapids	–	–	–	–	–	H	H	H	H	H	H	A	H	H	H	H	H	H	A	H	H	H
4 UnityPoint Health-Iowa Methodist Medical Center, Des Moines	–	–	–	–	–	H	H	H	H	H	H	A	A	H	H	H	H	H	H	H	H	H
5 Mercy Medical Center-Cedar Rapids	–	–	–	–	–	H	–	H	H	A	A	A	H	H	H	H	H	H	A	H	H	H
KANSAS																						
1 University of Kansas Hospital, Kansas City	N	N	H	5	2	H	H	H	H	H	H	H	H	H	H	H	H	H	H	H	H	H
2 Stormont Vail Hospital, Topeka	–	–	–	–	3	H	H	H	H	H	H	B	H	H	H	H	H	H	A	H	H	H
3 Advent Health Shawnee Mission	–	–	–	–	–	H	H	H	H	H	H	H	H	H	H	H	H	H	H	H	H	H
KENTUCKY																						
1 U. of Kentucky Albert B. Chandler Hospital, Lexington	N	–	H	–	3	H	H	H	H	H	H	A	H	H	H	H	H	H	A	H	A	H
2 St. Elizabeth Healthcare Edgewood & Covington Hosps.	–	–	–	–	–	H	H	H	H	H	H	A	H	H	H	H	H	H	A	H	H	H
3 Baptist Health Lexington	–	–	–	–	–	H	H	H	H	H	H	A	H	H	A	H	H	H	A	A	A	A
4 Baptist Health Louisville	–	–	–	–	–	H	H	H	H	A	A	A	H	H	A	H	H	H	A	A	A	A
5 Norton Hospital, Louisville	–	–	–	–	–	H	H	H	H	H	A	A	H	H	A	H	H	H	A	A	H	A
6 UofL Health-Jewish Hospital, Louisville	–	–	–	–	–	H	H	H	H	H	H	H	H	H	B	H	H	H	A	A	H	H
LOUISIANA																						
1 Ochsner Medical Center, New Orleans	–	–	–	1	1	H	H	H	H	H	H	H	H	H	H	H	H	H	H	H	H	H
2 Willis-Knighton Medical Center, Shreveport	–	–	–	–	–	H	H	H	H	H	H	A	H	H	H	H	H	H	A	H	H	H
3 Our Lady of the Lake Regional Medical Center, Baton Rouge	–	–	–	–	–	H	H	H	H	H	H	A	H	H	H	H	H	H	A	H	H	H
4 Tulane Medical Center, New Orleans	–	–	–	–	–	H	H	H	H	H	H	–	A	H	H	H	H	H	A	A	A	H
MAINE																						
1 Maine Medical Center, Portland	–	–	–	–	–	H	H	H	H	H	H	H	H	H	H	H	H	H	H	H	H	H
2 Eastern Maine Medical Center, Bangor	–	–	–	–	–	H	H	H	H	H	H	A	H	H	H	H	H	B	A	H	H	H
MARYLAND																						
1 Johns Hopkins Hospital, Baltimore	N	N	N	12	–	H	H	H	H	H	H	H	H	H	H	–	–	H	H	H	H	H
2 University of Maryland Medical Center, Baltimore	H	–	H	1	2	H	H	H	H	H	H	H	H	H	H	A	A	H	H	H	H	H
3 University of Maryland St. Joseph Medical Center, Towson	–	–	–	–	–	H	H	H	H	H	H	A	H	H	H	H	H	H	A	H	H	H
4 Greater Baltimore Medical Center	–	–	–	1	–	H	B	H	H	–	–	–	H	H	H	H	H	H	A	H	H	H
4 MedStar Union Memorial Hospital, Baltimore	–	–	H	–	–	–	–	H	H	H	H	A	H	H	H	H	H	H	A	H	H	H
6 Anne Arundel Medical Center, Annapolis	–	–	–	–	–	H	H	–	–	–	–	–	–	H	H	H	H	H	A	A	H	A
6 Johns Hopkins Bayview Medical Center, Baltimore	–	–	H	–	2	H	H	H	H	–	–	–	H	H	H	H	H	H	A	H	H	H
8 TidalHealth Peninsula Regional Hospital, Salisbury	–	–	–	–	–	H	–	H	H	A	B	–	H	H	H	H	H	H	A	A	H	A
8 Suburban Hospital, Bethesda	–	–	H	–	–	H	H	H	H	–	–	–	A	H	A	H	H	H	A	H	H	A
10 U. of Maryland Baltimore Washington Med. Ctr., Glen Burnie	–	–	–	–	–	H	–	H	H	A	A	–	H	H	A	H	H	H	A	A	A	A
11 Ascension St. Agnes Hospital-Baltimore	–	–	–	–	–	A	–	H	H	A	A	–	A	H	B	H	H	H	A	A	H	A
11 Howard County General Hospital, Columbia	–	–	–	–	–	A	–	A	–	–	–	–	H	H	A	H	H	H	A	A	H	A

In complex care specialties, (–) indicates hospital is not nationally ranked or high performing. In procedures and conditions, (–) indicates care not offered or hospital has too few Medicare patients to be rated. *TAVR: Transcatheter aortic valve replacement. *COPD: Chronic obstructive pulmonary disease

More @ usnews.com/bestregionalhospitals

BEST REGIONAL HOSPITALS

Legend:

COMPLEX SPECIALTY CARE
- ● (red) Nationally ranked
- ● (blue) High performing

COMMON PROCEDURES & CONDITIONS
- ● (blue) High performing
- ● (orange) Average
- ● (black) Below average

Column key (symbols used below): **R** = red (nationally ranked) · **●** = blue (high performing) · **○** = orange (average) · **■** = black (below average) · **—** = not ranked / not offered

State Rank	Hospital	Cancer	Cardiology & Heart Surgery	Orthopedics	Other Specialties (Nat'l Ranked)	Other Specialties (High Perf.)	Colon Cancer Surgery	Lung Cancer Surgery	Heart Attack	Heart Failure	Heart Bypass Surgery	Heart Valve Surgery	TAVR*	Abdominal Aortic Aneurysm	Stroke	Back Surgery	Hip Replacement	Knee Replacement	Hip Fracture	Diabetes	Kidney Failure	Pneumonia	COPD*
MARYLAND continued																							
11	UPMC Western Maryland, Cumberland	—	—	—	—	—	○	●	●	●	—	○	●	○	●	●	○	○	○	●	●	●	●
14	Holy Cross Hospital-Silver Spring	—	—	—	—	—	○	●	●	○	—	—	○	●	○	■	●	●	○	●	●	○	●
14	Sinai Hospital of Baltimore	—	—	—	—	—	○	●	●	○	—	●	■	●	●	●	○	●	○	●	●	●	●
MASSACHUSETTS																							
1	Massachusetts General Hospital, Boston[18]	R	R	R	11	—	●	●	●	●	●	●	●	●	●	●	●	●	●	●	●	●	●
2	Brigham and Women's Hospital, Boston[19]	R	R	●	9	—	●	●	●	●	●	●	●	●	●	●	●	●	●	●	●	●	●
3	Beth Israel Deaconess Medical Center, Boston	R	—	—	3	2	●	●	●	●	●	●	—	●	●	■	●	●	●	●	●	●	●
4	Lahey Hospital and Medical Center, Burlington	—	—	—	—	3	○	●	●	●	●	●	●	●	●	●	●	●	○	●	●	●	●
5	Baystate Medical Center, Springfield	—	●	—	—	—	○	●	●	●	○	—	—	●	●	●	●	●	●	●	●	○	●
6	Tufts Medical Center, Boston	—	—	—	—	1	●	●	●	●	●	●	●	—	●	●	●	●	●	●	●	●	●
6	UMass Memorial Medical Center, Worcester	—	—	—	—	—	●	●	●	●	●	●	—	—	●	●	●	●	●	●	●	●	●
8	South Shore Hospital-South Weymouth	—	—	—	—	1	○	●	●	●	—	—	—	●	●	○	●	●	●	●	●	●	●
9	Newton-Wellesley Hospital, Newton Lower Falls	—	—	—	—	—	●	●	●	●	—	—	—	●	●	○	●	●	●	●	●	●	●
9	Southcoast Hospitals-Fall River, New Bedford & Wareham	—	—	—	—	—	○	●	●	●	○	●	—	●	●	■	●	●	●	●	●	●	●
9	St. Vincent Hospital-Worcester	—	—	—	—	—	○	●	●	●	●	●	○	—	●	●	●	●	●	●	●	●	●
MICHIGAN																							
1	U. of Michigan Hospitals-Michigan Medicine, Ann Arbor	R	R	R	10	1	●	●	●	●	●	●	●	●	●	●	●	●	●	●	●	●	●
2	Beaumont Hospital-Royal Oak	●	R	R	6	1	●	●	●	●	●	●	●	●	●	●	●	●	●	●	●	●	●
3	Beaumont Hospital-Grosse Pointe	—	—	●	5	1	○	●	●	●	—	—	—	●	●	○	●	●	●	●	●	●	●
3	Beaumont Hospital-Troy	—	●	R	1	4	●	●	●	●	●	●	○	●	●	●	●	●	●	●	●	●	●
5	Spectrum Health-Butterworth & Blodgett, Grand Rapids	—	—	—	—	2	●	●	●	●	●	●	●	●	●	●	●	●	●	●	●	●	●
6	Munson Medical Center, Traverse City	—	—	—	—	—	●	●	●	●	●	●	—	●	●	●	●	●	●	●	●	●	●
7	St. Joseph Mercy Ann Arbor Hospital, Ypsilanti	—	—	—	—	—	○	●	●	●	○	○	●	●	●	●	●	●	●	●	●	●	●
8	Bronson Methodist Hospital, Kalamazoo	—	—	—	—	—	●	●	●	●	●	●	—	●	●	○	●	●	●	○	●	●	●
9	Henry Ford Hospital, Detroit	—	—	—	—	3	●	●	●	●	●	●	●	●	●	●	●	●	○	○	●	●	●
10	Ascension Providence Hospital-Southfield	—	—	●	—	—	●	●	●	●	●	●	○	●	●	●	●	●	●	●	●	●	●
10	Beaumont Hospital-Dearborn	—	—	—	—	—	●	●	●	●	●	●	○	○	●	●	●	●	●	●	●	●	●
12	Henry Ford West Bloomfield Hospital, West Bloomfield	—	—	●	—	—	●	—	●	—	—	—	—	●	●	●	●	●	●	●	●	●	●
13	Ascension Borgess Hospital, Kalamazoo	—	—	—	—	—	○	●	●	●	●	—	—	●	●	○	●	●	●	●	●	●	●
13	Ascension Genesys Hospital, Grand Blanc	—	—	—	—	—	○	●	●	●	■	●	—	●	●	○	●	●	●	●	●	●	●
13	Henry Ford Macomb Hospitals, Clinton Township	—	—	—	—	—	○	●	●	●	●	—	—	—	●	●	●	●	○	●	●	●	●
13	McLaren Northern Michigan Hospital, Petoskey	—	—	—	—	—	○	●	●	●	●	○	—	—	●	○	●	●	●	●	●	○	●
17	Ascension St. John Hospital, Detroit	—	—	—	—	—	○	●	●	●	●	●	○	●	●	■	●	●	●	●	●	●	●
17	Mercy Health St. Mary's Campus, Grand Rapids	—	—	—	—	—	○	●	●	●	—	—	—	●	●	○	●	●	●	●	●	●	●
17	MidMichigan Medical Center-Midland	—	—	—	—	—	○	●	●	●	●	○	—	—	●	●	●	●	○	●	●	●	●
17	St. Joseph Mercy Oakland, Pontiac	—	—	—	—	—	○	●	●	●	●	●	○	●	●	●	●	●	●	●	●	●	●
21	Henry Ford Allegiance Health-Jackson	—	—	—	—	—	○	●	●	●	●	●	○	—	●	●	●	●	○	●	●	●	●
22	Hurley Medical Center, Flint	—	—	—	—	—	○	—	●	●	—	—	—	●	●	■	●	●	○	●	●	●	●
23	McLaren Flint Hospital, Flint	—	—	—	—	—	—	—	■	●	●	—	●	—	●	■	●	●	■	○	●	●	●
MINNESOTA																							
1	Mayo Clinic, Rochester	R	R	R	11	1	●	●	●	●	●	●	●	○	●	●	●	●	●	●	●	●	●
2	Abbott Northwestern Hospital, Minneapolis[20]	—	R	●	1	5	●	●	●	●	●	●	●	●	●	●	●	●	●	●	●	●	○
3	St. Cloud Hospital, Saint Cloud	—	●	—	2	2	●	○	●	●	●	●	●	●	●	●	●	●	●	●	●	●	●

In complex care specialties, (—) indicates hospital is not nationally ranked or high performing. In procedures and conditions, (—) indicates care not offered or hospital has too few Medicare patients to be rated. *TAVR: Transcatheter aortic valve replacement. *COPD: Chronic obstructive pulmonary disease

A footnote indicates that another hospital's results are included, that the hospital has a different name in one or more areas of care, or both.
[18] Massachusetts Eye and Ear Infirmary. [19] Dana-Farber/Brigham and Women's Cancer Center. [20] Minneapolis Heart Institute at Abbott Northwestern Hospital.

ALWAYS ADVANCING
Our Expertise in Quality Care

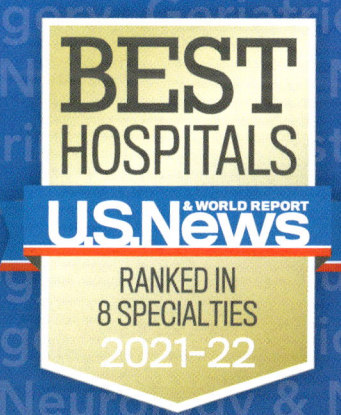
Beaumont Hospital, Royal Oak

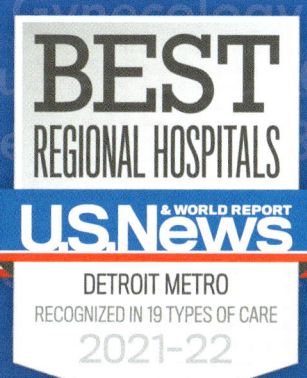
Beaumont Hospital, Troy

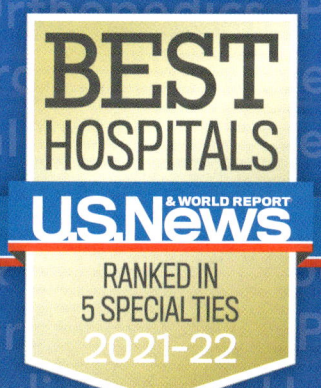
Beaumont Hospital, Grosse Pointe

Ranked among America's best hospitals by U.S. News & World Report

The most **NATIONALLY RANKED HOSPITALS** in Michigan

3 OF THE TOP 4 HOSPITALS in Michigan

24 specialty programs rated among the **TOP 10% IN THE COUNTRY**

Beaumont

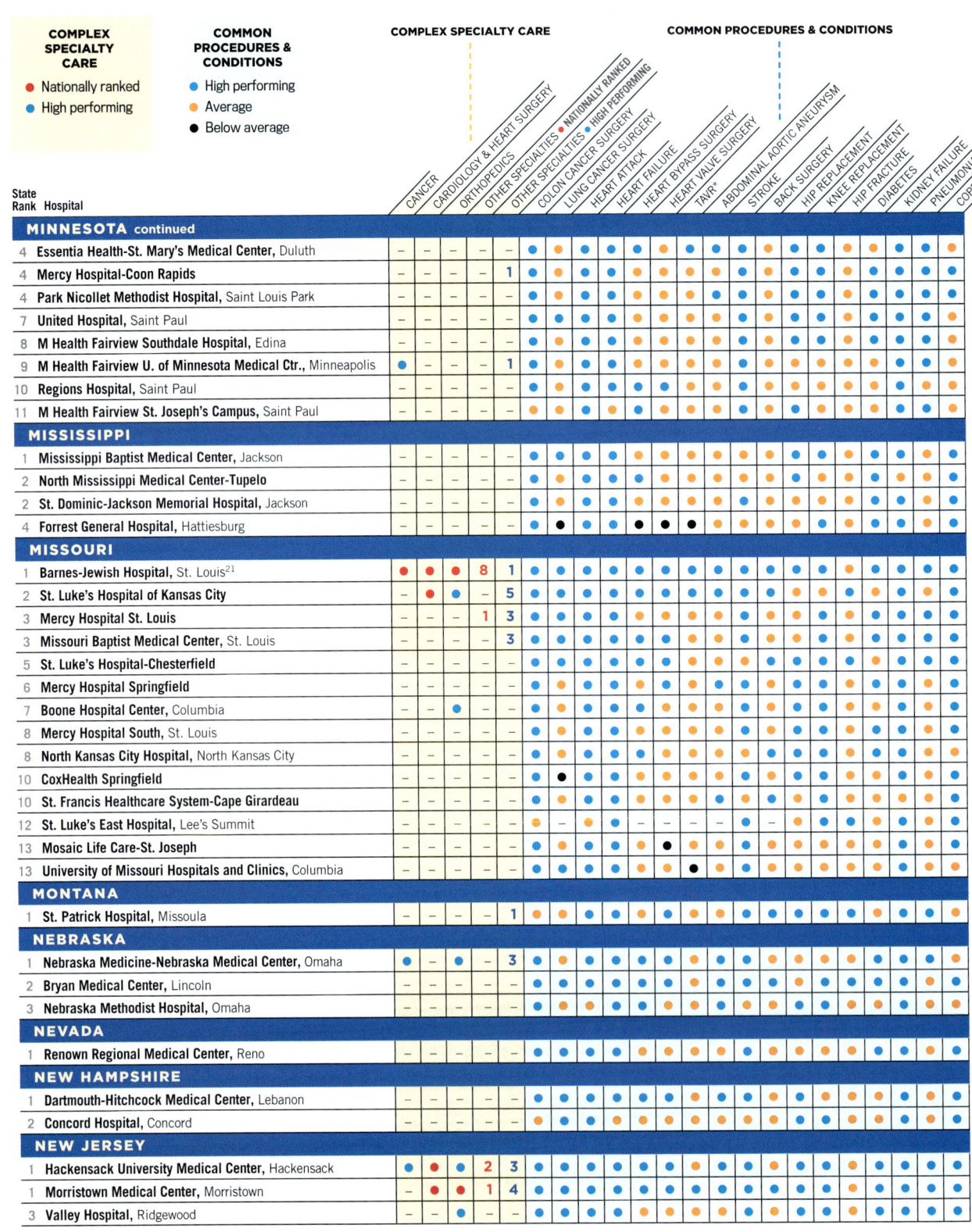

HACKENSACK UNIVERSITY MEDICAL CENTER

THE ONLY PLACE WITH NJ'S #1 ADULT AND CHILDREN'S HOSPITALS

We are honored that *U.S. News & World Report* has ranked Hackensack University Medical Center and Joseph M. Sanzari Children's Hospital as the #1 adult and children's hospitals* in New Jersey. Hackensack University Medical Center is also proud to be home to the state's best cancer center, and three specialties ranking in the top 50 nationally, including Cardiology & Heart Surgery, Neurology & Neurosurgery and Urology. And we're among the state's best for Geriatrics, Orthopedics and Gastroenterology & GI Surgery. Now more than ever, being recognized among the best only inspires us to keep getting better.

Learn more at HackensackMeridianHealth.org

*Tie 2021-2022

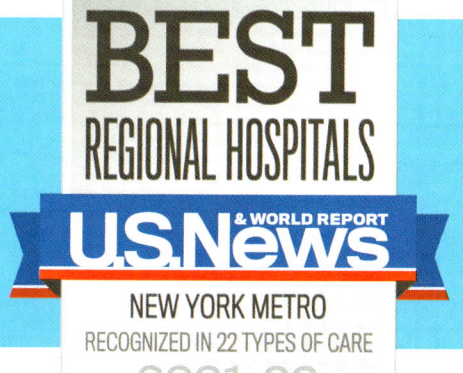
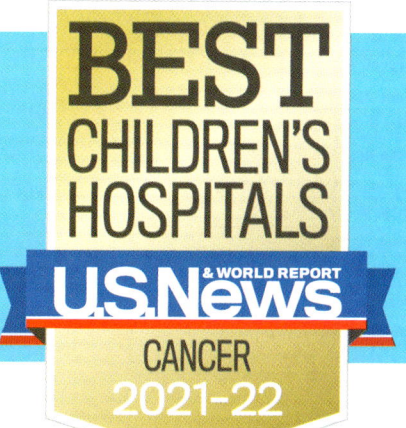

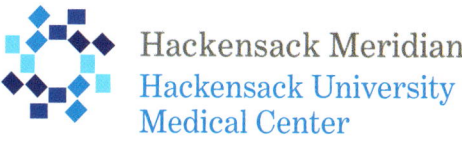
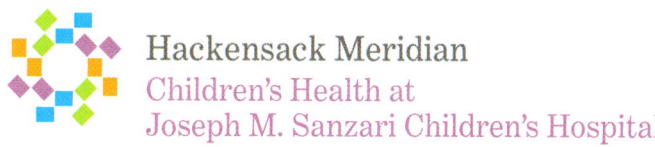

BEST REGIONAL HOSPITALS

COMPLEX SPECIALTY CARE
- 🔴 Nationally ranked
- 🔵 High performing

COMMON PROCEDURES & CONDITIONS
- 🔵 High performing
- 🟠 Average
- ⚫ Below average

Complex specialty care columns: Cancer, Cardiology & Heart Surgery, Orthopedics, Other Specialties (Nationally Ranked), Other Specialties (High Performing)

Common procedures & conditions columns: Colon Cancer Surgery, Lung Cancer Surgery, Heart Attack, Heart Failure, Heart Bypass Surgery, Heart Valve Surgery, TAVR*, Abdominal Aortic Aneurysm, Stroke, Back Surgery, Hip Replacement, Knee Replacement, Hip Fracture, Diabetes, Kidney Failure, Pneumonia, COPD*

State Rank	Hospital
	NEW JERSEY continued
4	Overlook Medical Center, Summit
5	Saint Barnabas Medical Center, Livingston
6	Robert Wood Johnson University Hospital, New Brunswick
7	AtlantiCare Regional Medical Center, Atlantic City
7	Cooper University Health Care-Camden
7	Jersey Shore University Medical Center, Neptune
10	Jefferson Hlth.-Stratford, Cherry Hill & Washington Twsp.
10	Our Lady of Lourdes Hospital, Camden
10	Virtua Voorhees, Voorhees
13	Riverview Medical Center, Red Bank
	NEW MEXICO
1	Presbyterian Hospital, Albuquerque
	NEW YORK
1	New York-Presbyterian Hospital-Columbia and Cornell
2	NYU Langone Hospitals, New York[22]
3	Mount Sinai Hospital, New York
4	Lenox Hill Hospital, New York[23]
5	North Shore University Hospital, Manhasset
6	St. Francis Hospital & Heart Center, Roslyn
7	Long Island Jewish Medical Center, New Hyde Park
7	Montefiore Medical Center, Bronx
9	Mount Sinai Morningside & Mount Sinai West Hosps., New York
10	Huntington Hospital, Huntington
10	New York-Presbyterian Brooklyn Methodist Hospital, Brooklyn
12	St. Peter's Hospital-Albany
12	Stony Brook University Hospital, Stony Brook
14	Albany Medical Center, Albany
15	Mount Sinai Beth Israel, New York
15	Northern Westchester Hospital, Mount Kisco
17	Buffalo General Medical Center
17	Rochester General Hospital, Rochester
17	St. Joseph's Health Hospital, Syracuse
17	Strong Memorial Hospital of the University of Rochester[24]
21	White Plains Hospital, White Plains
22	Southside Hospital, Bay Shore
23	Staten Island University Hospital, Staten Island
24	Garnet Health Medical Center-Catskills, Middletown
24	Mount Sinai South Nassau, Oceanside
24	New York-Presbyterian/Queens, Flushing
24	Upstate University Hospital, Syracuse
28	Good Samaritan Hospital-West Islip
28	Highland Hospital, Rochester
28	Mercy Hospital-Buffalo

In complex care specialties, (-) indicates hospital is not nationally ranked or high performing. In procedures and conditions, (-) indicates care not offered or hospital has too few Medicare patients to be rated. *TAVR: Transcatheter aortic valve replacement. *COPD: Chronic obstructive pulmonary disease

A footnote indicates that another hospital's results are included, that the hospital has a different name in one or more areas of care, or both.
[22]Perlmutter Cancer Center at NYU Langone Hospitals; NYU Langone Orthopedic Hospital; Rusk Rehabilitation at NYU Langone Hospitals.
[23]Manhattan Eye, Ear & Throat Hospital. [24]Wilmot Cancer Institute.

COMPLEX SPECIALTY CARE

- ● Nationally ranked
- ● High performing

COMMON PROCEDURES & CONDITIONS

- ● High performing
- ● Average
- ● Below average

State Rank Hospital	CANCER	CARDIOLOGY & HEART SURGERY	ORTHOPEDICS	OTHER SPECIALTIES (Nationally ranked)	OTHER SPECIALTIES (High performing)	COLON CANCER SURGERY	LUNG CANCER SURGERY	HEART ATTACK	HEART FAILURE	HEART BYPASS SURGERY	HEART VALVE SURGERY	TAVR*	ABDOMINAL AORTIC ANEURYSM	STROKE	BACK SURGERY	HIP REPLACEMENT	KNEE REPLACEMENT	HIP FRACTURE	DIABETES	KIDNEY FAILURE	PNEUMONIA	COPD*
NEW YORK continued																						
28 Vassar Brothers Medical Center, Poughkeepsie	–	–	–	–	–	●	●	●	●	●	●	●	●	●	●	●	●	●	●	●	●	●
32 Maimonides Medical Center, Brooklyn	–	–	–	–	–	●	●	●	●	●	●	●	●	●	●	●	●	●	●	●	●	●
33 Wyckoff Heights Medical Center, Brooklyn	–	–	–	–	●	–	●	–	–	–	–	–	●	–	–	●	●	●	●	●	●	●
34 Ellis Hospital, Schenectady	–	–	–	–	–	●	●	●	●	●	●	●	–	●	–	●	●	●	●	●	●	●
NORTH CAROLINA																						
1 Duke University Hospital, Durham	●	●	●	8	2	●	●	●	●	●	●	●	●	●	●	●	●	●	●	●	●	●
2 University of North Carolina Hospitals, Chapel Hill	●	–	–	4	1	●	●	●	●	●	●	●	●	●	●	●	●	●	●	●	●	●
3 Carolinas Medical Center, Charlotte[25]	●	–	●	–	2	●	●	●	●	●	●	●	●	●	●	●	●	●	●	●	●	●
3 UNC Rex Hospital, Raleigh	–	–	–	–	1	●	●	●	●	●	●	●	●	●	●	●	●	●	●	●	●	●
5 FirstHealth Moore Regional Hospital, Pinehurst	–	–	–	–	–	●	●	●	●	●	●	●	●	●	●	●	●	●	●	●	●	●
5 Vidant Medical Center, Greenville	–	–	–	–	2	●	●	●	●	●	●	●	●	●	●	●	●	●	●	●	●	●
7 Moses H. Cone Memorial Hospital, Greensboro	–	–	–	–	2	●	●	●	●	●	●	●	●	●	●	●	●	●	●	●	●	●
8 Wake Forest Baptist Medical Center, Winston-Salem	–	–	–	–	1	●	●	●	●	●	●	●	●	●	●	●	●	●	●	●	●	●
9 CarolinaEast Medical Center, New Bern	–	–	–	1	–	●	●	●	●	●	●	–	●	●	●	●	●	●	●	●	●	●
9 Duke Regional Hospital, Durham	–	–	–	1	–	●	–	●	●	–	–	–	●	●	–	●	●	●	●	●	●	●
11 New Hanover Regional Medical Center, Wilmington	–	–	–	–	–	●	●	●	●	●	●	●	●	●	●	●	●	●	●	●	●	●
12 Mission Hospital-Asheville	–	–	–	–	–	●	●	●	●	●	●	●	●	●	●	●	●	●	●	●	●	●
12 WakeMed Health and Hospitals, Raleigh Campus, Raleigh	–	–	–	1	–	●	●	●	●	●	●	●	●	●	●	●	●	●	●	●	●	●
14 CaroMont Regional Medical Center, Gastonia	–	–	–	–	–	●	●	●	●	●	●	●	●	●	●	●	●	●	●	●	●	●
14 Carolinas Healthcare Northeast, Concord	–	–	–	–	–	●	●	●	●	●	●	–	●	●	●	●	●	●	●	●	●	●
16 Carolinas Healthcare System Pineville, Charlotte	–	–	–	–	–	●	–	●	●	●	●	●	●	●	●	●	●	●	●	●	●	●
16 Novant Health Forsyth Medical Center, Winston-Salem	–	–	–	–	–	●	●	●	●	●	●	●	●	●	●	●	●	●	●	●	●	●
18 Cape Fear Valley Medical Center, Fayetteville	–	–	–	–	–	●	●	●	●	●	●	●	●	●	●	●	●	●	●	●	●	●
NORTH DAKOTA																						
1 Sanford Medical Center Fargo	–	–	–	–	1	●	●	●	●	●	●	●	●	●	●	●	●	●	●	●	●	●
2 Sanford Medical Center Bismarck	–	–	–	–	–	●	●	●	●	●	●	●	●	●	●	●	●	●	●	●	●	●
3 CHI St. Alexius Health-Bismarck	–	–	–	–	1	●	●	●	●	●	●	●	–	●	●	●	●	●	●	●	●	●
OHIO																						
1 Cleveland Clinic	●	●	●	10	–	●	●	●	●	●	●	●	●	●	●	●	●	●	●	●	●	●
2 Ohio State University Wexner Medical Center, Columbus[26]	●	●	–	8	1	●	●	●	●	●	●	●	●	●	●	●	●	●	●	●	●	●
3 University Hospitals Cleveland Medical Center[27]	●	●	–	3	3	●	●	●	●	●	●	●	●	●	●	●	●	●	●	●	●	●
4 Christ Hospital, Cincinnati	–	●	●	–	2	●	●	●	●	●	●	●	●	●	●	●	●	●	●	●	●	●
4 Cleveland Clinic Hillcrest Hospital	●	●	●	2	3	●	●	●	●	●	●	●	●	●	●	●	●	●	●	●	●	●
6 Cleveland Clinic Fairview Hospital	–	–	●	1	4	●	●	●	●	●	●	●	●	●	●	●	●	●	●	●	●	●
7 Cleveland Clinic Akron General, Akron	–	–	●	–	6	●	●	●	●	●	●	●	●	●	●	●	●	●	●	●	●	●
8 Miami Valley Hospital, Dayton	–	–	●	–	2	●	●	●	●	●	●	●	●	●	●	●	●	●	●	●	●	●
8 OhioHealth Riverside Methodist Hospital, Columbus	–	–	–	–	1	●	●	●	●	●	●	●	●	●	●	●	●	●	●	●	●	●
8 ProMedica Toledo Hospital, Toledo	–	–	–	–	–	●	●	●	●	●	●	●	●	●	●	●	●	●	●	●	●	●
11 Aultman Hospital, Canton	–	–	–	–	–	●	●	●	●	●	●	●	●	●	●	●	●	●	●	●	●	●
11 Kettering Medical Center, Kettering	–	–	–	–	–	●	●	●	●	●	●	●	●	●	●	●	●	●	●	●	●	●
13 Mount Carmel East and West Hospitals, Columbus	–	–	–	–	–	●	●	●	●	●	●	●	●	●	●	●	●	●	●	●	●	●
14 Mount Carmel St. Ann's, Westerville	–	–	–	–	–	●	●	●	●	●	●	–	●	●	●	●	●	●	●	●	●	●
14 St. Rita's Medical Center, Lima	–	–	–	–	1	●	●	●	●	●	●	●	●	●	●	●	●	●	●	●	●	●

In complex care specialties, (–) indicates hospital is not nationally ranked or high performing. In procedures and conditions, (–) indicates care not offered or hospital has too few Medicare patients to be rated. *TAVR: Transcatheter aortic valve replacement. *COPD: Chronic obstructive pulmonary disease

A footnote indicates that another hospital's results are included, that the hospital has a different name in one or more areas of care, or both.
[25] Levine Cancer Institute; Sanger Heart & Vascular Institute. [26] Ohio State University James Cancer Hospital. [27] University Hospitals Seidman Cancer Center.

BEST REGIONAL HOSPITALS

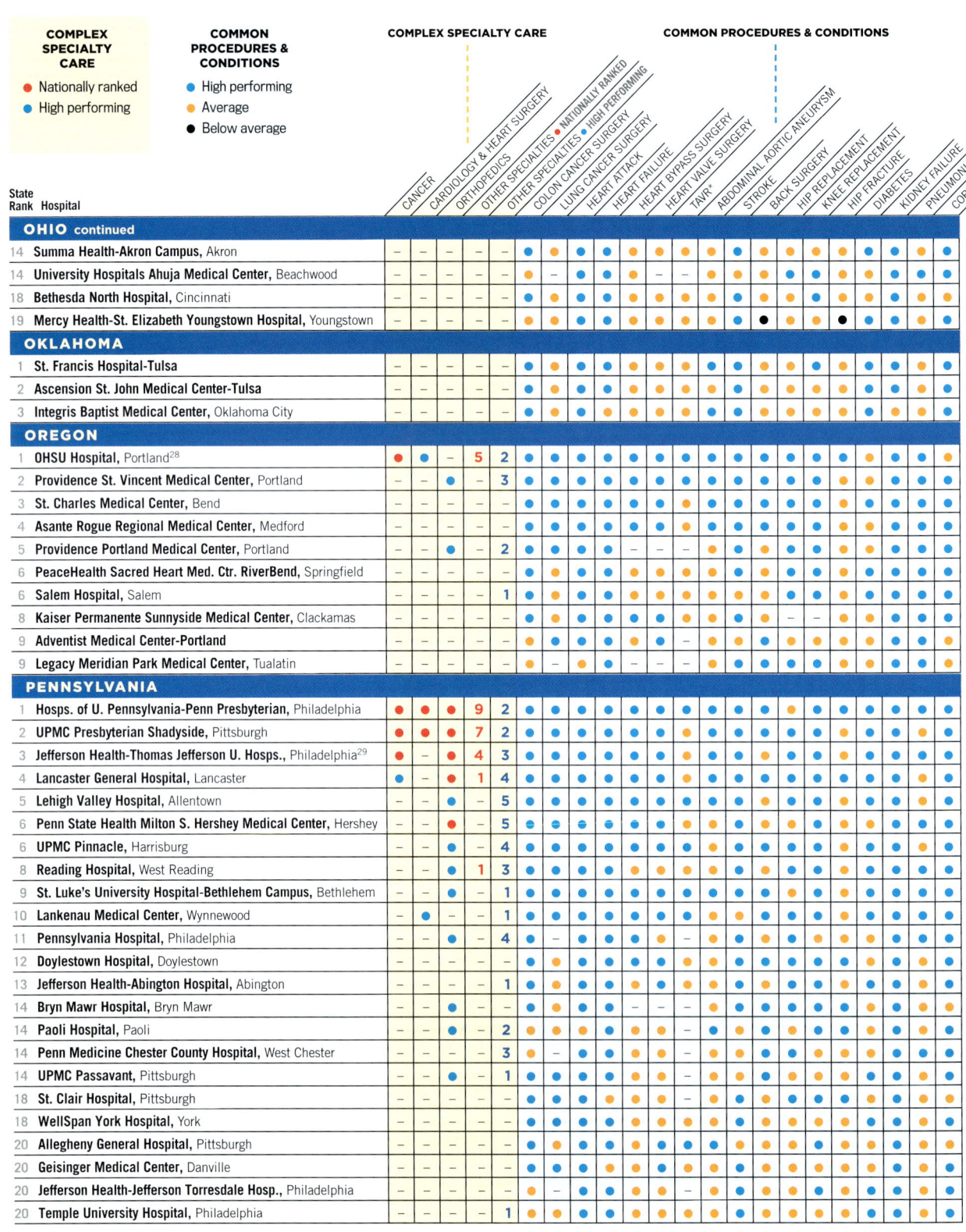

Legend:
- COMPLEX SPECIALTY CARE: ● Nationally ranked, ● High performing
- COMMON PROCEDURES & CONDITIONS: ● High performing, ● Average, ● Below average

State Rank	Hospital	Cancer	Cardiology & Heart Surgery	Orthopedics	Other Specialties	Other Specialties	Colon Cancer Surgery	Lung Cancer Surgery	Heart Attack	Heart Failure	Heart Bypass Surgery	Heart Valve Surgery	TAVR*	Abdominal Aortic Aneurysm	Stroke	Back Surgery	Hip Replacement	Knee Replacement	Hip Fracture	Diabetes	Kidney Failure	Pneumonia	COPD*
OHIO continued																							
14	Summa Health-Akron Campus, Akron	–	–	–	–	–	●	●	●	●	●	●	●	●	●	●	●	●	●	●	●	●	●
14	University Hospitals Ahuja Medical Center, Beachwood	–	–	–	–	–	●	–	●	●	–	–	●	●	●	●	●	●	●	●	●	●	●
18	Bethesda North Hospital, Cincinnati	–	–	–	–	–	●	●	●	●	●	●	●	●	●	●	●	●	●	●	●	●	●
19	Mercy Health-St. Elizabeth Youngstown Hospital, Youngstown	–	–	–	–	–	●	●	●	●	●	●	●	●	●	●	●	●	●	●	●	●	●
OKLAHOMA																							
1	St. Francis Hospital-Tulsa	–	–	–	–	–	●	●	●	●	●	●	●	●	●	●	●	●	●	●	●	●	●
2	Ascension St. John Medical Center-Tulsa	–	–	–	–	–	●	●	●	●	●	●	●	●	●	●	●	●	●	●	●	●	●
3	Integris Baptist Medical Center, Oklahoma City	–	–	–	–	–	●	●	●	●	●	●	●	●	●	●	●	●	●	●	●	●	●
OREGON																							
1	OHSU Hospital, Portland[28]	●	●	–	5	2	●	●	●	●	●	●	●	●	●	●	●	●	●	●	●	●	●
2	Providence St. Vincent Medical Center, Portland	–	–	●	–	3	●	●	●	●	●	●	●	●	●	●	●	●	●	●	●	●	●
3	St. Charles Medical Center, Bend	–	–	–	–	–	●	●	●	●	●	●	●	●	●	●	●	●	●	●	●	●	●
4	Asante Rogue Regional Medical Center, Medford	–	–	–	–	–	●	●	●	●	●	●	●	●	●	●	●	●	●	●	●	●	●
5	Providence Portland Medical Center, Portland	–	–	●	–	2	●	●	●	●	–	–	●	●	●	●	●	●	●	●	●	●	●
6	PeaceHealth Sacred Heart Med. Ctr. RiverBend, Springfield	–	–	–	–	–	●	●	●	●	●	●	●	●	●	●	●	●	●	●	●	●	●
6	Salem Hospital, Salem	–	–	–	–	1	●	●	●	●	●	●	●	●	●	●	●	●	●	●	●	●	●
8	Kaiser Permanente Sunnyside Medical Center, Clackamas	–	–	●	–	–	●	●	●	●	●	●	●	●	●	●	●	●	–	–	●	●	●
9	Adventist Medical Center-Portland	–	–	–	–	–	●	●	●	●	●	●	●	●	●	●	●	●	●	●	●	●	●
9	Legacy Meridian Park Medical Center, Tualatin	–	–	–	–	–	●	–	●	–	–	–	●	●	●	●	●	●	●	●	●	●	●
PENNSYLVANIA																							
1	Hosps. of U. Pennsylvania-Penn Presbyterian, Philadelphia	●	●	●	9	2	●	●	●	●	●	●	●	●	●	●	●	●	●	●	●	●	●
2	UPMC Presbyterian Shadyside, Pittsburgh	●	●	●	7	2	●	●	●	●	●	●	●	●	●	●	●	●	●	●	●	●	●
3	Jefferson Health-Thomas Jefferson U. Hosps., Philadelphia[29]	●	–	●	4	3	●	●	●	●	●	●	●	●	●	●	●	●	●	●	●	●	●
4	Lancaster General Hospital, Lancaster	●	–	●	1	4	●	●	●	●	●	●	●	●	●	●	●	●	●	●	●	●	●
5	Lehigh Valley Hospital, Allentown	–	–	●	–	5	●	●	●	●	●	●	●	●	●	●	●	●	●	●	●	●	●
6	Penn State Health Milton S. Hershey Medical Center, Hershey	–	–	●	–	5	●	●	●	●	●	●	●	●	●	●	●	●	●	●	●	●	●
6	UPMC Pinnacle, Harrisburg	–	–	●	–	4	●	●	●	●	●	●	●	●	●	●	●	●	●	●	●	●	●
8	Reading Hospital, West Reading	–	–	●	1	3	●	●	●	●	●	●	●	●	●	●	●	●	●	●	●	●	●
9	St. Luke's University Hospital-Bethlehem Campus, Bethlehem	–	–	●	–	1	●	●	●	●	●	●	●	●	●	●	●	●	●	●	●	●	●
10	Lankenau Medical Center, Wynnewood	–	●	–	–	1	●	●	●	●	●	●	●	●	●	●	●	●	●	●	●	●	●
11	Pennsylvania Hospital, Philadelphia	–	–	●	–	4	●	●	●	●	●	–	●	●	●	●	●	●	●	●	●	●	●
12	Doylestown Hospital, Doylestown	–	–	–	–	–	●	●	●	●	●	●	●	●	●	●	●	●	●	●	●	●	●
13	Jefferson Health-Abington Hospital, Abington	–	–	●	–	1	●	●	●	●	●	●	●	●	●	●	●	●	●	●	●	●	●
14	Bryn Mawr Hospital, Bryn Mawr	–	–	●	–	–	●	●	●	●	–	–	●	●	●	●	●	●	●	●	●	●	●
14	Paoli Hospital, Paoli	–	–	●	–	2	●	●	●	●	●	●	●	●	●	●	●	●	●	●	●	●	●
14	Penn Medicine Chester County Hospital, West Chester	–	–	–	–	3	●	–	●	●	–	–	●	●	●	●	●	●	●	●	●	●	●
14	UPMC Passavant, Pittsburgh	–	–	●	–	1	●	●	●	●	●	●	●	●	●	●	●	●	●	●	●	●	●
18	St. Clair Hospital, Pittsburgh	–	–	–	–	–	●	●	●	●	●	●	●	●	●	●	●	●	●	●	●	●	●
18	WellSpan York Hospital, York	–	–	–	–	–	●	●	●	●	●	●	●	●	●	●	●	●	●	●	●	●	●
20	Allegheny General Hospital, Pittsburgh	–	–	–	–	–	●	●	●	●	●	●	●	●	●	●	●	●	●	●	●	●	●
20	Geisinger Medical Center, Danville	–	–	–	–	–	●	●	●	●	●	●	●	●	●	●	●	●	●	●	●	●	●
20	Jefferson Health-Jefferson Torresdale Hosp., Philadelphia	–	–	–	–	–	●	●	●	●	–	–	●	●	●	●	●	●	●	●	●	●	●
20	Temple University Hospital, Philadelphia	–	–	–	–	1	●	●	●	●	●	●	●	●	●	●	●	●	●	●	●	●	●

In complex care specialties, (–) indicates hospital is not nationally ranked or high performing. In procedures and conditions, (–) indicates care not offered or hospital has too few Medicare patients to be rated. *TAVR: Transcatheter aortic valve replacement. *COPD: Chronic obstructive pulmonary disease

A footnote indicates that another hospital's results are included, that the hospital has a different name in one or more areas of care, or both.
[28] OHSU Hospital-Knight Cancer Institute; OHSU Hospital-Harold Schnitzer Diabetes Health Center; OHSU Hospital-Knight Cardiovascular Institute. [29] Thomas Jefferson University Hospitals-Sidney Kimmel Cancer Center; Thomas Jefferson University Hospitals-Vickie and Jack Farber Institute for Neuroscience; Rothman Orthopaedics at Thomas Jefferson University Hospitals; Thomas Jefferson University Hospitals-Jane and Leonard Korman Respiratory Institute.

Legend

COMPLEX SPECIALTY CARE
- ● Nationally ranked
- ● High performing

COMMON PROCEDURES & CONDITIONS
- ● High performing
- ● Average
- ● Below average

Best Hospitals

State Rank Hospital	CANCER	CARDIOLOGY & HEART SURGERY	ORTHOPEDICS	OTHER SPECIALTIES NATIONALLY RANKED	OTHER SPECIALTIES HIGH PERFORMING	COLON CANCER SURGERY	LUNG CANCER SURGERY	HEART ATTACK	HEART FAILURE	HEART BYPASS SURGERY	HEART VALVE SURGERY	TAVR*	ABDOMINAL AORTIC ANEURYSM	STROKE	BACK SURGERY	HIP REPLACEMENT	KNEE REPLACEMENT	HIP FRACTURE	DIABETES	KIDNEY FAILURE	PNEUMONIA	COPD*
PENNSYLVANIA continued																						
24 Riddle Hospital, Media	–	–	–	–	–	●	–	●	●	–	–	–	–	●	●	●	●	●	●	●	●	●
24 St. Mary Medical Center-Langhorne	–	–	–	–	–	●	●	●	●	●	●	●	●	●	●	●	●	●	●	●	●	●
24 UPMC Hamot, Erie	–	–	–	–	–	●	●	●	●	●	●	●	●	●	●	●	●	●	●	●	●	●
27 Einstein Medical Center Philadelphia	–	–	–	–	–	●	●	●	●	●	–	–	●	●	●	●	●	●	●	●	●	●
28 UPMC Altoona, Altoona	–	–	–	–	–	●	●	●	●	●	●	–	●	●	●	●	●	●	●	●	●	●
RHODE ISLAND																						
1 Miriam Hospital, Providence	–	–	●	–	2	●	●	●	–	●	●	●	●	●	●	●	●	●	●	●	●	●
2 Rhode Island Hospital, Providence	–	–	–	–	–	●	●	●	●	●	●	●	●	●	●	●	●	●	●	●	●	●
SOUTH CAROLINA																						
1 MUSC Health-University Medical Center, Charleston	●	–	●	2	3	●	●	●	●	●	●	●	●	●	●	●	●	●	●	●	●	●
2 Bon Secours St. Francis Health System-Greenville	–	–	–	–	–	●	●	●	●	●	●	●	●	●	●	●	●	●	●	●	●	●
3 McLeod Regional Medical Center, Florence	–	–	–	–	–	●	●	●	●	●	●	●	●	●	●	●	●	●	●	●	●	●
3 Spartanburg Medical Center, Spartanburg	–	–	–	–	–	●	●	●	●	●	●	●	●	●	●	●	●	●	●	●	●	●
5 Lexington Medical Center, West Columbia	–	–	–	–	–	●	●	●	●	●	●	●	●	●	●	●	●	●	●	●	●	●
6 Roper Hospital, Charleston	–	–	–	–	–	●	●	●	●	●	●	●	●	●	●	●	●	●	●	●	●	●
7 AnMed Health Medical Center, Anderson	–	–	–	–	–	●	●	●	●	●	●	●	●	●	●	●	●	●	●	●	●	●
8 Grand Strand Regional Medical Center, Myrtle Beach	–	–	–	–	–	●	●	●	●	●	●	●	●	●	●	●	●	●	●	●	●	●
SOUTH DAKOTA																						
1 Sanford USD Medical Center, Sioux Falls	–	–	●	–	2	●	●	●	●	●	●	●	●	●	●	●	●	●	●	●	●	●
2 Avera McKennan Hospital and U. Health Center, Sioux Falls	●	–	–	1	1	●	●	●	●	–	–	–	●	●	●	●	●	●	●	●	●	●
TENNESSEE																						
1 Vanderbilt University Medical Center, Nashville	●	●	●	7	3	●	●	●	●	●	●	●	●	●	●	●	●	●	●	●	●	●
2 Baptist Memorial Hospital-Memphis	–	–	–	–	–	●	●	●	●	●	●	●	●	●	●	●	●	●	●	●	●	●
2 CHI Memorial Hospital, Chattanooga	–	–	–	–	–	●	●	●	●	●	●	●	●	●	●	●	●	●	●	●	●	●
2 University of Tennessee Medical Center, Knoxville	–	–	–	–	–	●	●	●	●	●	●	●	●	●	●	●	●	●	●	●	●	●
5 Ascension Saint Thomas Hospital West, Nashville	–	–	–	–	–	●	●	●	●	●	●	●	●	●	●	●	●	●	●	●	●	●
6 Methodist Hospitals of Memphis	–	–	–	–	–	●	●	●	●	●	●	●	●	●	●	●	●	●	●	●	●	●
7 Fort Sanders Regional Medical Center, Knoxville	–	–	–	–	–	●	●	●	●	●	–	–	●	●	●	●	●	●	●	●	●	●
8 Parkwest Medical Center, Knoxville	–	–	–	–	–	●	●	●	●	●	●	●	●	●	●	●	●	●	●	●	●	●
8 TriStar Centennial Medical Center, Nashville	–	–	–	–	–	●	●	●	●	●	●	●	●	●	●	●	●	●	●	●	●	●
10 Erlanger Medical Center, Chattanooga	–	–	–	–	–	●	●	●	●	●	●	●	●	●	●	●	●	●	●	●	●	●
TEXAS																						
1 Houston Methodist Hospital	●	●	●	7	–	●	●	●	●	●	●	●	●	●	●	●	●	●	●	●	●	●
2 UT Southwestern Medical Center, Dallas	●	●	●	7	–	●	●	●	●	●	●	●	●	●	●	●	●	●	●	●	●	●
3 Baylor St. Luke's Medical Center, Houston[30]	●	●	–	3	2	●	●	●	●	●	●	●	●	●	●	●	●	●	●	●	●	●
4 Memorial Hermann-Texas Medical Center, Houston	●	●	–	1	5	●	●	●	●	●	●	●	●	●	●	●	●	●	●	●	●	●
5 Baylor University Medical Center, Dallas[31]	●	–	●	2	3	●	●	●	●	●	●	–	●	●	●	●	●	●	●	●	●	●
6 Memorial Hermann Greater Heights Hospital, Houston	–	–	●	–	4	●	●	●	●	●	●	●	●	●	●	●	●	●	●	●	●	●
6 Memorial Hermann Memorial City Medical Center, Houston	–	–	●	–	–	●	●	●	●	●	●	●	●	●	●	●	●	●	●	●	●	●
8 Ascension Seton Medical Center Austin	–	–	–	–	1	●	●	●	●	●	●	●	●	●	●	●	●	●	●	●	●	●
8 Baylor Scott and White Medical Center-Temple	–	–	●	–	1	●	●	●	●	●	●	●	●	●	●	●	●	●	●	●	●	●
8 Houston Methodist Sugar Land Hospital, Sugar Land	–	–	–	1	3	●	●	●	●	–	●	●	●	●	●	●	●	●	●	●	●	●
11 St. David's Medical Center, Austin	–	–	–	1	–	●	–	●	●	●	●	●	●	●	●	●	●	●	●	●	●	●

In complex care specialties, (-) indicates hospital is not nationally ranked or high performing. In procedures and conditions, (-) indicates care not offered or hospital has too few Medicare patients to be rated. *TAVR: Transcatheter aortic valve replacement. *COPD: Chronic obstructive pulmonary disease

A footnote indicates that another hospital's results are included, that the hospital has a different name in one or more areas of care, or both.
[30] Dan L Duncan Comprehensive Cancer Center at Baylor St. Luke's Medical Center; Texas Heart Institute at Baylor St. Luke's Medical Center.
[31] Baylor University Medical Center and Baylor Scott and White Heart and Vascular Hospital-Dallas.

BEST **REGIONAL** HOSPITALS

COMPLEX SPECIALTY CARE
- ● (red) Nationally ranked
- ● (blue) High performing

COMMON PROCEDURES & CONDITIONS
- ● (blue) High performing
- ● (orange) Average
- ● (black) Below average

COMPLEX SPECIALTY CARE: Cancer through Other specialties ● high performing. COMMON PROCEDURES & CONDITIONS: Colon cancer surgery through COPD*.

State Rank	Hospital	Cancer	Cardiology & Heart Surgery	Orthopedics	Other Specialties ● Nationally Ranked	Other Specialties ● High Performing	Colon Cancer Surgery	Lung Cancer Surgery	Heart Attack	Heart Failure	Heart Bypass Surgery	Heart Valve Surgery	TAVR*	Abdominal Aortic Aneurysm	Stroke	Back Surgery	Hip Replacement	Knee Replacement	Hip Fracture	Diabetes	Kidney Failure	Pneumonia	COPD*
	TEXAS continued																						
12	**Christus Mother Frances Hospital-Tyler**	–	–	blue	–	–	blue	orange	blue	blue	orange	orange	orange	blue	blue	orange	orange	blue	orange	blue	blue	orange	blue
12	**Houston Methodist Willowbrook Hospital**	–	–	blue	–	1	orange	orange	blue	blue	orange	–	–	orange	blue	blue	orange	orange	orange	blue	blue	blue	blue
12	**Texas Health Presbyterian Hospital Dallas**	–	–	blue	1	–	blue	orange	blue	blue	orange	orange	orange	orange	blue	orange	blue	blue	orange	blue	blue	orange	blue
15	**Medical City Dallas**	–	–	–	–	–	orange	blue	blue	blue	blue	orange	orange	orange	blue	orange	orange	blue	orange	orange	blue	orange	blue
15	**Methodist Hospital-San Antonio**	–	–	–	–	–	blue	orange	blue	blue	orange	orange	orange	orange	blue	orange	orange	blue	orange	blue	blue	orange	blue
15	**Texas Health Harris Methodist Hospital Fort Worth**	–	–	–	–	–	blue	orange	blue	blue	blue	orange	orange	orange	blue	orange	orange	orange	orange	blue	blue	orange	blue
18	**BSA Hospital,** Amarillo	–	–	–	–	–	blue	orange	blue	blue	orange	orange	–	orange	blue	blue	black	orange	orange	blue	blue	orange	blue
18	**Baptist Medical Center,** San Antonio	–	–	–	–	–	blue	blue	blue	blue	orange	orange	black	orange	orange	orange	blue	blue	orange	blue	blue	orange	orange
18	**Covenant Medical Center-Lubbock**	–	–	–	–	–	blue	black	blue	blue	orange	orange	orange	orange	blue	orange	orange	blue	orange	blue	blue	blue	orange
18	**Texas Health Harris Methodist Hosp. Southwest,** Fort Worth	–	–	blue	–	–	orange	–	orange	blue	–	–	–	–	orange	blue	blue	blue	orange	orange	blue	orange	blue
22	**Baylor Scott and White All Saints Med. Center-Fort Worth**	–	–	–	–	–	blue	–	blue	blue	orange	orange	orange	orange	orange	orange	orange	orange	orange	orange	blue	blue	blue
22	**Baylor Scott and White Medical Center-Round Rock**	–	–	–	–	–	orange	orange	blue	blue	orange	orange	–	–	blue	blue	orange	orange	orange	orange	blue	blue	orange
22	**East Texas Medical Center Tyler**	–	–	–	–	–	blue	orange	blue	blue	orange	orange	orange	orange	blue	orange	orange	orange	orange	orange	blue	orange	blue
22	**University Medical Center-Lubbock**	–	–	–	–	–	orange	orange	blue	blue	orange	orange	orange	orange	blue	orange	orange	orange	orange	orange	blue	blue	blue
26	**HCA Houston Healthcare Clear Lake,** League City	–	–	–	–	–	orange	orange	blue	blue	orange	black	black	orange	blue	orange	orange	orange	orange	blue	blue	orange	blue
26	**Methodist Dallas Medical Center**	–	–	–	–	–	blue	orange	orange	blue	orange	black	orange	orange	blue	orange	orange	orange	orange	orange	blue	blue	blue
26	**South Texas Health System-Edinburg**	–	–	–	–	–	orange	–	blue	blue	orange	black	–	orange	blue	black	–	orange	orange	blue	blue	blue	blue
29	**Las Palmas Medical Center,** El Paso	–	–	–	–	–	orange	orange	blue	blue	black	black	–	orange	blue	orange	orange	orange	orange	blue	blue	orange	blue
29	**Texoma Medical Center,** Denison	–	–	–	–	–	orange	black	blue	blue	orange	black	orange	orange	blue	orange	orange	orange	orange	blue	blue	orange	blue
29	**University of Texas Medical Branch,** Galveston	–	–	–	–	–	orange	orange	blue	blue	orange	black	orange	orange	blue	orange	black	orange	orange	orange	blue	blue	blue
	UTAH																						
1	**University of Utah Hospital,** Salt Lake City[32]	red	–	–	1	3	blue	blue	blue	blue	blue	orange	blue	blue	blue	blue	blue	blue	blue	orange	blue	blue	orange
2	**Intermountain Medical Center,** Murray	–	–	–	–	1	orange	orange	blue	blue	blue	blue	blue	blue	blue	blue	orange	orange	orange	blue	blue	blue	blue
3	**Intermountain St. George Regional Hospital,** Saint George	–	–	–	–	–	orange	orange	blue	blue	blue	orange	orange	blue	blue	blue	blue	blue	blue	orange	blue	blue	orange
4	**Utah Valley Regional Medical Center,** Provo	–	–	–	–	–	orange	orange	blue	blue	blue	blue	–	blue	blue	blue	orange	blue	orange	orange	blue	blue	orange
5	**McKay-Dee Hospital Center,** Ogden	–	–	–	–	–	orange	orange	blue	orange	orange	orange	orange	blue	blue	blue	orange	blue	orange	orange	blue	blue	orange
	VERMONT																						
1	**University of Vermont Medical Center,** Burlington	–	–	–	–	–	blue	orange	blue	blue	orange	orange	orange	orange	blue	orange	blue	orange	orange	orange	blue	blue	orange
	VIRGINIA																						
1	**Inova Fairfax Hospital,** Falls Church	–	blue	blue	1	6	blue	blue	blue	blue	blue	blue	blue	blue	blue	blue	blue	blue	orange	blue	blue	blue	blue
2	**University of Virginia Medical Center,** Charlottesville	blue	–	blue	–	4	blue	blue	blue	blue	blue	blue	orange	blue	blue	blue	blue	blue	orange	blue	blue	blue	blue
3	**Sentara Norfolk General Hospital,** Norfolk[33]	–	–	–	1	2	orange	blue	blue	blue	blue	blue	blue	orange	blue	orange	–	–	orange	blue	blue	blue	blue
3	**VCU Medical Center,** Richmond	blue	blue	blue	–	2	blue	blue	blue	blue	blue	orange	orange	orange	blue	orange	orange	orange	orange	orange	blue	blue	blue
3	**Winchester Medical Center,** Winchester	–	–	–	–	2	blue	blue	blue	blue	blue	blue	orange	orange	blue	orange	orange	blue	orange	blue	blue	blue	blue
6	**Carilion Roanoke Memorial Hospital,** Roanoke	–	–	–	–	–	blue	blue	blue	blue	blue	blue	blue	orange	blue	orange	blue	blue	orange	blue	blue	orange	blue
6	**Centra Lynchburg General Hospital,** Lynchburg	–	–	–	–	2	blue	blue	blue	blue	orange	orange	orange	orange	blue	orange	blue	blue	orange	blue	blue	orange	blue
8	**Virginia Hospital Center,** Arlington	–	–	blue	–	–	blue	blue	blue	blue	orange	orange	orange	orange	blue	orange	blue	blue	blue	orange	blue	orange	blue
9	**Sentara RMH Medical Center,** Harrisonburg	–	–	–	–	1	blue	orange	blue	blue	orange	orange	orange	orange	blue	orange	blue	orange	orange	blue	blue	blue	blue
10	**Inova Fair Oaks Hospital,** Fairfax	–	–	–	–	1	blue	–	orange	blue	–	–	–	orange	orange	blue	blue	blue	orange	orange	blue	blue	blue
10	**Mary Washington Hospital,** Fredericksburg	–	–	–	–	–	blue	blue	orange	blue	orange	orange	orange	orange	blue	orange	blue	blue	orange	blue	blue	orange	blue
10	**Sentara Martha Jefferson Hospital,** Charlottesville	–	–	–	–	1	blue	blue	orange	blue	–	–	–	orange	blue	orange	orange	blue	orange	orange	blue	blue	blue
13	**Inova Alexandria Hospital,** Alexandria	–	–	–	–	–	blue	–	orange	blue	–	–	–	orange	blue	orange	orange	blue	orange	blue	blue	blue	blue
13	**Inova Loudoun Hospital,** Leesburg	–	–	–	1	3	orange	–	orange	blue	–	–	–	–	orange	orange	orange	orange	orange	orange	blue	orange	blue

In complex care specialties, (-) indicates hospital is not nationally ranked or high performing. In procedures and conditions, (-) indicates care not offered or hospital has too few Medicare patients to be rated. *TAVR: Transcatheter aortic valve replacement. *COPD: Chronic obstructive pulmonary disease

A footnote indicates that another hospital's results are included, that the hospital has a different name in one or more areas of care, or both.
[32]Huntsman Cancer Institute at the University of Utah.
[33]Sentara Norfolk General Hospital-Sentara Heart Hospital.

More @ usnews.com/bestregionalhospitals

COMPLEX SPECIALTY CARE
- 🔴 Nationally ranked
- 🔵 High performing

COMMON PROCEDURES & CONDITIONS
- 🔵 High performing
- 🟠 Average
- ⚫ Below average

Legend codes used below: N = Nationally ranked (red), H = High performing (blue), A = Average (orange), L = Below average (black), – = not ranked / not rated

State Rank	Hospital	Cancer	Cardiology & Heart Surgery	Orthopedics	Other Specialties (Nat'l Ranked)	Other Specialties (High Perf)	Colon Cancer Surgery	Lung Cancer Surgery	Heart Attack	Heart Failure	Heart Bypass Surgery	Heart Valve Surgery	TAVR*	Abdominal Aortic Aneurysm	Stroke	Back Surgery	Hip Replacement	Knee Replacement	Hip Fracture	Diabetes	Kidney Failure	Pneumonia	COPD*
VIRGINIA continued																						
13	Sentara Leigh Hospital, Norfolk	–	–	H	–	–	H	A	H	A	H	–	–	–	H	–	H	H	H	H	A	H	H
16	Chippenham Hospital, Richmond	–	–	–	–	–	A	A	A	A	A	A	A	A	A	A	A	A	A	A	A	A	A
16	Sentara Princess Anne Hospital, Virginia Beach	–	–	H	–	–	H	A	–	–	–	–	–	A	H	A	H	H	H	H	H	H	H
18	Augusta Health-Fishersville	–	–	–	–	–	H	A	H	A	A	–	–	A	H	A	H	H	H	A	A	H	H
19	Chesapeake Regional Healthcare, Chesapeake	–	–	–	–	–	H	A	H	A	–	–	–	A	H	L	A	A	A	A	A	A	A
WASHINGTON																						
1	University of Washington Medical Center, Seattle[34]	N	–	N	4	5	H	H	A	A	A	H	H	A	H	H	A	A	H	H	H	H	H
2	Virginia Mason Medical Center, Seattle	–	–	H	–	4	H	H	H	A	H	H	H	H	H	H	H	H	H	A	A	A	H
3	Providence St. Peter Hospital, Olympia	–	–	–	–	1	H	A	A	A	H	–	–	A	H	A	H	H	H	A	A	A	H
4	Legacy Salmon Creek Medical Center, Vancouver	–	–	–	–	1	H	–	A	A	–	–	–	A	H	H	H	H	H	H	A	H	H
4	Providence Sacred Heart Med. Ctr. & Children's, Spokane	–	–	–	–	–	H	A	H	A	H	H	–	A	H	A	H	H	A	A	A	A	A
6	EvergreenHealth Kirkland	–	–	–	–	1	H	A	H	A	–	–	–	A	H	H	H	H	H	H	A	H	H
6	Providence Regional Medical Center Everett	–	–	–	–	–	H	A	A	A	H	H	–	A	H	A	H	H	A	A	A	A	A
6	St. Joseph Medical Center-Tacoma	–	–	–	–	–	H	A	A	A	H	H	–	H	H	A	H	H	A	A	A	A	A
9	Overlake Medical Center, Bellevue	–	–	–	–	–	H	H	A	A	A	A	–	A	H	A	H	H	A	A	A	A	A
10	PeaceHealth Southwest Medical Center, Vancouver	–	–	–	–	–	H	A	A	A	H	A	–	A	H	A	H	H	A	A	A	A	A
10	PeaceHealth St. Joseph Medical Center, Bellingham	–	–	–	–	–	H	A	A	A	H	A	–	A	H	A	H	H	A	A	A	A	A
12	Swedish Medical Center-First Hill, Seattle	–	–	–	–	–	H	H	H	A	H	H	–	–	H	A	H	H	A	A	A	A	A
13	Harrison Medical Center, Bremerton	–	–	–	–	–	H	H	A	A	H	–	–	L	H	A	H	H	A	A	A	A	A
13	MultiCare Tacoma General Hospital, Tacoma	–	–	–	–	–	H	A	A	A	H	H	–	A	H	A	H	H	A	A	A	A	A
13	Swedish Medical Center-Cherry Hill, Seattle	–	–	–	1	–	–	–	A	A	H	A	H	A	H	A	–	–	A	A	A	A	A
13	UW Medicine/Valley Medical Center, Renton	–	–	–	–	1	A	–	A	H	–	–	–	–	H	A	A	A	A	A	A	A	A
WEST VIRGINIA																						
1	West Virginia University Hospitals, Morgantown[35]	–	–	H	–	3	H	A	H	H	H	H	H	H	H	H	H	H	H	H	H	H	H
2	Charleston Area Medical Center, Charleston	–	–	–	–	–	H	A	A	A	H	H	H	A	H	A	H	H	A	A	A	A	A
3	St. Mary's Medical Center-Huntington	–	–	–	–	–	H	A	A	A	H	A	–	A	H	A	H	H	A	A	A	A	A
WISCONSIN																						
1	University of Wisconsin Hospitals, Madison	H	H	N	6	1	H	H	H	H	H	H	H	H	H	H	H	H	H	A	H	H	H
2	Froedtert Hosp. & the Med. College of Wisconsin, Milwaukee	–	–	H	3	3	H	H	H	A	H	H	H	H	H	H	H	H	H	A	H	H	H
3	Aurora St. Luke's Medical Center, Milwaukee	–	H	–	–	2	H	A	H	A	H	H	H	H	H	H	H	H	A	A	A	A	A
4	Mayo Clinic Eau Claire	–	–	–	–	1	H	A	A	A	H	H	–	A	H	A	H	H	A	A	A	A	A
5	Aurora Medical Center-Grafton	–	–	–	–	–	H	A	A	A	H	–	–	A	H	A	H	H	A	A	A	A	A
6	Aspirus Wausau Hospital, Wausau	–	–	–	–	–	H	A	A	A	H	A	–	A	H	A	H	H	A	A	A	A	A
6	Aurora Medical Center-Summit	–	–	–	–	–	H	A	A	A	–	–	–	–	H	A	H	H	A	A	A	A	A
6	Bellin Memorial Hospital, Green Bay	–	–	–	–	–	H	A	A	A	H	A	–	A	H	A	H	H	A	A	A	A	L
6	Marshfield Medical Center, Marshfield	–	–	–	–	1	H	A	A	A	H	A	H	A	H	H	H	H	A	A	A	A	A
6	SSM Health St. Mary's Hospital-Madison	–	–	–	–	–	H	A	A	A	H	A	H	A	H	A	H	H	A	A	A	A	A
11	Aurora BayCare Medical Center, Green Bay	–	–	–	–	–	H	A	A	A	H	A	–	A	H	A	H	H	A	A	A	A	A
11	Gundersen Health System-La Crosse	–	–	–	–	–	H	A	A	A	H	A	–	A	H	A	H	H	A	A	A	A	A
13	Ascension Columbia St. Mary's Hospital Milwaukee	–	–	–	–	–	A	A	A	A	H	A	–	L	–	A	H	H	A	A	A	A	A

In complex care specialties, (-) indicates hospital is not nationally ranked or high performing. In procedures and conditions, (-) indicates care not offered or hospital has too few Medicare patients to be rated. *TAVR: Transcatheter aortic valve replacement. *COPD: Chronic obstructive pulmonary disease

A footnote indicates that another hospital's results are included, that the hospital has a different name in one or more areas of care, or both.
[34] Seattle Cancer Care Alliance/University of Washington Medical Center.
[35] WVU Cancer Institute; WVU Heart & Vascular Institute; WVU Rockefeller Neuroscience Institute.

More @usnews.com/bestregionalhospitals

Best Regional Children's Hospitals

For good reasons, parents of kids who need specialty care tend to seek a hospital close to home, usually within the state where they live or in a neighboring state. Designed to help families identify top pediatric centers near home, the region-by-region rankings below compare children's hospitals on overall performance across 10 pediatric specialties

● NATIONALLY RANKED

Rank	Hospital	CANCER	CARDIOLOGY & HEART SURGERY	DIABETES & ENDOCRINOLOGY	GASTROENTEROLOGY & GI SURGERY	NEONATOLOGY	NEPHROLOGY	NEUROLOGY & NEUROSURGERY	ORTHOPEDICS	PULMONOLOGY & LUNG SURGERY	UROLOGY
NEW ENGLAND • Connecticut • Maine • Massachusetts • New Hampshire • Rhode Island • Vermont											
1	Boston Children's Hospital[1]	●	●	●	●	●	●	●	●	●	●
2	Yale New Haven Children's Hospital, New Haven, Conn.	–	–	●	●	●	●	●	–	●	–
3	Connecticut Children's Medical Center, Hartford	–	–	●	●	●	–	–	●	–	●
3	MassGeneral Hospital for Children, Boston	–	–	●	●	●	–	–	–	●	●
MID-ATLANTIC • Delaware • District of Columbia • Maryland • New Jersey • New York • Pennsylvania • Virginia • West Virginia											
1	Children's Hospital of Philadelphia	●	●	●	●	●	●	●	●	●	●
2	Children's National Hospital, Washington, D.C.	●	●	●	●	●	●	●	●	●	●
3	UPMC Children's Hospital of Pittsburgh[2]	●	●	●	●	●	●	●	●	●	●
4	Johns Hopkins Children's Center, Baltimore	●	●	●	●	●	●	●	●	●	●
5	Cohen Children's Medical Center, New Hyde Park, N.Y.	●	–	●	●	●	●	●	●	●	●
6	New York-Presbyterian Hospital-Columbia and Cornell, New York	●	●	●	●	●	●	●	–	●	●
7	Children's Hospital at Montefiore, New York	●	–	●	–	●	●	●	–	–	–
7	Penn State Children's Hospital, Hershey, Pa.	●	●	–	–	●	–	●	–	●	–
7	University of Virginia Children's Hospital, Charlottesville	–	●	●	●	●	●	–	–	●	–
10	Children's Hospital of Richmond at VCU, Va.	●	–	–	–	–	●	●	–	●	●
10	Mount Sinai Kravis Children's Hospital, New York	–	–	●	–	●	●	–	–	–	–
10	Nemours Alfred I. duPont Hospital for Children, Wilmington, Del.	●	–	–	●	–	–	–	●	●	●
13	Children's Hospital at St. Peter's University Hospital, New Brunswick, N.J.	–	–	–	–	●	–	–	–	–	–
13	Inova Children's Hospital, Falls Church, Va.	–	–	–	–	●	–	–	–	–	–
13	Joseph M. Sanzari Children's Hospital at Hackensack University Medical Center, Hackensack, N.J.[3]	●	–	–	–	–	–	–	–	–	–

(–) indicates hospital is not nationally ranked.

A footnote indicates that another hospital's results are included, that the hospital has a different name in one or more areas of care, or both.
[1] Dana-Farber/Boston Children's Cancer and Blood Disorders Center [2] UPMC Children's Hospital of Pittsburgh-Shriners Hospitals for Children
[3] Hackensack Meridian Health Sanzari and Hovnanian Children's Hospitals

● NATIONALLY RANKED

Rank	Hospital	Cancer	Cardiology & Heart Surgery	Diabetes & Endocrinology	Gastroenterology & GI Surgery	Neonatology	Nephrology	Neurology & Neurosurgery	Orthopedics	Pulmonology & Lung Surgery	Urology
MID-ATLANTIC continued											
13	University of Maryland Children's Hospital, Baltimore	–	●	–	–	–	–	–	–	–	–
13	University of Rochester-Golisano Children's Hospital, N.Y.	–	–	–	–	●	–	–	–	–	–
13	West Virginia University Children's Hospital, Morgantown	–	–	–	–	–	–	–	–	–	●
SOUTHEAST • Alabama • Arkansas • Florida • Georgia • Louisiana • Mississippi • North Carolina • South Carolina • Tennessee											
1	Children's Healthcare of Atlanta	●	●	●	●	●	●	●	●	●	●
1	Monroe Carell Jr. Children's Hospital at Vanderbilt, Nashville, Tenn.	●	●	●	●	●	●	●	●	●	●
3	Children's Hospital of Alabama at UAB, Birmingham	●	●	–	●	●	●	●	●	●	●
3	Duke Children's Hospital and Health Center, Durham, N.C.	●	●	●	●	●	●	●	●	●	●
5	Johns Hopkins All Children's Hospital, St. Petersburg, Fla.	●	–	●	–	●	●	●	●	●	●
5	Levine Children's Hospital, Charlotte, N.C.	●	●	–	●	●	●	●	●	●	–
5	UF Health Shands Children's Hospital, Gainesville, Fla.	●	●	●	●	–	●	●	–	●	●
8	Le Bonheur Children's Hospital, Memphis, Tenn.	–	●	●	●	–	–	●	–	●	–
8	North Carolina Children's Hospital at UNC, Chapel Hill	●	–	●	●	●	●	●	–	●	–
10	Arnold Palmer Hospital for Children, Orlando	–	●	–	–	●	–	●	–	–	●
10	Nicklaus Children's Hospital, Miami	–	●	–	–	–	–	●	●	●	–
12	Arkansas Children's Hospital, Little Rock	–	●	–	–	–	●	–	–	●	●
12	MUSC Shawn Jenkins Children's Hospital, Charleston, S.C.[4]	●	–	–	●	–	●	–	–	–	–
14	Joe DiMaggio Children's Hospital at Memorial, Hollywood, Fla.	–	●	–	–	–	–	–	●	–	–
14	Wolfson Children's Hospital, Jacksonville, Fla.	–	–	●	–	–	–	–	●	–	–
16	AdventHealth for Children, Orlando	–	–	–	–	–	●	–	–	–	–
16	Holtz Children's Hospital at UM-Jackson Memorial Medical Center, Miami	–	–	●	–	–	–	–	–	–	–
16	Ochsner Hospital for Children, New Orleans	–	●	–	–	–	–	–	–	–	–
MIDWEST • Illinois • Indiana • Iowa • Kansas • Kentucky • Michigan • Minnesota • Missouri • Nebraska • North Dakota • Ohio • South Dakota • Wisconsin											
1	Cincinnati Children's Hospital Medical Center[5]	●	●	●	●	●	●	●	●	●	●
2	Nationwide Children's Hospital, Columbus, Ohio	●	●	●	●	●	●	●	●	●	●
3	Ann and Robert H. Lurie Children's Hospital of Chicago[6]	●	●	●	●	●	●	●	●	●	●
3	C.S. Mott Children's Hospital-Michigan Medicine, Ann Arbor	●	●	●	●	●	●	●	●	●	●
3	Cleveland Clinic Children's Hospital	●	●	●	●	●	●	●	●	●	●
3	St. Louis Children's Hospital-Washington University[7]	●	●	●	●	●	●	●	●	●	●
7	Children's Mercy Kansas City, Mo.	●	●	●	●	–	●	●	●	●	●
7	Riley Hospital for Children at IU Health, Indianapolis	●	●	●	●	●	●	●	–	●	●
9	Mayo Clinic Children's Center, Rochester, Minn.[8]	●	●	●	●	●	–	●	●	–	●
9	Rainbow Babies and Children's Hospital, Cleveland	●	–	●	●	●	●	–	●	●	●
11	Spectrum Health Helen DeVos Children's Hospital, Grand Rapids, Mich.	●	●	–	–	●	–	●	●	–	–
12	Children's Hospital of Michigan, Detroit	–	●	–	●	–	●	●	●	–	–
12	Children's Hospital of Wisconsin, Milwaukee	●	–	●	–	●	●	●	●	●	–
12	SSM Health Cardinal Glennon Children's Hospital-St. Louis University, St. Louis	●	●	–	●	●	–	–	–	●	–
15	University of Iowa Stead Family Children's Hospital, Iowa City	–	–	●	–	●	●	●	●	–	–
16	Akron Children's Hospital, Ohio	–	–	●	–	●	–	●	●	●	–
16	Children's Hospital and Medical Center, Omaha	–	●	–	●	–	●	–	–	●	–
18	M Health Fairview University of Minnesota Masonic Children's Hospital, Minneapolis[9]	–	–	–	–	●	–	–	–	–	–
19	Children's Minnesota, Minneapolis	–	–	●	–	–	–	–	–	●	–
19	Dayton Children's Hospital, Ohio	–	–	–	–	–	–	–	●	–	–
19	Norton Children's Hospital, Louisville, Ky.	–	–	●	–	–	–	–	–	–	–
19	University of Chicago Comer Children's Hospital	–	–	●	●	–	–	–	–	–	–
23	Advocate Children's Hospital, Oak Lawn, Ill.[10]	–	●	–	–	–	–	–	–	–	–
23	American Family Children's Hospital, Madison, Wis.	–	●	–	–	–	–	–	–	–	–

(-) indicates hospital is not nationally ranked.

A footnote indicates that another hospital's results are included, that the hospital has a different name in one or more areas of care, or both.
[4]MUSC Children's Heart Network of South Carolina [5]Cincinnati Children's and Kentucky Children's Hospital Joint Heart Program [6]Ann and Robert H. Lurie Children's Hospital-Prentice Women's Hospital [7]St. Louis Children's Hospital-Washington University/Shriners Hospital [8]Mayo Clinic Children's Minnesota Cardiovascular Collaborative [9]University of Minnesota Masonic Children's Hospital-Children's Minnesota [10]Advocate Children's Heart Institute; Advocate Children's Hospitals, Oak Lawn and Park Ridge

BEST REGIONAL HOSPITALS

● NATIONALLY RANKED

Rank	Hospital	CANCER	CARDIOLOGY & HEART SURGERY	DIABETES & ENDOCRINOLOGY	GASTROENTEROLOGY & GI SURGERY	NEONATOLOGY	NEPHROLOGY	NEUROLOGY & NEUROSURGERY	ORTHOPEDICS	PULMONOLOGY & LUNG SURGERY	UROLOGY
MIDWEST continued											
23	Kentucky Children's Hospital, Lexington, Ky.[11]	–	–	–	–	–	–	–	●	–	–
23	OSF HealthCare Children's Hospital of Illinois, Peoria	–	–	–	–	●	–	–	–	–	–
ROCKY MOUNTAIN • Colorado • Idaho • Montana • Nevada • Utah • Wyoming											
1	Children's Hospital Colorado, Aurora	●	●	●	●	●	●	●	●	●	●
2	Intermountain Primary Children's Hospital-University of Utah, Salt Lake City[12]	●	●	●	●	–	●	●	●	●	●
SOUTHWEST • Arizona • New Mexico • Oklahoma • Texas											
1	Texas Children's Hospital, Houston	●	●	●	●	●	●	●	●	●	●
2	Children's Medical Center Dallas[13]	●	●	●	●	●	●	●	●	●	●
2	Phoenix Children's Hospital	●	●	●	●	●	●	●	●	●	●
4	Children's Memorial Hermann Hospital, Houston	–	●	–	–	–	●	–	–	–	–
4	Cook Children's Medical Center, Fort Worth	–	–	●	–	–	–	–	–	–	–
PACIFIC • Alaska • California • Hawaii • Oregon • Washington											
1	Children's Hospital Los Angeles	●	●	●	●	●	●	●	●	●	●
2	Lucile Packard Children's Hospital Stanford, Palo Alto, Calif.	●	●	●	●	●	●	●	●	●	●
3	Rady Children's Hospital, San Diego	●	●	●	●	●	●	●	●	●	●
3	Seattle Children's Hospital	●	●	●	●	●	●	●	●	●	●
3	UCSF Benioff Children's Hospitals, San Francisco and Oakland	●	●	●	●	●	●	●	●	●	●
6	CHOC Children's Hospital, Orange, Calif.	●	–	●	●	●	●	–	●	●	●
6	Valley Children's Healthcare and Hospital, Madera, Calif.	–	–	●	●	●	●	–	●	●	●
8	UCLA Mattel Children's Hospital, Los Angeles	●	–	–	●	●	●	●	●	–	–
9	Doernbecher Children's Hospital at Oregon Health and Science University, Portland, Ore.[14]	●	–	●	–	●	●	●	–	–	–
10	UC Davis Children's Hospital, Sacramento, Calif.[15]	–	–	–	–	●	●	–	●	–	●
11	Loma Linda University Children's Hospital, Loma Linda, Calif.	–	●	–	–	–	–	–	–	–	–
11	MemorialCare Miller Children's & Women's Hospital Long Beach, Calif.	–	–	–	–	–	–	–	–	●	–

(–) indicates hospital is not nationally ranked.

A footnote indicates that another hospital's results are included, that the hospital has a different name in one or more areas of care, or both.
[11]Kentucky Children's Hospital-Shriners Hospitals for Children [12]Intermountain Primary Children's Hospital-Shriners Hospitals for Children-University of Utah
[13]Children's Medical Center Dallas-Texas Scottish Rite Hospital for Children [14]OHSU Doernbecher Children's Hospital/Shriners Hospitals for Children Portland
[15]UC Davis Children's Hospital/Shriners Hospitals for Children-Northern California

CHILDREN'S HOSPITAL LOS ANGELES

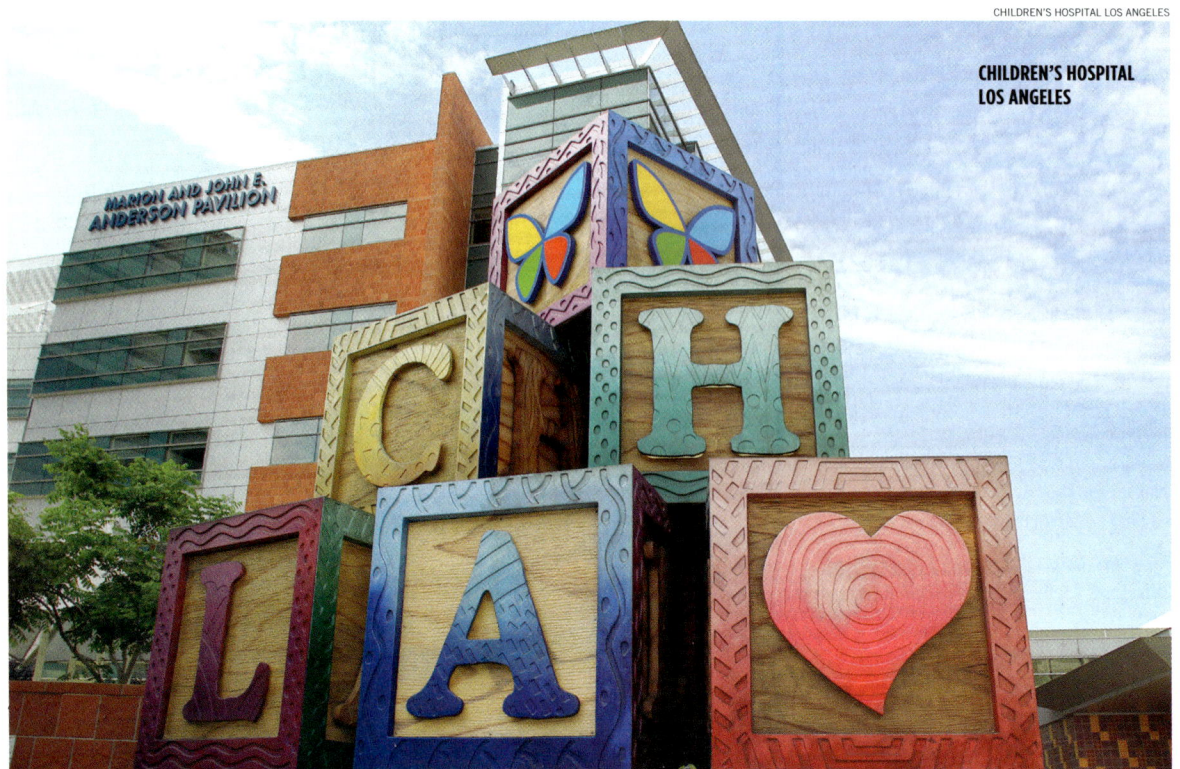

CHILDREN'S HOSPITAL LOS ANGELES

WHEN IT COMES TO **SPINE CARE,** OUR DOCTORS ARE AHEAD OF THE CURVE.

At Och Spine Hospital, we've recruited many of the world's finest orthopedic and neurosurgical spine surgeons.

They're part of a collaborative team treating children and adults with spine problems from the simple to the complex. Offering advanced imaging and the latest non-surgical therapies.

Together, their work is nothing short of amazing.

And it's all backed by NewYork-Presbyterian Hospital, ranked #1 in New York, and powered by the brains of two leading medical schools.

But you don't need to have an extraordinary condition to get extraordinary spine care.

Come see us.

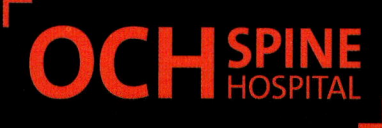

Make an appointment at **nyp.org/Och**

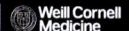

NewYork-Presbyterian Hospital as ranked by U.S. News & World Report 2021–22

We treat the most important cancer: Yours.

While Memorial Sloan Kettering is proud to be named one of the top cancer centers in the nation, we're still focused on what got us here: giving you and your loved ones the benefits of breakthrough research and world-class care.

Call us today at 833-990-2418 or visit msk.org/NearYou

Memorial Sloan Kettering
Cancer Center

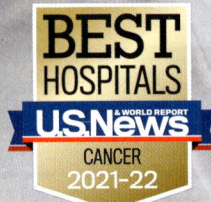

Lisa DeAngelis, MD
Physician-in-Chief

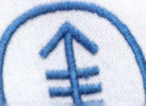

©2021 Memorial Sloan Kettering Cancer Center. All rights reserved.

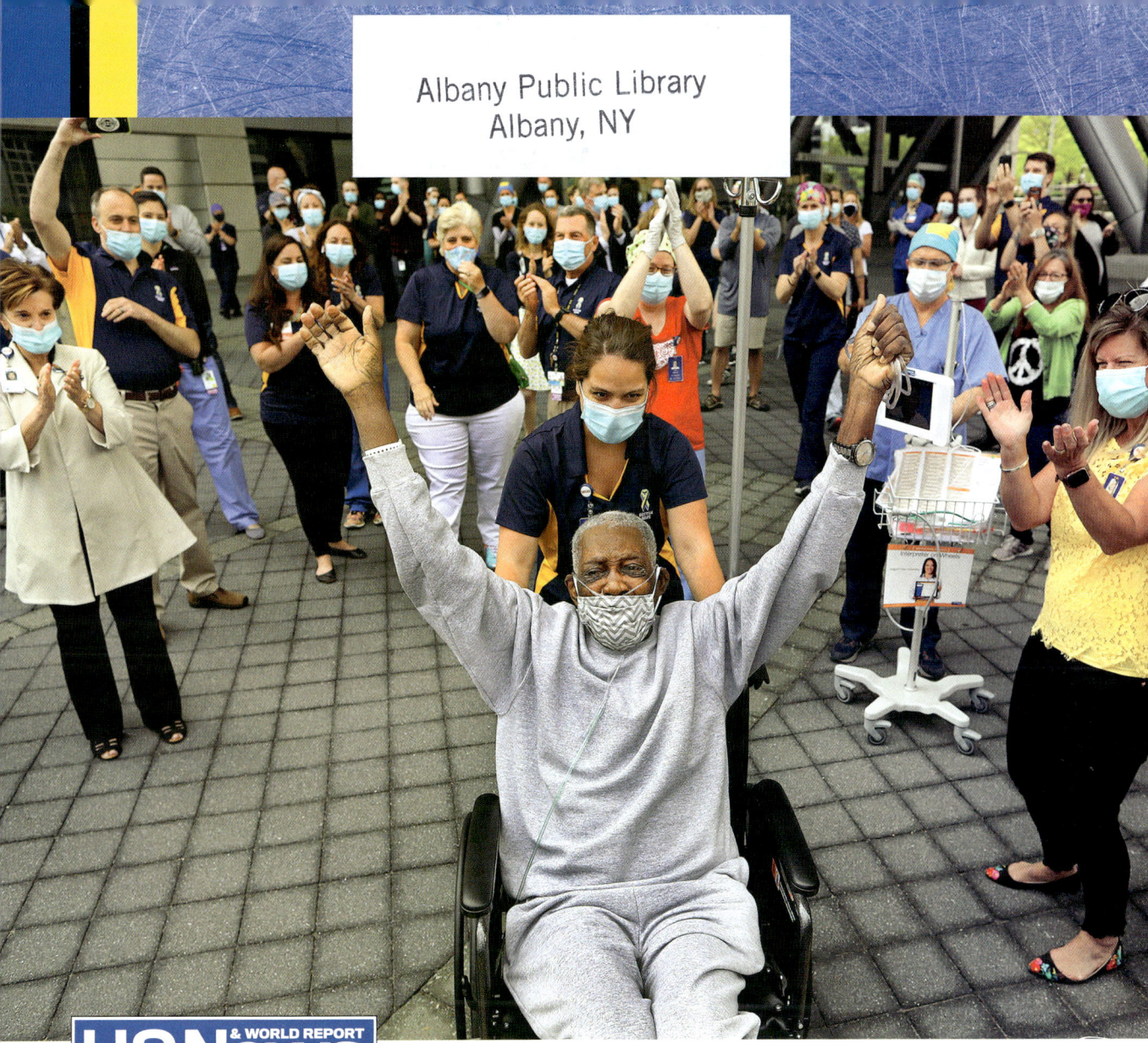

U.S. News & WORLD REPORT
2022 EDITION

Best Hospitals

Copyright © 2021 by U.S. News & World Report L.P.
1050 Thomas Jefferson Street, N.W., Washington, D.C. 20007-3837, 978-1-931469-97-5.
All rights reserved. Published by U.S. News & World Report L.P., Washington, D.C.

IN JUNE 2020, THE LAST PATIENT LEAVING THE FIELD HOSPITAL AT THE BOSTON CONVENTION CENTER GETS A FAREWELL.
JOHN TLUMACKI – THE BOSTON GLOBE VIA GETTY IMAGES

CONTENTS

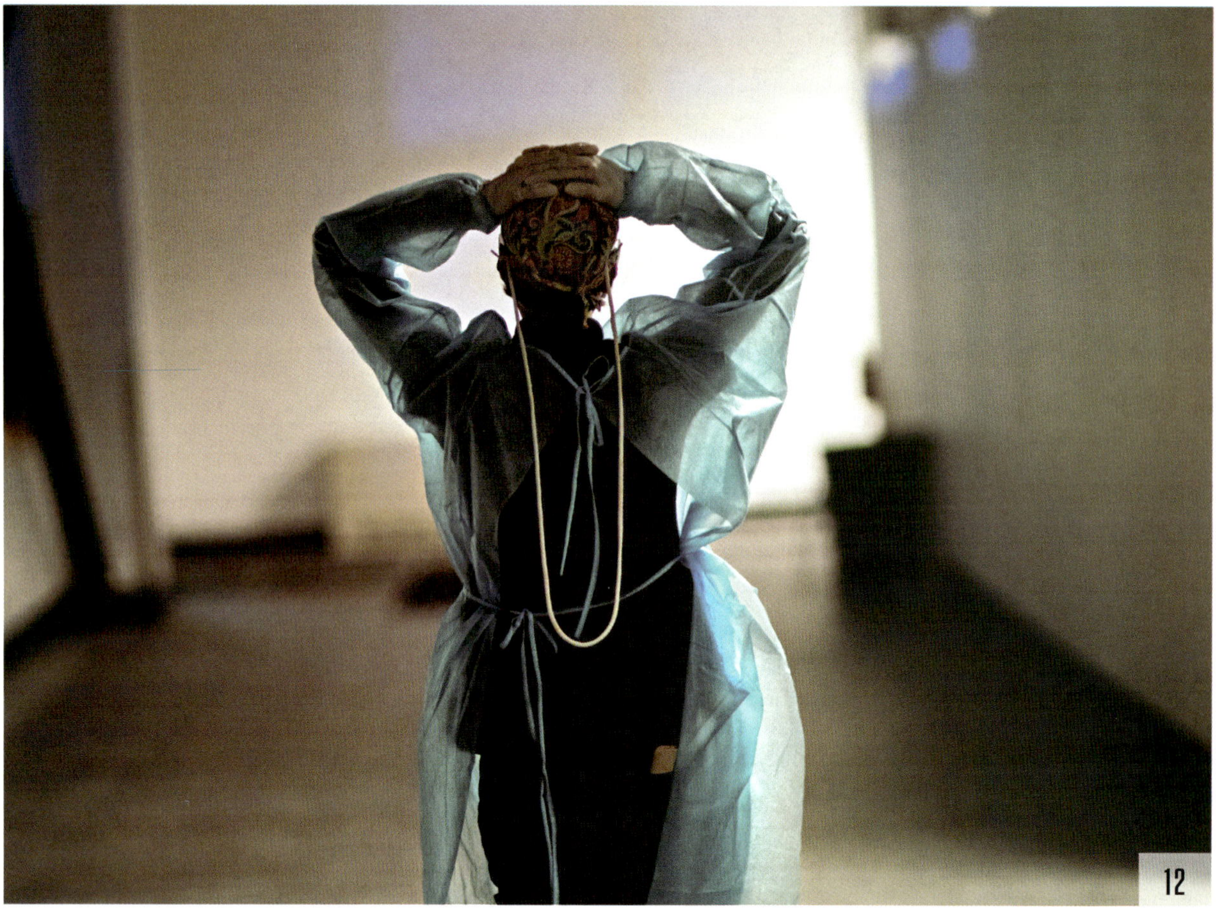

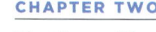

CHAPTER ONE
On Medicine's Front Lines

12 Weighing COVID's Heavy Toll
The hit to the nation's health – and health system – goes far beyond the effects of the virus itself.

22 Photo Essay: A Look Back
Revisit a few moments, from around the country, of these difficult times.

30 Virtual Care's Post-pandemic Role
Experts think that as much as half of care could be delivered remotely.

52 Searching for Ways to Close Health Gaps
Providers are getting serious about addressing patients' social needs and tackling health disparities.

58 On the Cutting Edge of Cancer Care
Four leading experts discuss the latest advances.

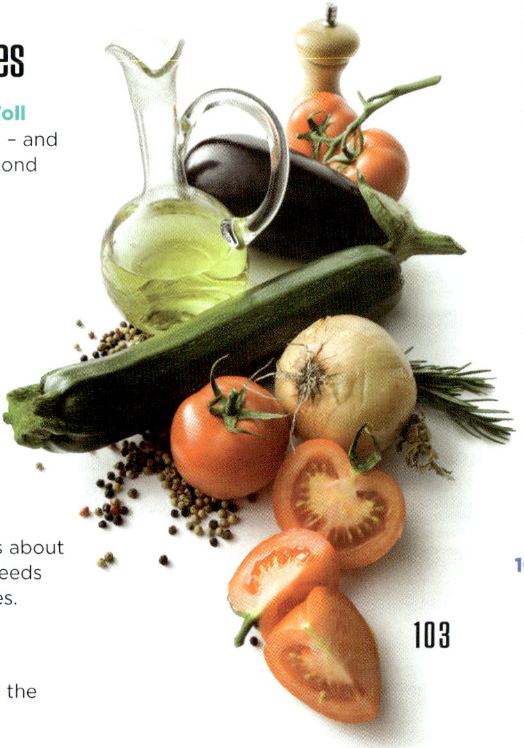

CHAPTER TWO
Patient Power

66 The Plight of the COVID Long Haulers
There's still much to learn about the serious, lasting symptoms.

89 Strengthened Defenses
Long term, here's what you can do to boost your immune system.

92 Measuring Cancer's Unequal Impact
Overall, the prospects may be brighter – but not for everyone.

96 Building Strength With a Purpose
Functional fitness training is a way to improve your performance.

100 Best Diets: Which Ones Work?
Our panel of experts weighed in on the merits of 39 eating plans.

CONTENTS CONTINUED ON PAGE 4

COVER: GETTY IMAGES

FROM TOP: DAVID GOLDMAN – AP; GETTY IMAGES